Living with Hearing Difficu

Dedication

We dedicate this book to Patricia Kerr who provided many of the ideas behind it, but was unable to participate in its writing because of health problems.

Living with Hearing Difficulties: the process of enablement

Dafydd Stephens FRCP
Honorary Professor of Audiological Medicine
Cardiff University
Cardiff
Wales

Sophia E. Kramer PhD
Senior Researcher and Psychologist
Department of ENT/Audiology
EMGO Institute for Health and Care Research
VU University Medical Centre
Amsterdam
Netherlands

WILEY-BLACKWELL

A John Wiley & Sons, Ltd., Publication

Library of Congress Cataloging-in-Publication Data

Stephens, Dafydd.
  Living with hearing difficulties: the process of enablement / Dafydd Stephens and
Sophia E. Kramer.
      p. ; cm.
  Includes bibliographical references and index.
  ISBN 978-0-470-01985-6 (pbk. : alk. paper)   1. Hearing impaired–Rehabilitation.
I. Kramer, Sophia.   II. Title.
  [DNLM: 1. Hearing Loss–rehabilitation.   2. Adult.   3. Quality of Life.   4. Rehabilitation
of Hearing Impaired. WV 270 S833L 2010]
  HV2380.S74 2010
  362.4′28–dc22

                                                                              2010011963

A catalogue record for this book is available from the British Library.

Set in 9.5 on 11.5 pt Palatino by SNP Best-set Typesetter Ltd., Hong Kong

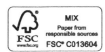

Contents

Foreword

Hearing loss began to be a nuisance to me, rather than just an occasional inconvenience, in my early forties. I was sitting on a government Council at the time, and finding the august debates round the long table were tapering off into gobbledegook. My GP, as always, refused to take the tragic view. I was, he said in his letter to the consultant, simply finding that 'their lordships are whispering a little *too* confidentially'. I got my first hearing aids a few weeks later. But the wording of that irreverent referral helped every bit as much. Ever since, I've tried to take a comic view of hearing loss, to view it not as a unmitigated disaster but as something to tack round, to use as a jumping-off point for new ideas and improvisations.

Some years later, I put together a 'field aid' for boosting birdsong beyond what my conventional aids could achieve. Kitted up with an all-directional gun mike and heavy-duty headphones, I looked like a walking radio station. But it worked, and was a wonderful conversation opener. It made me begin to wonder whether the whole tone of the 'hearing compensation' business – the stress on discretion, on the exquisite delicacy and camouflage of the aids, on the let's-try-and-act-as-if-nothing-is-amiss approach – was counter-productive. I'd had more embarrassment around dinner tables – and in close relationships – pretending I was coping than if I'd been upfront about my problem from the outset. I would have fared much better if I'd come out brandishing an ear trumpet.

Hearing loss is always a *social* as well as a personal challenge. It's mapped more accurately by the disruption it causes in your relationships than by any objective audiometric tests. So it makes sense to seek solutions in those relationships as much as, so to speak, in the ear. I've always had trouble with TV sound. American movies and soft-voiced presenters are more or less incoherent, and no loop systems or sophisticated digital aid settings help. Having the volume high is unacceptable unless you're alone. I found the answer in the subtitle option, and was delighted to discover that films still had plots as well as action. There was a bonus, too. For all news and live programmes, the broadcasting companies rely on automatic voice-recognition software to turn the spoken words into text. The software is, understandably, as unreliable as any dodgy human ear, and every so often gets things wrong – wonderfully, hilariously wrong. I'd long looked on what I call 'creative mishearing' as the best, frustration-dissolving antidote to hearing confusion. Now here was a machine not only experiencing all my own difficulties with lost consonants and eccentric accents but also making better puns from them than I ever had. When, in the heat of the US election campaign, it rendered Barack Obama's name first as 'back the bomber' and then, trying to be fair, as 'back the barman', I knew I'd found the most reassuring hearing aid on the planet.

At their root, most of the problems associated with hearing loss are to do with language. Those with reduced hearing quickly learn how much language is necessary for purely functional communication and how much is concerned with nuance and subtlety and detail. But that's surely a hopeful lesson. Language is a fluid, living entity, constantly being reshaped by *all* the people who use it. I often feel that those of us with reduced hearing abilities are like early humans on the edge of language use, playing with half-finished words and imperfect meanings. A fuller language only emerged because these embryonic sounds were being continuously experimented with socially. This rich book is about coping strategies, so I'd recommend this as one: bring those you communicate with into your social language, as much as trying to enter theirs. You may find you are not a hearing-loss statistic, but an aural poet.

Richard Mabey
Writer

Preface

The origins of this book go back to 1980, when David Goldstein and Dafydd Stephens spent many months discussing the integration of the different aspects of the enablement (rehabilitation) process and how it could be made more relevant to the needs of our patients. Such ideas resulted in our publication of a 'management model' of audiological rehabilitation, presenting our key ideas (Goldstein and Stephens, 1981). This has been widely cited, and led to the idea of our writing a book to draw our ideas together for a wider audience. This was perhaps rather premature at that time and the idea was gradually shelved as we both became preoccupied with a number of other professional activities.

In the 1990s, following her PhD on the experiences of people with severe acquired hearing impairment in Belfast, Patricia Kerr together with Dafydd Stephens extended this work with an examination of the development of *primary* and *secondary handicap* with the World Health Organization's *International Classification of Impairments, Disabilities and Handicaps* (ICIDH; WHO, 1980; Stephens and Hétu, 1991) as a starting point. This brought in the work of Patricia Kerr on the role of positive experiences in adjusting to hearing impairment and led to further joint studies on that topic (e.g. Stephens and Kerr, 2003).

It also led to new plans to include these ideas in a more comprehensive book. Much of this book was planned before Patricia developed a chronic illness, which prevented her from taking any further part in the project, which was subsequently put on a back burner once more.

In the meantime Sophia Kramer had been working on assessing the effects of hearing impairment on people and its measurement (e.g. Kramer *et al.*, 1996) and we began to collaborate following the Eriksholm workshop on 'Self-report outcome measures in audiological rehabilitation' (Cox *et al.*, 2000). This began with the European Union's GENDEAF project working group on the 'Psychosocial aspects of genetic hearing impairment', which emphasised the importance of taking a broad approach to the experiences of people with hearing problems (e.g. Kramer *et al.*, 2006a, 2006b).

As a result of such collaboration, we felt the need to highlight the different aspects of this field, particularly within the context of having a patient-centred approach to the process of audiological enablement, building as well on some of the ideas of enablement in the field of neurological rehabilitation, developed by Derrick Wade (e.g. Wade, 2006). This ultimately led to the writing of the present book.

We have aimed to make this book accessible and relevant to both professionals and to people with hearing difficulties themselves in a non-prescriptive manner, highlighting the concepts of audiological enablement being an interactive process with active involvement of both the clinician and the patient. The term 'deaf' has variously been used to refer to people with a pre-lingual, profound hearing impairment through to those with a post-lingual, usually moderate or severe, hearing impairment. As such, we do not find the term helpful and have avoided it. 'Deaf' (uppercase 'D') is used to refer to and by those people who use sign language as their first or preferred form of communication, do not perceive their deafness as a medical disability and define themselves as part of a cultural and linguistic group, often referred to as the 'Deaf community'. In addition we have also emphasized the role of significant others, mainly family and friends.

In this context, we follow the philosophy of the Serenity Prayer, which has been popularised in songs, books and as part of twelve-step programmes (such as Alcoholics Anonymous):

> Learn to change the things you can
> Learn to accept the things you cannot change
> Have the wisdom to know the difference.

To this, we would add:

> Involve those around you in the process so that they can support what you are doing.

Some believe that the prayer is predated by a version of Mother Goose from 1695:

> For every ailment under the sun
> There is a remedy, or there is none;
> If there be one, try to find it;
> If there be none, never mind it.

What we understand by 'things' or 'ailments' in this context are very much the *participation restrictions* of the individual – in other words, what their hearing impairment stops them doing. This, in turn, should have a knock-on effect on the psychological consequences of their condition. In describing the process of addressing such problems, we have consciously adopted the term *enablement*, involving active participation by patient, professional and others, rather than the traditional term *rehabilitation*, which implies merely service provision. This is discussed further in Chapter 1.

We start with four chapters dealing with the general background to the problems which the individual may experience. The first is an introductory chapter dealing with the terminology which we use as well as considering the bases of our holistic approach in relation to other ways of addressing hearing difficulties which have been used in the past.

The next three chapters cover the individual's entry into the process, the type of hearing impairment which they may have and other related conditions which may influence the impact of their hearing loss on the individual.

Entry into the process (Chapter 2) involves a number of hurdles which, while relatively easy to overcome, stand between the individual and the provision of help for their difficulties. This is reflected by the fact that only about a quarter of those with significant hearing impairment have hearing aids or other forms of appropriate support. Some will not be aware of or admit to their hearing impairment, even if it is impacting on their families. Others will be aware of it and not have done anything about it, and yet others will have been dissuaded by their primary physician or other 'gatekeepers' from seeking appropriate help.

The type of hearing impairment which the individual has will influence its impact on the individual and this is discussed in Chapter 3. Chapter 4 considers how such impacts can be affected both by other conditions which may be associated with the hearing impairment, such as tinnitus or vertigo, and also by factors which may or may not have a direct aetiological relationship with the condition. These include any visual impairment, the person's cognitive status, as well as other factors such as any neuromuscular or arthritic disorders which they also have.

The next five chapters deal with the ways in which the individual's hearing impairment can influence different aspects of their life, touching on how such impacts can be reduced. Chapter 5 deals with the basis of communication, particularly as a two-way process, influenced in part by the individual's cognitive abilities.

Chapter 6 deals with the social and emotional impact of the hearing impairment, which can vary considerably from individual to individual, and can be influenced by a range of factors. Related to this is Chapter 7, which deals with the impact of the hearing impairment on the family and relationships within the family. The role of family members and their attitudes can be a key area here.

Chapters 8 and 9 deal with specific aspects of the individual's life, namely in the work situation and in their leisure activities. The attitudes of significant others, such as colleagues and superiors, can play a major role in the work situation, and how this can be approached is considered. In the context of leisure, while many decisions as to the choice of activities depend on the individual, such choices are also often dependent on the cooperation of those around the person with hearing difficulties.

Chapters 10 to 12 present an overall view of how we see the different aspects of the process of audiological enablement, bringing in and drawing together elements of the earlier chapters. The philosophy behind this approach is that it should be applicable to any sociomedical system and relevant to individuals with all types of hearing problems. This is also highlighted in our concluding chapter, which emphasizes the main concepts behind the book and their implementation.

Along with this book, readers may find the *Living with Hearing Difficulties* web site (http://www.wiley.com/go/stephens) a valuable resource. It contains additional documents, for example some of the questionnaires that we refer to in this book, which readers may find useful. The web site also demonstrates the concept of the signal-to-noise ratio. The documents may be freely downloaded.

We are grateful to our colleague Louise Hickson, Professor of Audiology at the University of Queensland, Australia, for writing an appendix based on work which we did together and which highlights the dynamic and changing nature of hearing problems, even for the same individual.

Finally, we return to the beginning and the excellent foreword written by Richard Mabey, a leading author and naturalist, who really emphasises the importance of taking a positive approach to overcoming any hearing problems.

Acknowledgements

We acknowledge the enormous contribution of our teachers and colleagues to the development of our ideas. We are also deeply indebted to many of our patients with whom we had long discussions which helped us maintain our perspective and led to the clarification of many of the concepts expressed in this book.

Among our teachers, Dafydd acknowledges William Burns, who first triggered his interest in hearing, Scott Reger who encouraged him into audiology and, in particular, Ronald Hinchcliffe, his professional 'godfather' throughout his career. In addition, Ole Bentzen and Bjørn Blegvad stimulated his interest in rehabilitation/enablement, which was honed during long discussions with David Goldstein over the years.

Sophia is grateful to Theo Kapteyn, who introduced her to the field of audiology. His inspiring enthusiasm, creativity and support created the basis for her scientific work. Sophia also acknowledges Dafydd Stephens for his tremendous support throughout the years and for the opportunities he offered. She has been delighted to collaborate with him on a range of projects, a collaboration that she has always greatly enjoyed.

We very much appreciate the contributions to this book from our colleague Louise Hickson and from Richard Mabey. Louise wrote the appendix, which reflects many of the ideas that we developed together. Richard is the leading natural history writer in the United Kingdom, best known for his books *Food for Free*, *Flora Britannica* and *Nature Cure*, among many others, and wrote the Foreword, based on his own experiences with hearing impairment.

Last, but not least, we are indebted to our spouses, Janig and José, for their tolerance and encouragement during the writing of this book.

Dafydd Stephens, Sophia Kramer

1 Introduction

The need for this book

There is a wide range of books currently available which cover different aspects of audiological rehabilitation/enablement, so the question arises: 'Why yet another book?' We would argue that almost all existing books are orientated towards specific aspects of the rehabilitative process (such as hearing aids, cochlear implants or speechreading/lip-reading), at rehabilitation specific to one particular sociomedical system (e.g. private practice in the Unite States) or, at best, reflect an approach related to the perspective of concerned professionals.

While we would be the last to deny the influence of our backgrounds as a retired audiological physician and an active psychologist working in the field, we try to approach the problems and needs from the standpoint of what the patient/client is seeking rather from what we, as professionals, can provide. In order to do this we shall call upon autobiographical accounts, the general rehabilitative and health psychology literature as well as the audiological literature and our own experience.

In this way, we hope to provide an intellectual and practical source book for a range of professionals who may encounter and be called upon to support individuals with hearing difficulties as well as making it accessible to individuals with hearing difficulties themselves. In the last context, it must be remembered that only a minority of people with hearing difficulties seek rehabilitative help (Davis, 1995; see also Chapter 2). Thus, we would hope that, by making relevant information easily available, this might encourage some of those individuals, reluctant to seek help, to present to rehabilitation departments earlier, and so reduce some of the problems experienced by themselves and by those around them.

Our approach has always been one of problem-solving, aimed at addressing particular and often specific needs experienced by people with hearing difficulties, rather than trying to fit the individual to a particular service model or set of devices. We shall therefore emphasise repeatedly the need to discuss their particular problems with the individual, their reaction to such problems and the reasons behind such reactions. In this context, it is always important to consider the role, attitudes and reactions of the individual's significant others (e.g. spouse, partner, child, friend), while being sure that the interests of the individual with the hearing difficulties has the dominant role in any rehabilitative approach.

In addition, we are aware that problems experienced by individuals with hearing difficulties will change as a result of any rehabilitative intervention and changes in lifestyle and experiences. We shall consider how this may be addressed and present some preliminary results in this domain collected by some members of the International Collegium of Rehabilitative Audiology in the Appendix.

Most of this book is concerned with individuals experiencing acquired hearing difficulties, from mild to profound, but we shall not neglect those born with such problems. Many such individuals with pre-lingual hearing impairment opt to lead their lives within the Deaf community and are, often justifiably, loath to seek help from health care professionals. However, some Deaf individuals may seek help at certain periods of their lives, such as if they have hearing children whom they want to support orally at critical stages of their lives, or if they find themselves in a particularly difficult employment environment. Even in other situations, they may find aspects of the rehabilitative process, such as updating of environmental aids (assistive listening devices) and help with new legislative arrangements, relevant and important.

Finally, we have taken the decision to restrict the scope of the book to adults with hearing disabilities rather than including all from birth to old age. The balance of hearing problems (e.g. severe vs moderate) and the fact that most affected children have never experienced normal hearing has led us to this decision, although much of what we include will be relevant to the audiological enablement of many children. In addition, we shall include in our text our experiences with hearing impaired school leavers, many of whom had hearing impairments dating from birth. Furthermore, we have excluded a specific section on the impact and needs of ethnicity and religious beliefs, beyond considering them in general terms as they influence the rehabilitative/enablement process. We accept that this may be an increasing problem in a world with more and more population movements, but here we are aiming to propose a universal approach which can encompass any and all such belief groups. For a more detailed discussion of specific needs and problems arising in immigrant groups, the reader is referred to Ahmad *et al.* (1998) and Jones *et al.* (2006).

Terminology

Enablement

The most commonly used terms for what we are broadly addressing in this book are *audiological rehabilitation* or *aural rehabilitation*. These terms have been generally accepted, but have a number of philosophical limitations. These are centred around the fact that they are based on the function of the ears or of the auditory system on one hand rather than on the 'complete' individual, and second that they give the impression of a system into which the person with hearing difficulties is fitted. Early definitions of such processes were along the lines of '*Auditory Rehabilitation* implies the return of persons to a former state of "normalcy", but is used here to describe the treatment and training of all persons with hearing too impaired to permit adequate effectiveness in auditory communication' (Bergman, 1950). We prefer the following definition: 'A problem-solving process aiming to minimise the disablements experienced by individuals with hearing disorders and to maximise their quality of life' (Stephens, 2003), but this still has the negative implications associated with the term *rehabilitation*.

The audiological rehabilitative literature states two goals of rehabilitation:

1. To furnish the individual with the communication tools with which to offset their impairment to an optimum degree
2. To help them gain insight into their disability and the problems it raises (Pauls and Hardy, 1948).

In the general rehabilitative literature, they have been defined as:

1. To optimise social participation of the patient
2. To maximise the well-being of the patient
3. To minimise stress on and distress of relatives.

(Wade, 2005)

The term *enablement* has been used in the neurological rehabilitation literature (Wade, 2003, 2006) and has the implications of helping individuals to do what they would like to do, to the extent that their inherent functional limitations allow. Wade argues that this refers to the *facilitation* of the patient. It is 'Not a passive process' and could refer to 'the patient achieving or having:

▪ More skills, a wider behavioural repertoire
▪ A better environment and
▪ More appropriate expectations'.

Thus, we propose to use within this book the term *audiological enablement*, which we define as a problem-solving process aimed at:

▪ enhancing the activities and participation of an individual with hearing difficulties
▪ improving their quality of life
▪ minimising any effect on significant others
▪ facilitating their acceptance of any residual problems.

Hearing impairment

While most patients presenting with hearing problems have an acquired disorder and hence *hearing loss*, we do not wish to exclude consideration of those with a congenital disorder, who have never 'lost' any hearing, and so prefer to use the term *hearing impairment*. In addition, this overcomes the problems with the inclusion of patients with King-Kopetzky syndrome (Hinchcliffe, 1992) who, while having hearing disability, have essentially normal hearing audiometrically, and hence no 'loss' of hearing. However, as shown by Zhao and Stephens (2000), on sensitised audiometric testing, most of such individuals have some degree of impairment, so may be regarded as being within the boundaries of *hearing impaired*.

In this context, we follow the recommendations of the European Work group on the Genetics of Hearing Impairment (Stephens, 2001) in which a number of relevant audiometric terms are defined. Following those recommendations, we also eschew the term *deafness* except in the context of the Deaf community, where the word has sociocultural connotations. We are aware that certain people within that community dislike the terms *impairment* and *impaired*, but we would argue that it is a valid term to use in people who have a measurable deficit in their hearing. Such people may, however, neither have a disability nor be disabled.

The terms *disability* and *handicap* will be discussed below in the context of the World Health Organization's (WHO) classifications. At this stage, we would argue that *handicap* is a confusing term, with many different connotations and uses, while the implications of *disability* have changed even within the two major WHO definitions (WHO, 1980, 2001).

'Patients', 'clients' or 'people with hearing impairments'

We have thought much about this aspect of terminology, namely the people whom we are dealing with and trying to help. As we have both worked within medical environments and the individuals with whom we are concerned have either a demonstrable pathological lesion or psychological problems, we have opted to use the term *patient*. We accept that some people will be uneasy with this 'medicalisation' of the problem but, as we shall show, we reject the simplistic medical model of disease and disability.

   We are unhappy with the term *client*, which implies a financial relationship to the service provider, one alien to the sociomedical environments in which we live and work. *People with hearing impairments*, and its acronym PHI, apart from being a clumsy term, implies that the individual with whom we are concerned must have a demonstrable impairment of function. While this is true for the vast majority of those with whom we are concerned, it is a term which excludes those complaining of hearing difficulties but who have no such demonstrable impairment. Like Wade (2006), we would argue that such individuals require rehabilitative help as much as those with clear impairments do, and that the enablement process should be able to encompass both groups.

Environmental aids/assistive listening devices (ALDs)

The role of environmental devices in the enablement process has received increasing attention (e.g. Lesner, 2003). While the term *assistive listening devices* is widely used, particularly in North America, and some of them such as television amplifiers and electromagnetic loop systems may be specifically concerned with listening, others such as flashing light doorbells and vibrator alarms are not. Further, the terminology including such devices in the *International Classification of Functioning, Disability and Health* (ICF; WHO, 2001) of 'Assistive products and technology for *personal* use in daily living' misses the point, as most of such devices, as opposed to hearing aids or cochlear implants, may be used by several people with hearing problems at the same time. We would therefore argue that the term *environmental aids*, used for a number of years in the rehabilitation literature, would be most appropriate, as it implies that they are devices which may help a range of people with hearing problems in a particular environment in which they might expect to have difficulties hearing what they would like to hear.

Layout of the book

We divide the main body of the book into four main sections, which broadly follow the categories of the WHO's ICF (2001).

   In the first section (Chapters 2–4), we cover entry into the process and the underlying dysfunctions found in affected individuals, including non-auditory factors which impact upon them. This has implications both for the affected individual and for those concerned with facilitating their entry into the process of enablement.

The second section (Chapters 5–6) will deal with the effect of such impairments of communication and emotional functions of the individual. It will also examine how the individual's other characteristics (e.g. attitudes, personality and non-auditory disabilities) as well as those around the individual can influence the difficulties which they experience.

The third main section (Chapters 7–9) will consider the individual in their environment, within their family, in work, as well as in broader leisure and other situations. Again, this will cover ways in which the individuals achieving their desired participation in such situations can be facilitated.

The fourth section (Chapters 10–12) provides a discussion of the process of enablement, the factors within the patient which need to be taken into account and what can be done to address the various problems experienced. In addition, we shall examine how these individuals can be helped to accept the fact that there will remain certain situations in which they will be unable to participate despite optimal facilitation approaches.

The World Health Organization classifications

Phillip Wood, a rheumatologist, was the first to propose the concept of a defined terminology for the consequences of disease (Wood, 1980), which was subsequently adopted by the WHO (1980). Previously, a range of terms including *disability* and *handicap* had been used in a variety of different ways by different groups of professionals and in different countries, and it had become clear that a widely agreed classification was going to be necessary if different professional were going to be able to communicate with each other in a meaningful way.

Within this classification – the *International Classification of Impairments, Disabilities and Handicaps* (ICIDH; WHO, 1980) – the three levels of consequence of impairment, disability and handicap were defined (Figure 1.1).

These manifestations were subsequently classified according to whether they referred to:

1. a loss or abnormality of psychological, physiological or anatomical structure or function – *impairment*
2. a restriction or lack of ability to perform an activity in the manner or within the range considered normal for a human being – *disability*
3. a disadvantage for an individual that limits or prevents the fulfilment of a role that is normal for that individual – *handicap*.

Thus, *impairments* represent disturbances at an organ level, *disabilities* at the level of the person and *handicaps* reflect interaction with and adaptation to the individual's surroundings.

The overall relationship between these aspects is shown in Figure 1.2

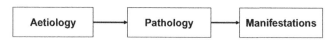

Figure 1.1 The consequences of disease.

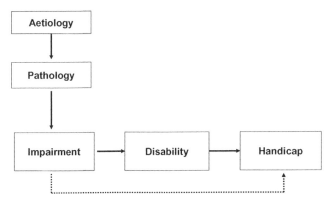

Figure 1.2 The basic classification embodied in ICIDH (1980).

It subsequently became apparent that this model could not cope with various aspects, particularly of the generation of handicap, and that it had a number of internal weaknesses from an audiological point of view. A variety of attempts was made by different authors (e.g. Stephens and Hétu, 1991) to address ways in which the model could be modified to allow for secondary handicaps and the influences of rehabilitative interventions.

Through the late 1990s and into 2001 a number of draft amendments to the ICIDH model were developed by the WHO, taking into account the various criticisms and suggestions made in the intervening years. This led to the publication in 2001 of the *International Classification of Functioning, Disability and Health* (ICF). Apart from changes in terminology, this had a number of key differences from the ICIDH.

1. There was a change from the presentation of the negative consequences of disease (what individuals cannot do) to its positive aspects (what individuals can do). Thus, broadly, 'impairment' was replaced by 'structure and function', 'disability' by 'activities' and 'handicap' by 'participation'. Negative aspects of these are termed 'impairment' (as before), 'activity limitation' and 'participation restriction'.
2. The concept of *contextual factors* – both environmental and personal – was introduced. These are factors around and within the individual, respectively, which can influence the activity or participation within an individual with a certain condition.
3. The third change lies in the fact that an alteration in one element (function, activity or participation) as a result of changes in contextual factors or from some form of intervention can influence those elements which precede it as well as those which follow it. That is, the model does not have just a simple left–right progression, but can show changes in any direction. This includes contextual factors, which can be altered by changes in activity or participation as well as altering them. The overall model is shown in Figure 1.3.

Both models have a number of key features in common. They each have three components of the consequences of the health condition, the first based on effects on the organ or system, the second on effects on the individual per se and the third on the effects on the individual within their environment/society. Second, while there

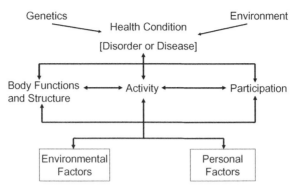

Figure 1.3 A modified version of ICF, including aetiological factors.

are exceptions, the general principle is that the health condition will lead to changes in structure or function, which in turn affect activity, while this modifies participation. Third, while the underlying condition may result in a number of individual effects, there is no attempt to determine an overall impact on the individual, which, for example, Wade (2003) proposes as 'wellness' and elsewhere as 'quality of life' (Wade and Halligan, 2003).

There are a number of specific weaknesses to the model when applied to particular domains, and a number of these have been highlighted by Wade and Halligan (2003) in a general context and by Stephens and Danermark (2005) in the context of people with hearing problems. Thus, Wade and Halligan (2003) highlight the need to specify more about 'the person' (i.e. the individual being considered) in their environment, their society, their body and their organ, and also include a section on the individual's choice: 'free will'. Elsewhere, Wade and de Jong (2000) point out that the model fails to take into account patient's subjective experiences.

Stephens and Danermark (2005) focus on the weaknesses of the ICF term *personal factors*, which, they argue, is poorly defined, and suggest that a well-defined, two-way interaction between *personal factors* and both *activity* and *participation* could overcome many of the problems. They also point out weaknesses from a hearing point of view in the classification of listening activities and of attempts within ICF to provide quantitative assessments of impairments. Wade and Halligan (2003) further argue that there should be more integration of ICF with ICD-10, the *International Statistical Classification of Diseases and Related Health Problems* – 10th Revision (ICD-10) (WHO, 1992), and also that the concept of *time* be applied to disabilities, which may have changed markedly since the onset of the individual's current set of problems.

However, despite these weaknesses, ICF remains a valuable model in the context of considering the impact of disorders such as hearing impairments. It is a model which will guide many aspects of the present book, even if we ignore its putative quantitative elements.

Within ICF, activity limitation and participation are lumped together under the collective term *disability*, which thus has a new definition and replaces the collective term *disablement*, used in ICIDH. The separation of activity and participation is generally based on 'what the person *can* do' for activity and 'what the person *does* do' for participation. However, ICF, in its Annex 3 describes alternative classifications based on a division of the disabilities into a group of 'tasks or actions that an individual does' as activities and 'involvement in life situations' as participations. In practice, there is relatively little difference in the practical outcome of the two classifications, and this will be discussed further in Chapter 10.

Theoretical/management models in the general rehabilitation literature

Katz *et al.* (1997), in the post-ICIDH era, describe the 'traditional approach' of three stages of 'Functional assessment' (the patient's disorder at a single moment), 'Diagnosis' (merely listing impairments and disabilities) and 'Treatment planning' (concerned with the management of functional problems at the time of assessment). They replace this with their Neurologic Model of Rehabilitation, comprising 'Diagnosis', involving assessment of the underlying brain disorder in relation to the disablements, 'Prognosis', dependent on personal and environmental factors as well as the natural history of the disease, and 'Treatment planning', involving the interactive process of recovery. This is illustrated in the model shown in Figure 1.4.

It may be seen that it emphasises the role of personal, social and environmental factors in interacting with the interventional process, which they call 'Learning'. This, in turn, is superimposed on the natural recovery process, which they argue is influenced by personal and environmental factors.

A similar approach is incorporated in the biopsychosocial model, which has been widely used in the context of pain management (e.g. McMahon and Koltzenburg, 2005) and the management of gastrointestinal disorders (Drossman, 1998). Drossman contrasts it with the previously used biomedical model, which fails to take into account psychosocial factors in the development of *illness* (Figures 1.5a and 1.5b). He argues that the biopsychosocial model takes these factors into account and explains the various psychosomatic disorders. Thus, comparing Figures 1.5a and 1.5b, it may be seen that the biopsychosocial model incorporates psychological predisposing factors with the biological ones as the starting point. The relationship between disease (pathology) and illness (perceived lack of wellness) becomes a two-way process, the balance of which may be changed by psychological modifiers. They, in turn, can be

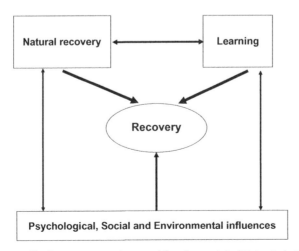

Figure 1.4 Factors contributing to recovery (summarising the model of Katz *et al.*, 1997).

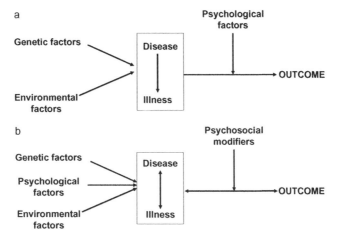

Figure 1.5 a Representation of the biomedical model. **b** Representation of the biopsychosocial model.

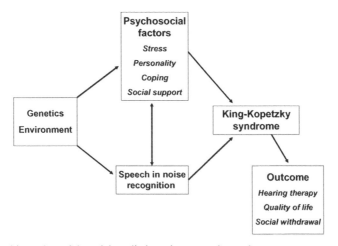

Figure 1.6 The biopsychosocial model applied to King-Kopetzky syndrome.

affected by the disease/illness process. Drossman (1998) argues that this involves a return to the holistic approach, integrating the psyche and physical factors, which characterised Greek medicine.

As an example, Figure 1.6 shows an application of the psychosocial model to King-Kopetzky syndrome, based on Drossman's application to irritable bowel syndrome. Pryce and Wainwright (2008) indicate that this condition comes within the same category of 'medically unexplained symptoms'.

Wade has developed various models of neurological rehabilitation (Wade, 2005, 2006b), considering different aspects of the process. Their focus is predominantly on activity limitations, whereas much of audiological rehabilitation is more orientated towards overcoming aspects of participation restrictions. However, many of the concepts Wade introduces are very relevant to the audiological field.

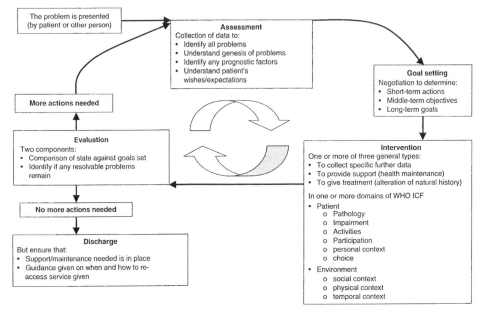

Figure 1.7 The rehabilitation process. (*Source:* derived from Wade, 2005, with permission.)

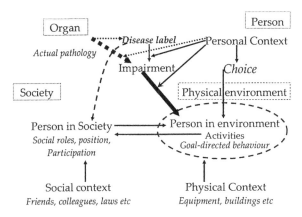

Figure 1.8 WHO ICF rehabilitation analysis of illness. (*Source:* derived from Wade, 2006b, with permission.)

Figure 1.7 shows an overview of the rehabilitation process, developed in the context of neurological rehabilitation, which may be seen as a cyclical process which continues until the evaluation indicates that no further actions are needed (Wade, 2005). At the same time, the model allows for re-entry into the system, should further support be required at a later stage. This reflects, in several ways the model of audiological rehabilitation described by Kiessling *et al.* (2003). It thus demonstrates the existence of many commonalities in the process of rehabilitation applied to different systems, even though details of the interventions will obviously differ. One important aspect of this model is the consideration of short-, medium- and long-term goals.

Elsewhere Wade (2006b) emphasises the importance of considering in the rehabilitation process those individuals presenting to health care services who have no underlying pathology. He argues that the rehabilitation process should be equally relevant to such individuals as to those with a clear pathology. There may be analogies there with the management of King-Kopetzky syndrome, in which many individuals have no clear auditory pathology. In addition, Wade argues that individuals simulating or exaggerating their symptoms could be considered in this context, even if the approach to their detailed management might be different.

In this context, he developed a modification of ICF analysis of illness, taking into account the aspects of personal choice. This is shown in Figure 1.8, which illustrates how the 'person', with their characteristics and attitudes, interacts with other elements of ICF.

Models of audiological enablement

Prior to the end of World War Two, there was little attempt to integrate the different aspects of rehabilitative provision for adults with hearing impairments, with leading authors in Europe and America considering instrumental and non-instrumental support under very separate headings (e.g. Bunch, 1943; Ewing, 1944). The major changes with attempts to provide an integrated service came after that war with the Veterans Association in the United States (e.g. Bergman, 1950) and the establishment of rehabilitation departments in the new National Health Service provisions in the United Kingdom (e.g. Whetnall, 1951) and Scandinavia (e.g. Ewertsen, 1976).

Rehabilitation programmes developed by Bergman (1950) and lasting either four weeks or two and a half days are shown in his Figures 5 and 6. These cover most of the components of clinical audiological rehabilitation currently considered, even if they are not presented in relationship to each other. In addition, auditory assessments are assumed to have been completed prior to the rehabilitative process, and so are not specifically included within it. The total plan of the programme, however, including both assessment and remediation (from Bergman's Figure 6, p. 49) is shown in Figure 1.9. All the components of Bergman's model took place within the institutions of the Veteran's Administration.

Bergman's model (1950) represents a detailed functional descriptive approach to the rehabilitative process, rather than a conceptual or analytical model. Markides (1977a) adopted an approach similar to Bergman's in his comprehensive description of the Danish state rehabilitative system and included external sources of support for people with hearing difficulties, such as voluntary organisations, church and further education. His organisational chart is shown in Figure 1.10. The top half of the chart broadly represents services provided within the institutions and the lower half within the patient's home.

These two models draw together most of the major components of the rehabilitative process but do not specifically address the question of fitting the process to the patient's needs. This is also a criticism which may be made of some of the more recent models, although, on the whole, they do try to address this problem.

The first serious attempts to provide a flow diagram of the process of rehabilitation came with the work of Alpiner (1978) and Walden (1980). Interestingly, Walden's approach is based, like Bergman's (1950), on his experience in the US Veterans Administration.

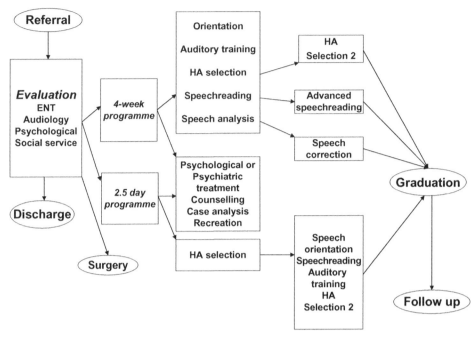

Figure 1.9 Rehabilitation programme developed by Bergman. (*Source:* adapted from Bergman, 1950, p. 49. Reproduced by permission of the author.)

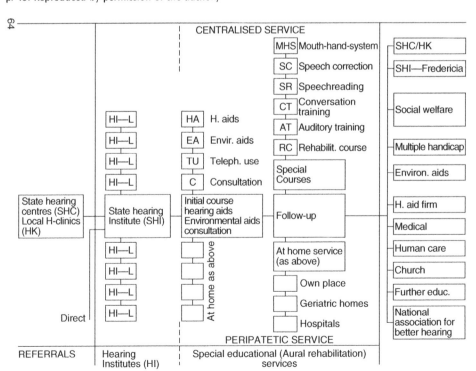

Figure 1.10 Rehabilitative organisational chart for services in Denmark. (*Source:* from Markides, 1977. Reproduced by permission of the author.)

Within his approach, Walden (1980) does consider psychosocial factors, in particular 'Problem awareness' and 'Situation control' and 'Adjustment problems', in both the audiological diagnosis and rehabilitative intervention but does not present them in a specific goal-setting context. In addition, the main elements of the process are the clear audiological components, although he does recommend 'Environmental control training' for those with 'Situation control problems' (identification and assertiveness) and counselling for those with adjustment problems (social, vocational and emotional).

The Goldstein–Stephens model

Goldstein and Stephens (1980, 1981) developed a management model, which they proposed would:

1. highlight the many components which constitute the entirety of the process being considered (in this, we tried to make explicit some of the subtle parameters of the 'clinical art' so that they could be more rationally evaluated)
2. consider the sequences and interaction of these components
3. provide guidance in the training of audiologists.

It aimed to be general and not system-specific, particularly given the different backgrounds of its authors, one a university-clinic-based American audiologist within the US sociomedical system and the other an audiological physician within the UK National Health Service. It was thus broad and independent of setting and philosophy.

Goldstein and Stephens deliberately, however, avoided any consideration of factors which might have determined whether an individual with hearing problems enters the rehabilitation system and also any consideration of the 'completeness' or final outcome of the rehabilitative process. These will be addressed in the present book in a later section in which we consider our present working model (Chapter 10).

The overall model comprising the various components is shown in Figure 1.11. The three columns show different degrees of elaboration of the process, from the basic elements of evaluation and remediation on the left through to the more specific components, such as the individual elements of communication status on the right.

Goldstein and Stephens emphasise the elements of evaluation which were relevant to the rehabilitative process and argue that different components of the evaluation should be assessed in ways appropriate to the particular component. Thus, auditory function should be assessed by formal and relevant audiometric tests, whereas certain other components could be assessed by interview or observation. This has been considered in more detail elsewhere (e.g. Stephens, 1982, 1987a) and we shall return to this question in Chapter 10.

In addition, in their presentation of the model, Goldstein and Stephens discussed ways that each individual component could be elaborated, using computer flow diagrams, similar to those used by Walden (1980). Examples of these are shown in Goldstein and Stephens (1980, 1981), and a more extended elaboration in the context of hearing aid selection was presented in Stephens (1984).

Evaluation

Returning to the basic model, Goldstein and Stephens that, while the communication status of the individual was a key area in the evaluation of the patient presenting for

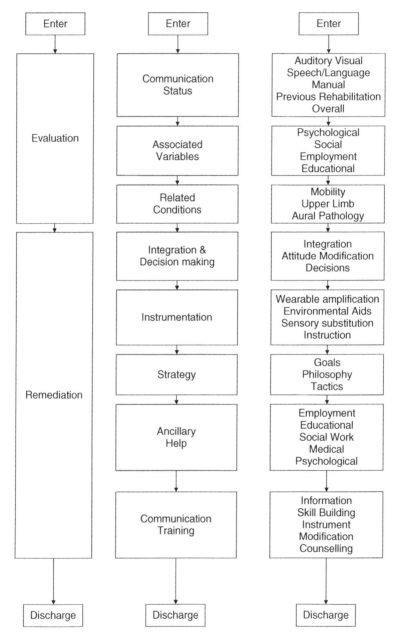

Figure 1.11 Goldstein and Stephens' (1981) model outlined with each column showing increasing detail. (Reproduced with permission.)

rehabilitation, it was only one of several key areas. The other two areas which they identified there were what they call 'Associated variables' and 'Related conditions'. The first of these, associated variables, comprises what may be broadly considered as the psychosocial elements of the process, involving both patients and those around them. The second, related conditions, comprises a variety of other elements of the patient that may complicate the rehabilitative process.

In general terms, communication status comprises the raw materials with which the audiologist has to work, associated variables govern the overall approach to be adopted with the patient and significant others, and related conditions determine detailed aspects of the approach to be followed. Elements of the last comprise, for example, whether the individual is bed-bound or house-bound, whether they have severe tremors and whether they have tinnitus or discharging ears.

Remediation

The first element of remediation is labelled 'Attitude'. This comprises three major components: first, the drawing together of information obtained in the evaluation process, and, second, some preliminary modification of the patient's acceptance, understanding and expectations of the rehabilitative process and third an initial triage of the patients. This last has important implications for the rehabilitative process and has four categories ranging from 'keen and straightforward' through to 'rejecting any rehabilitative intervention'.

This triage/classification of patients has withstood the tests of time for over a quarter of a century, although the proportions in the different categories may vary according to the age breakdown and population under consideration (e.g. Stephens, 1982; Stephens and Meredith, 1991a). However, in all reports, some 90% of individuals come in attitudes/rehabilitation types 1 and 2. A brief description of the four types is shown in Table 1.1.

Type 1 patients are the most common among the younger age bands and require relatively limited resources in terms of ongoing support and pass quickly through the system, returning of their own volition should they have any further problems. Type 2 patients are positively motivated but additional problems may be anticipated. This may be because they have severe/profound hearing loss or a very mild loss,

Table 1.1 Rehabilitation types.

Rehabilitation type	Description
1	**Positively motivated without complicating factors** will accept relevant instrumental intervention and pass rapidly and effectively through the system
2	**Positively motivated with complicating factors** will require more attention with regard to specific instrumentation and handling, communication skills and tactics
3	**Want help, but reject a key component** will require careful handling with counselling and involvement of significant others
4	**Deny any problems** no intervention for the patient, but the significant others may require support and advice

they may have an audiogram which may be difficult to fit with hearing aids (e.g. a low-frequency sensory loss), or they may have other complicating factors such as tinnitus, otorrhoea, severe tremor etc. Type 3 patients genuinely want help but may reject a particular element which might be most appropriate for them, such as a hearing aid. Alternatively, they may have inappropriate expectations of a hearing aid, thinking it will solve all their psychosocial problems, when in fact counselling is what is needed. Both types 2 and 3 will generally require considerably more time and effort from the rehabilitative service. Subsequently, Piercy and Goldstein (1994) subdivided type 3 patients into 3A, negative about hearing aids, and 3B, expecting hearing aids to solve all their problems.

Type 4 patients are usually persuaded to seek help by long-suffering significant others and will deny any disability even though they patently have marked hearing difficulties. They will never wear a hearing aid if fitted and will reject all other aspects of the rehabilitative process. Little is to be gained by either the patient or the audiologist in continuing with the rehabilitative process, even if it were ethically justified. The patient is usually informed that they have a hearing loss and that they can return to the system if they change their mind and feel that they need help. At the same time, it can be helpful to separately provide the significant other, often at the end of their tether, with advice regarding communication tactics and environmental aids which they could introduce unobtrusively in order to make their life more tolerable.

The main elements of the immediate remedial intervention are covered by 'Instrumental 1', 'Strategy' and 'Ancillary', with 'Communication training' often being a longer-term component, particularly with rehabilitation Types 2 and 3. Instrumental 1 covers the initial approach to instrumental help for the individual, including both personal (e.g. hearing aids, cochlear implants) and general, covering environmental aids. In both cases, an important element comprises instructing the patient as to how to derive most benefit from the instrument concerned.

In 'Strategy' they attempted to break with the 'one size fits all' approach to hearing tactics by first considering, in conjunction with the patient, the goals which were both important for the patient and potentially achievable. Further, in the choice of appropriate hearing tactics, it was also essential to take into account the personality and life philosophy of the individual and select tactics in accord with that. Thus, for example, a shy introvert would never adopt highly assertive tactics.

The 'Ancillary' section admits that, as audiologists, whatever our background, we are rarely able to meet all the patients' needs by ourselves. This section is therefore concerned with the involvement of relevant external professionals, physicians, psychologists, social workers, employment support workers etc., who can complement the audiologist in enabling patients to function to the best of their abilities.

Unlike these three components, which are essentially short-term from the audiologist's standpoint, 'Communication training' is an ongoing process which may take just one or two sessions, but which in other patients may continue for months or even years. In all cases, it comprises activities under the four headings of 'Information (provision)', 'Skill-building', 'Instrumental 2 (modification)' and 'Counselling'. We are not prescriptive here, but it is essential to consider under these headings the ongoing needs of the patient. Thus, for example, the skill-building may range from patiently teaching an older patient how to fit their hearing aid to their ear through to training a patient with a cochlear implant in telephone use.

The initial flow diagram with decision boxes for this process is shown in Figure 1.12. Within this, for example, Rehabilitation type 1 patients may pass through quickly

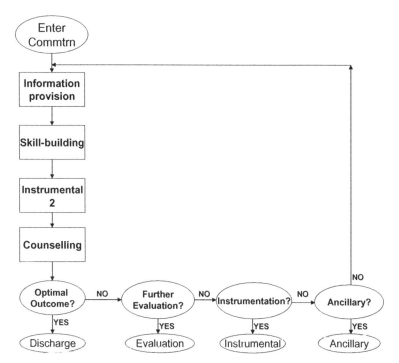

Figure 1.12 Flow diagram for communication training block. (*Source*: adapted from Goldstein and Stephens, 1981, with permission.)

with just some fine adjustments of their hearing aid(s) and further advice on environmental aids. Type 2 patients, on the other hand may require elements of several of the components, and Type 3 patients a considerable input from Counselling, possibly in a group context where they may accept suggestions and criticisms from their peers better than from professionals.

The model continued to retain the same format over the years, although minor changes were made. The first significant change came in the conference proceedings of 'Psychological and psychosocial approaches to adult hearing loss' (Stephens, 1996). Within this, elements of the WHO's *International Classification of Impairments, Disabilities and Handicaps* (ICIDH; WHO, 1980) were incorporated into the model, following some development of the concepts applied to that framework by Stephens and Hétu (1991).

Thus, in this version of the model, the first block of 'Communication Status' was preceded by a block 'Disability and handicap', in order to increase the emphasis on the problems which the individual was experiencing, and we discussed the role of *positive experiences* in the development of *handicap*. (This will be discussed further in a later section of the present chapter.) Following the work of Hallberg and Barrenäs (1993) and of Hétu and Getty (1991), the role of significant others was enhanced in the discussion of the development of handicap and in the 'associated variables' section of the model.

The next change was to separate the block 'Attitude', in which elements of the evaluation were brought together, from the remediation process and have it as a separate block between evaluation and remediation, and renamed 'Integration and decision-making'. While it remains generally the same, an element of preliminary

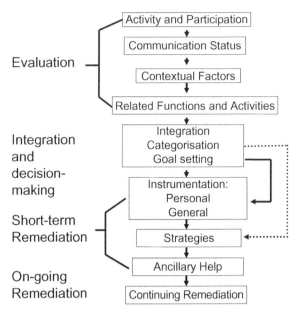

Evaluation
- Activity and Participation
- Communication Status
- Contextual Factors
- Related Functions and Activities

Integration and decision-making
- Integration Categorisation Goal setting
- Instrumentation: Personal General

Short-term Remediation
- Strategies

On-going Remediation
- Ancillary Help
- Continuing Remediation

Figure 1.13 Updated model of audiological rehabilitation. (*Source:* adapted from Stephens, 2003.)

goal-setting was incorporated into this block, which would then lead into the Remediation process.

The only other change, a minor one, was to separate the 'communication training' block into 'Ongoing remediation', leaving the three other components as 'Short-term remediation'.

Subsequent changes came with the publication of the WHO's *International Classification of Functioning, Disability and Health* (ICF; WHO, 2001), which led to the incorporation of the terminology of that framework into the model (Stephens, 2003). This is shown in Figure 1.13.

Thus, 'Handicap' and 'Disability' become 'Activity' and 'Participation', and 'Communication status' remains unchanged. 'Associated variables' becomes 'Contextual factors'. This maintains the element of 'psychological factors' in the ICF listing of 'Personal factors'. Social factors include ICF's 'Support and Relationships' as well as 'Attitudes, values and beliefs', which are classified there as 'Environmental Factors'. However, 'Products and technology', including existing environmental aids and hearing aids, are now brought into this section, with 'Services, systems and policies' covering the background provisions which may be available for the individual.

'Related functions and activities' replaces 'Related factors' and covers within it 'Mental functions; Sensations associated with hearing and vestibular function; Touch function; Manipulative activities; and Walking activities'. Most elements are broadly similar to the previous components of 'Related conditions' except for the inclusion of 'Mental functions', which, in this context, covers mainly the intellectual, attention, cognitive and memory functions of the patient. These will obviously have an impact on how the remediation process is implemented.

The four components of remediation remain largely unchanged, although the role of significant others (secondary to that of the patient) is given more emphasis in the

'Strategy' box. In addition, the role of voluntary organisations and self-help groups is brought into the 'Ancillary' section. Within 'Continuing remediation' renamed from 'Communication training', the concept of 'Changes to the physical and cultural environment' is also introduced. This implies involvement of the patient, employers, colleagues, family, caregivers and educators as well as the audiology professionals in an effort to ameliorate the acoustical, visual and stress-related situations confronting the patient.

The most recent proposed model incorporating many of these concepts was described by Kiessling *et al.* (2003) and arose from an Eriksholm symposium on 'Candidature and delivery of audiological services: special needs of older people'. While maintaining much of Stephens' (2003) model, it incorporates the concept of *instrumental* and *non-instrumental rehabilitation* as presented in a parallel way, and includes a section on 'Outcome measurement'.

Earlier, the model had demonstrated the applicability of the original model to specific patient groups, including older people (Stephens and Goldstein, 1983) to individuals with central auditory dysfunction (Fourcin *et al.*, 1985) and to those with profound hearing loss (Stephens, 1988). Furthermore, it has been adopted in a number of contexts by Smaldino and Traynor (1982), Schow and Nerbonne (1995, 2007) and others. Within their latest publication, Schow and Nerbonne (2007) have also attempted to modify the model within the context of ICF, although their approach is somewhat different from those described above.

Further interesting approaches along broadly similar lines have been proposed by Hyde and Riko (1994) in their Decision-Analytic approach and by Tye-Murray (1998), among others.

The role of positive experiences associated with hearing impairment

Anecdotal accounts of positive experiences associated with hearing impairment date back several centuries. Thus, for example, the English portrait painter and founder of the Royal Academy, Joshua Reynolds (1723–1792), alluded to it in his correspondence, and as reported by a biographer: 'Reynolds did not let his deafness worry him, it assisted his natural gift for reading character' (Hudson, 1958). Other anecdotal accounts, discussed by Kerr and Stephens (1997) mention the 'development of personal attributes', 'social contacts' and 'contacts with other hearing-impaired groups'.

Systematic investigation of the impact of positive experiences in systemic diseases such as neoplasia, HIV infections and cardiovascular disease date back only to the 1980s and have been discussed by Kerr and Stephens (2000). Such effects include changes in existential values, increased self-knowledge and relationship change.

The first study in the hearing field arose from the PhD study by Patricia Stewart-Kerr (1992) when, investigating handicap in adults with severe acquired hearing impairment, she identified as separate themes 'stronger religious feelings', a 'better understanding of human nature', 'positive experiences of communication' and 'practical and social support from hearing people'. She found that 'positive experiences of communication' and 'stronger religious feelings' were the two which had the strongest positive impact on people's lives.

This work was extended in two qualitative and one quantitative study on patients attending rehabilitation clinics in Cardiff (Kerr and Stephens, 1997, 2000; Stephens and Kerr, 2003). In the qualitative studies, patients were asked to list, in order of importance, any positive experiences which they may have had as a result of their

Table 1.2 Main positive themes identified by Kerr and Stephens (1997, 2000).

Theme	Number of respondents	
	1997 study	*2000 study*
Reduced disturbance from unwanted sounds	26	43
Successful communication strategies	24	24
Affinity to other deaf and disabled people	17	15
Perceived self-development	13	14
Using deafness to self-advantage	10	6
Communicative support from hearing people	9	6
Technical aids (e.g. Teletext)	1	7

hearing loss. This questionnaire was administered to consecutive series of first-time hearing aid candidates and, in the first study, Kerr and Stephens (1997) sought to determine the proportion of patients listing one or more positive experiences and the main experiences listed. Some 22% listed positive experiences and the main experiences listed are shown in Table 1.2.

The second qualitative study (Kerr and Stephens, 2000) obtained positive responses from some 40% of hearing aid candidates, and these responses followed a very similar pattern to that found in the first study (Table 1.2). When Kerr and Stephens demographic predictors of whether an individual was able to identify one or more positive experiences, we found that this was independent of the severity of hearing impairment, gender and the duration of hearing impairment. However, younger patients, those of non-manual social classes and those who had had previous hearing aids were more likely to report positive experiences.

On the basis of these two qualitative studies, Stephens and Kerr (2003) a quantitative questionnaire with 48 statements to which the respondents were required to state whether a particular experience was often, sometimes, rarely or never true for them. From this, they identified eight themes using a factor analysis. They comprised 'Cognitive changes to self-perception', 'Successful communication behaviours', 'Technical facilitators of communication', 'Using hearing loss to self-advantage', 'Effort in communication', 'Social support', 'Social contact' and 'Resignation'.

On this basis, the questionnaire was reduced to 20 questions and presented this together with a number of outcome measures to a further group of patients. This identified six main factors, three of which were predominantly auditory and three non-auditory. These are shown in Table 1.3.

Among the possible demographic predictors, the only one to relate to the total score, and also to the non-auditory factors, was the age of the individual, younger people perceiving more positive experiences. The only other relationship of note was that 'Using hearing loss to self-advantage' related to the duration of the reported hearing loss.

In this study, there was only a limited relationship with other measures including the Satisfaction with Life Scale (Diener et al., 1985) and the more specific Hearing Disability and Handicap Scale (Hétu et al., 1994). The two measures 'Cognitive changes to self perception' and 'Using hearing loss to self advantage' related positively to the handicap measure (basically psychological impact), and the two com-

Table 1.3 Main positive factors identified by Stephens and Kerr (2003).

Factor	Auditory factors	Non-auditory factors	Total variance (%)
1		Cognitive changes to self-perception	14.7
2	Use hearing loss to self-advantage		13.5
3	Successful communication behaviours		9.4
4		Resignation	8.4
5		Effort in communication	7.3
6	Technical facilitators of communication		7.3

Table 1.4 Questions loading on 'Successful communication behaviour' factor.

Questions	Loading
Have enjoyable conversations	0.71
Clinic staff understanding	0.61
Feel important to family	0.57
Take part in leisure activities	0.52
Have own ways of coping	0.40

(*Source:* adapted from Stephens and Kerr, 2003.)

munication based positive factors (factors 3 and 5) related negatively to this measure. Factor 3 also correlated positively with the Satisfaction with Life Scale.

It is thus interesting to note that a perception of successful communication has a positive effect on these approaches to quality of life. Specific questions loading on this factor are shown in Table 1.4.

In addition, it is interesting to note that Dibb and Yardley (2006), studying patients with Menière's disorder, found a significant relationship between a 'Downwards Positive Social Comparison' (e.g. 'When I read about others who experience more difficulties than I do, I am relieved about my own situation') and quality of life as assessed by the SF-36 Health Survey Standard Version. However, it showed no significant relationship with further changes over a 10-month period. Furthermore, no studies have so far been made on the impact of positive experiences on the outcome of audiological rehabilitation.

Relevant measures in assessing patients' needs and the outcomes of interventions

This section is meant as an introduction to a theme to which we shall return at various stages throughout the book. It is a topic essential to any serious consideration of possible benefits of audiological enablement and the demonstration of the effectiveness of different elements of it and their benefits to the patient. There is an extensive literature in this field (e.g. Noble, 1998; Bentler and Kramer, 2000), but what concerns us here is measures which are relevant to the individual with hearing problems. In

Table 1.5 Goals of outcome measures in audiology.

Goal	Goal
1	To assess the rehabilitative outcomes for an individual hearing impaired person
2	To assess the effectiveness of the services provided by a particular clinical unit or agency
3	To assess the effectiveness of new hearing aid technologies
4	To assess the effectiveness of hearing rehabilitation services on quality of life

(*Source:* derived from Cox *et al.*, 2000.)

particular, we are concerned with the definition of the needs of the patient at the beginning of the process of enablement and then an assessment of how well these needs are met when we approach the end of the process. In addition, there will be, inevitably, some measures as to how well the patient perceives that the process has succeeded for them, given the fact that, prior to intervention, they will be unaware of all the implications of the enablement process.

Cox *et al.* (2000) discuss the various purposes of outcome measures. These are shown in Table 1.5. While we shall consider Goals 2–4 where they are relevant to other discussions within this book, in this and later chapters most emphasis will be put on Goal 1. In this context, we shall take the article by Cox *et al.* as our starting point. These goals are discussed further in Chapter 12.

In this context, Cox *et al.* start with the general recommendation that this 'should be designed to facilitate assessing the client's needs and preferences' and later continue that the 'measure should primarily be based on individualized self-report, in which the nature of the assessing items or listening situations is determined by each client rather than being standardized across clients'.

They continue to suggest that both activity limitations and participation restrictions should, optimally, be included in the assessment as well as soliciting reports from significant others. They then give some examples of potentially relevant tools.

We are happy with this general approach, and indeed were contributors to the paper, but some recent studies suggest that the approach needs to be extended, and this will be discussed at different points throughout this book. Some missing aspects include the individual's ability to cope with their hearing problems as well as their satisfaction with the treatment which they have received. Furthermore, it needs to be emphasised that the patient, rather than the significant other, is the subject of the enablement process, and while invaluable information may be obtained from significant others, ultimate decisions must always rest with the patient.

Cox *et al.* (2000) very reasonably suggest that the Client-Oriented Scale of Improvement (COSI; Dillon *et al.*, 1997) is a valuable starting point in such assessment. Prior to intervention, the audiologist determines the hearing problems most important to the individual and, after intervention, the improvement and residual elements of such problems.

One of the problems which need to be addressed is how we determine the input to COSI in terms of the patient's problems and how we elicit their real problems. An early intervention study (Stephens *et al.*, 1991a) found that it is the effects on the individual of their hearing impairment (participation restriction and emotional effects) rather than their activity limitations which determine help-seeking. We have long advocated use of the Barcham and Stephens (1980) Problem Questionnaire as a starting point into defining the patient's real problems, supplemented by further

Table 1.6 Mean number of responses per subject in ICF domains elicited using different open-ended questions.

WHO ICF category	Difficulties question (number of respondents)	Life-effects question (number of respondents)
Functional impairments	0.26	0.11
Activity limitations	1.77	1.48
Participation restrictions	0	1.24
Environmental factors	0.12	0.39
Personal/psychological factors	0.08	0.88

(*Source:* adapted from Stephens *et al.*, 2001.)

questioning at interview. However, this approach would appear to be relatively ineffective at eliciting participation restrictions (Cox *et al.*, 2000; Stephens *et al.*, 2000), and Cox argues that this is an area which needs to be addressed.

This was addressed in a subsequent paper (Stephens *et al.*, 2001) in which the original wording of 'Please make a list of all the difficulties which you have because of your hearing loss' was replaced with 'Please make a list of the effects your hearing problems have on your life. Write down as many as you can think of.'

When we used this approach, the number of participation restrictions and psychological factors which were elicited increased considerably and this is shown in Table 1.6.

It may be seen that there were marked differences (significant at $P < 0.01$ or better) in all WHO ICF domains apart from activity limitations. It may thus be argued that this 'life effects' question sent to the patients prior to their clinic visit is useful in eliciting a range of relevant consequences of the individual's hearing impairment. It should always be supplemented by further questioning and clarification during the clinic visit which will then lead to the establishment of the appropriate input to COSI or an equivalent approach and also to goal-setting in the enablement process.

The one potential problem with the use of such open-ended patient questionnaires, and which can generally be clarified at interview, is that it is sometimes unclear as to whether the patient is referring to an activity limitation (what they *can* do) or to a participation restriction (what they *do* do). To clarify this, Stephens *et al.* (2001) examined an alternative classification (WHO, 2001, Annex 3, p. 234) in which the first four disability domains ('Learning and applying knowledge', 'General tasks and demands', 'Communication', 'Mobility') are regarded as activities and the last five ('Self-care', 'Domestic life', 'Interpersonal interactions', 'Major life areas', 'Community, social and civic life') as participations.

This was performed as a retrospective analysis of 100 older patients attending a rehabilitation clinic where activity limitations and participation restrictions had been elicited by means of the Problem Questionnaire and by interview. The results are shown in Figure 1.14, which shows no significant difference in the number of responses regardless of which categorisation of activities and participations was used.

While the most widely used approach to outcome assessment using such personalised measures are used to input to COSI, an alternative approach is to use them with visual analogue scales (VAS). Although COSI is the most appropriate and straightforward approach for most patients with hearing difficulties, for those in whom a number of repeat measures may be required, such as patients with cochlear

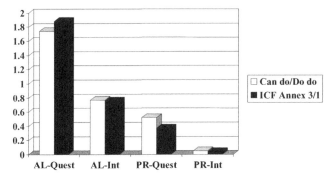

Figure 1.14 Mean number of responses in different categories using the traditional (Can do/Do do) classification of activities and participations versus the separation by disability types (Annex 3/1). AL = activity limitations, PR = participation restrictions, Quest = questionnaire, Int = interview.

implants, the VAS approach may be more appropriate, examples of this approach are given by Andersson *et al.* (1995a), Stephens and Zhao (2002) and Bai and Stephens (2005).

The open-ended questionnaire approach can also be effectively used with significant others of patients who can be asked about both the impact of the patient's hearing impairment on themselves as well as on the patient (e.g. Stephens *et al.*, 1995). There do not, however, appear to have been any quantitative studies using this approach.

Benefits and limitations of audiological interventions can also be used in a personalised way. Thus, Tyler and Kelsay (1990) asked patients who had received cochlear implants to list all the advantages that 'you believe a cochlear implant has provided. List them in order of importance starting with the greatest advantage, list as many as you can.' Their second question used the same format but with 'disadvantage' substituted for 'advantage'. A similar approach was independently introduced by Stephens and Meredith (1991b) in the context of hearing aids. However, the reliability of a quantitative approach to such a measure remains to be investigated.

Finally, an approach to how the patient is coping with their hearing problems needs to be defined on an individual basis. While Andersson *et al.* (1994) developed a 'Hearing coping assessment', the use of a patient-specific visual analogue or categorical scale could be a valuable alternative, which needs to be explored further.

Development of a preliminary model appropriate to hearing impairment

Coming from the earlier consideration of different models, it would seem appropriate to conclude this chapter with an outline of the position from which we are working. Figure 1.15 gives an outline of the stages through which the individual within the community who experiences hearing problems may pass. There will be detailed decision boxes with a range of factors influencing them at different stages and these will be considered in the next and subsequent chapters.

At the present stage, it is premature to consider further details of these, beyond emphasising the paramount importance of the input from the patient in proceeding

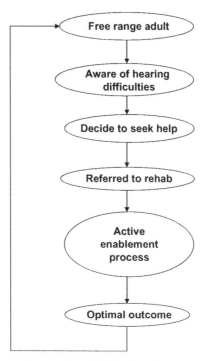

Figure 1.15 An outline of the main stages in audiological enablement.

from one stage to the next. There will, obviously, be various feedback loops at different stages and these will be considered further in Chapter 10.

For a number of reasons, the more detailed model of the active enablement process will follow the earlier version of the model illustrated in Figure 1.13, rather than that proposed by Kiessling *et al.* (2003). One of the main reasons behind such a decision is that we feel the need to separate the short-term elements of enablement which are applicable to almost all patients from many of the longer-term aspects which will be relevant only to a minority. Furthermore, we would argue that the provision of the 'Surveillance and maintenance' feedback loop will not be relevant to a significant proportion of patients. Thus, while it may be offered to all, the decision to accept/ participate in this must rest with the individual patient.

Conclusion

The term *enablement* is more appropriate to a patient-centred approach, involving participation by the patient and significant others, than the more traditional term *rehabilitation*. Our model of enablement is based on a combination of WHO's ICF and Goldstein and Stephens' (1980, 1981) Management Model. This model is presented in relation to other models in audiology. On the basis of a number of our studies, the importance of highlighting the positive experiences of patients reporting hearing difficulties is emphasised. We also argue the importance of having patient-friendly and relevant outcome measures for the assessment of the efficacy of the process, such as Dillon's (1997) Client-Oriented Scale of Improvement (COSI).

2 Seeking help

Introduction

The main thrust of this chapter is to determine why some people seek help for their hearing difficulties when they have little or no hearing loss whereas others with a moderate to severe loss may take no action. It has been well established in a number of studies that only about a quarter or less of those people who might benefit from a hearing aid or aids actually have one (Humphrey et al., 1981; Davis, 1995). The UK Medical Research Council's survey of ear, nose and throat problems (MRC–ENT) showed that, while some 20% of individuals indicated hearing difficulties ('problems hearing TV' 18.8%, 'difficulties with conversation in noise' 21.4%), only 3.4% currently had hearing aids (Davis et al., 2007). The survey also showed that among those who found their hearing difficulties severely annoying only 48% had hearing aids (Figure 2.1).

When evaluating the efficacy of a speech-in-noise test for self-testing of hearing over the telephone, Smits et al. (2006a) found that only 42% of those with 'Poor' speech recognition had hearing aids. This signal/noise ratio (>5.6 dB) at which these subjects, aged 60 years and over, could not recognise speech was broadly equivalent to a hearing level of 46 dB averaged over 0.5–4 kHz (Smits et al., 2006b).

In addition, and related to this, is the fact that the average patient seeking a hearing aid for the first time has had hearing problems for some 10–20 years before taking such a help-seeking decision (Brooks, 1976; Thomas and Gilhome Herbst, 1980).

The hurdles (or *filters*) which need to be overcome in the process of help-seeking are discussed elsewhere (Stephens, 1983a) as are the factors which determine whether individuals achieve their goals of acquiring rehabilitative support (Stephens, 1983b). The major factors involved in this process are shown in Table 2.1 and will be discussed further within this chapter.

Help-seeking starts with the individual becoming conscious that there are certain things which they have difficulty hearing, particularly in noisy circumstances. The next stage will be deciding to take some action or help to overcome this difficulty. Engelund (2006) describes this process as 'Time for hearing', and argues that the role of stigma is less important than suggested by other authors.

Such help-seeking may be initially with their partner or alternative significant other, who may or may not encourage them to seek professional help. Early intervention programmes have been proposed and piloted to encourage such individuals to seek help at an earlier stage, and we shall discuss the effectiveness and ethical aspects of such programmes.

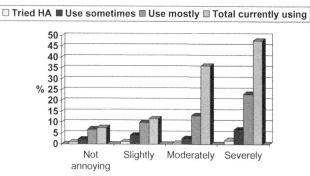

Figure 2.1 Hearing aid possession by annoyance caused by hearing difficulties. (*Source:* derived from Davis *et al.*, 2007.)

Table 2.1 Factors influencing whether an individual seeks rehabilitative help.

1	The physical status of the individual
2	Their psychological status
3	Social factors
4	Educational and vocational influences
5	The accessibility of the rehabilitative facilities
6	The attitude of professional encountered
7	Experiential factors

(*Source:* derived from Stephens, 1983b.)

When the individuals do decide to seek help, they must convince their primary carer or primary physician that they need such help and to send/refer them to the appropriate provider of rehabilitative support. Whatever the system, with state or private provision, there are further hurdles to be overcome here and perseverance is necessary to ensure appropriate referral.

On arrival at a centre which may offer appropriate enablement, there remain a number of problems, the first of which is for the professionals to define what the patient's main problems are and how these can best be overcome. This will depend not only on the characteristics of the patient and their significant others but also on the background and professional skills of the audiological professional concerned. For all good professionals this will entail an interactive process with the patient and their significant others, and indeed, this may take place in the patient's home prior to attendance at the clinic, as advocated by Brooks (1989).

Finally, on the web site related to this book (http://www.wiley.com/go/stephens), we shall include some appendices covering the most commonly posed questions and answers from this stage of the process, difficulties to be considered and further sources of information.

Becoming aware of hearing difficulties

Before anyone can seek hearing help, they must become aware that they have difficulties with their hearing. It might seem that there was a simple relationship between

Table 2.2 Factors which may influence the awareness of hearing problems.

1	Age
2	Gender
3	Rate of onset
4	Related symptoms
5	Psychological factors
6	Role models
7	Significant others
8	Lifestyle
9	Work situations
10	Linguistic situation
11	Cognitive factors
12	Presence of other disabilities

some criterion of hearing impairment and an awareness of hearing problems, but a number of studies have shown that this is not a simple one-to-one relationship. Thus, for example, Merluzzi and Hinchcliffe (1973) found that the degree of hearing loss which an individual must have (in decibels) before they report that their hearing is 'not as good as it used to be' increases markedly with age. Thus, for 30-year-olds, such a threshold is 5 dB, rising to 30 dB for 70-year-old people.

In a similar vein, Gilhome Herbst *et al.* (1991) investigated individuals over the age of 70 years in general practices in Islington, London and Glyncorrwg, Wales, whose mean hearing level in their better hearing ears was 35 dB or worse. In the London sample, 26% reported no hearing difficulties, and 25% of the Welsh sample denied any problems. More recently, Duijvestijn *et al.* (2003) investigated individuals over the age of 55 years who participated voluntarily in a driving test and health check. Their mean age was 66.7 years (range 55–91) and their criterion of impairment was a better ear hearing level >30 dB averaged across 500 Hz to 4 kHz. They found 23% of those meeting this criterion rated their hearing as good.

At the opposite end of the spectrum are individuals with King-Kopetzky syndrome, who complain of hearing difficulties, particularly hearing speech in noise, in the absence of any significant elevation of their pure tone threshold. Zhao and Stephens (2000) found that, even using sensitised audiometric tests of peripheral and central auditory function, some 20% had no significant auditory abnormality, and higher percentages were found in other studies which they examined. Price and Wainwright (2008) argue that this tendency to regard minimal difficulties hearing in background noise as being abnormal is a function of the individual's 'illness perception'

If we return to those people who have a significant hearing impairment, but are not aware of any hearing difficulties, it is important to consider what factors might influence whether such an individual has any problems. Such potential factors are presented in Table 2.2.

The role of age in this context is shown by Merluzzi and Hinchcliffe (1973), as mentioned earlier. They argue that the role of age in the perception of hearing difficulties may be due to the insidious onset of the hearing impairment generally associated with age-related factors rather than the fact that what they term 'auditory handicap' is age-dependent. However, Gatehouse (1991) has subsequently shown that older people report less hearing difficulties for a given degree of impairment than do younger people. Interestingly, he also found this to be related to the subject's neuroticism, although there does not appear to be any information regarding personality measures and the perception of hearing difficulties. Gatehouse's findings have been supported in a number of subsequent studies reviewed by Kricos (2000).

The results of Merluzzi and Hinchcliffe (1973) suggest a possible gender effect, with their Figure 3 indicating relatively better thresholds for hearing difficulty with increasing age in males than in females. However, they argue that this may be due to the different configurations of age-related hearing impairment in the two sexes. Furthermore, Kricos (2000) suggests that women are more sensitive to other health-related concerns than are men, and implies that this situation would extend to hearing difficulties.

Merluzzi and Hinchcliffe (1973) argue that a reason for the age effect might be the gradual onset of most age-related hearing impairment, so that the individual is not aware of their gradually deteriorating hearing. Thus, a sudden deterioration of hearing to the same level would be more noticeable to the individual.

Similarly, if the onset of the hearing impairment were related to other symptoms, such as tinnitus or pressure sensation in the ears, this would focus the individual's attention on their ears. Arguably, this would then make them more aware of any hearing impairment which might also be present.

The question of possible psychological factors can be addressed only indirectly. Intuitively, one would expect these to have a major influence on anxious or depressed individuals, who might be more sensitive to possible hearing difficulties. This concept is supported in terms of patients with King-Kopetzky syndrome, who tend to be more anxious and depressed than matched normally hearing controls (Saunders and Haggard, 1989; King and Stephens, 1992).

In the context of effects on self-report scales, as referred to above, Kricos (2000) concluded, from her analysis of a range of studies, that anxious individuals yield higher 'handicap' ratings than less anxious people. Cox et al. (1999) also provide some evidence that extraverts report more problems in an unaided situation. St Claire and He (2009) adduce evidence that self-categorisation (how individuals define themselves) can have an important influence on reported participation restrictions.

The question of the influence of role models is, perhaps, more controversial. If the individual is aware of someone with hearing impairment among their family and friends who copes well with their problems, they are more likely to be prepared to admit or accept that they have hearing difficulties themselves. However, if such a role model has reacted badly to their difficulties, the individual will be more reluctant to admit that they have hearing problems too, attributing their mishearing, for example, to the fact that 'people don't speak as clearly as they used to'.

The limited evidence comes from an analysis of the impact of having a family history on the relationship between response to the question 'Do you have a hearing loss?' and the hearing thresholds in the Blue Mountains study. An analysis of these results indicated that those who reported normal hearing, and whose parents had a hearing impairment, had more sensitive thresholds than those whose parents did not have a hearing impairment (Stephens, 2007, Figure 10.3). This implies that they were more likely to report hearing difficulties with less hearing impairment if their parents were hearing impaired.

Whereas the above may relate to role models who are no longer alive, such as parents of the individuals who took part in the Blue Mountains study, significant others may have an effect on those same individuals because they are with them on a regular basis. These will generally be partners, children or carers. Such individuals will be affected by difficulties which the individual with hearing impairments has, and which will also impact on them. Hence, they may well be more likely to draw the hearing difficulties to the attention of the person and, subsequently, encourage them to seek professional help.

However, in some cases, the significant other may attribute the problems to the age or senility of the person affected and reassure them that they do not really have any hearing difficulties. The different attitudes of spouses in regard to the hearing difficulties of their partners has been discussed by Hallberg and Barrenäs (1993) and others.

The lifestyle of the individual will undoubtedly have an impact on such awareness. While, as a generalisation, those gregarious individuals who enjoy widespread social contacts may become aware of hearing problems at an earlier stage, it is important not to forget the quieter, more withdrawn people who may be lovers of music or radio enthusiasts and so will be sensitive to changes in the quality of the sounds to which they listen.

Some individuals work in more auditorily focused occupations and so may become aware of problems at an earlier stage. Examples of this are musicians and sound engineers, as well as teachers working in noisy and reverberant classrooms with poorly articulating children. The hearing difficulties for these individuals are inevitably greater than for those in less acoustically stressful environments and, consequently, they are more likely to become aware of hearing deterioration at an earlier stage. Indeed, such individuals may also present with King-Kopetzky syndrome in the absence of significant audiological abnormalities, and it has been found that in some 40% of such patients this was a contributory factor (Rendell and Stephens, 1988).

A similar group who have been shown to have such problems comprises those who find themselves in a difficult communicative or educational situation. There, the fact that they have less knowledge of the system language than native speakers will increase their difficulties. They may be immigrants with relatively little of the language of their new country, or may have been there for a number of years, but when their hearing begins to deteriorate, they find considerable problems understanding the language of their adopted country in which, for them, there is less redundancy. Again, this is a contributory factor in King-Kopetzky syndrome. Another example, cited elsewhere (Stephens and Rendell, 1988), is that of the case of a student from a Welsh-speaking family and community who had her primary and secondary education through the medium of Welsh but later found herself in a higher education situation where the medium was English.

Cognitive factors such as intellectual changes associated with old age may well have an impact on awareness of hearing difficulties. Thus, people with some cognitive deterioration may either be unaware of any hearing problems or, alternatively, attribute part or all of their cognitive difficulties to some hearing problems, hence being more sensitive to their hearing loss. While there is a degree of parallelism between hearing changes and cognitive deterioration in older people (Gilhome Herbst and Humphrey, 1980), there is little evidence to suggest a causative relationship, in that hearing impairment may result in dementia. It may, however, aggravate the possible signs of dementia.

Other disabilities, such as motor, cardiac, visual as well as cognitive, may also impact on awareness of hearing problems in different ways. From a communicative standpoint, people with severe visual impairment will be more dependent on their hearing and hence more sensitive to any deterioration in it. In other conditions, particularly those in which the individual's mobility and so opportunity to meet other people is limited, there may be less stress on their auditory communication and hence less consciousness of any hearing impairment. This may change, however, if they find themselves in hospital or care centres with poor acoustical environments and unfamiliar voices.

The decision to seek help

Edgett (2002) argues that this process can be broken down into four stages:

1. Understanding hearing loss
2. Personal experience
3. Interaction with society
4. Taking action.

Engelund subsequently (2006) proposed the stages, involving more internalisation, of:

1. Attracting attention
2. Becoming suspicious
3. Sensing tribulation
4. Jeopardising fundamental self.

However, many of the factors which influence this process are similar to those influencing the perception of hearing disabilities. In addition, there are the important components of the stigma associated with hearing disabilities and the accessibility of rehabilitative help. Among older people, Humphrey et al. (1981) found that 34% of those with better ear hearing of 35 dB or worse in London did not seek help for their condition. A subsequent study in Wales found that 25% came within this category (Gilhome Herbst et al., 1991). In the Netherlands, Van den Brink et al. (1996) found 27% within this category. However, when the basis of the calculations was changed to a mean hearing level across 1, 2 and 4 kHz, the proportion not seeking help rose to 38%. Subsequently, Duijvestijn et al. (2003) found the proportion of those reporting hearing problems and who had not sought help was 30%.

In the MRC–ENT survey (Davis et al., 2007) of those who admitted any problems with their hearing, only 22.4% had been seen by their primary physician or in hospital about it in the previous 12 months. This percentage increases with the degree of annoyance caused by the hearing disability, but even among those who reported their hearing problems to be extremely annoying only 47.4% had been seen in that period. These results and those for people seen by their GP alone are shown in Figure 2.2.

Factors which may influence the process of help-seeking (Box 2.1) have been discussed elsewhere (Stephens, 1983b; Van den Brink et al., 1996).

The physical status of the individual encompasses a range of general health factors. Some may act in a negative way, making the individual less likely to seek rehabilitative help, whereas others, such as severe visual impairment, may result in help-seeking being more likely. Such factors may work in complex ways, certain aspects of the condition making the individual more concerned to seek help and other aspects resulting in their being less concerned.

Thus, for example, an individual with a severe incapacitating illness such as a metastatic neoplasm or cerebrovascular accident may consider that their hearing problems are trivial in comparison with their primary disease and not worth bothering about. However, the condition may bring them into contact with new carers or

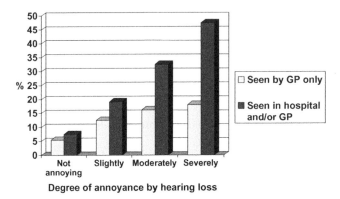

Figure 2.2 Percentage of people consulting about hearing problems by degree of annoyance caused. (*Source:* derived from Davis *et al.*, 2007.)

Box 2.1 Factors influencing help-seeking by individuals with hearing problems.

The physical status of the individual
Their psychological status
Social factors
Attitude of significant others
Demographic factors
Vocational influences
The accessibility of the rehabilitative facilities
The attitude of professional encountered
Experiential factors

(*Source:* derived from Stephens, 1983b; Van den Brink, 1995.)

health professionals who they have difficulty hearing, which, in turn, will make them more likely to seek rehabilitative help.

Individuals who have conditions that affect their ability to communicate, such as speech and language disorders and visual impairment, are more likely to seek help. However, in patients with refractive problems of their vision, their communication may be more helped by correcting such a visual problem than by audiological intervention.

The psychological status of the individual is likely to influence help-seeking in various ways. Thus, an anxious individual might consult their health care service as soon as they become aware of any problems, whereas a more placid individual may not do so until their difficulties become more pronounced.

Cox *et al.* (2005) investigated patients seeking hearing aids at both private practice and Veterans Administration clinics and compared them with population norms on a number of measures. Both groups were found to have lower openness scores on the NEO Five-Factor Inventory (Costa and McCrae, 1992) than the normal population. In addition, both groups scored higher in terms of 'Internal locus of control and less use of social support coping'. Furthermore, a number of significant differences were found between the private patients and the veterans. Cox *et al.* (2005) maintain that there is no difference between those seeking hearing aids for the first time and those seeking new hearing aids and that hearing impaired individuals within the general population do not differ from age- and sex-matched non-impaired individuals. Overall, these results suggest that help-seekers are those who look to themselves rather than to those around them for ways of overcoming their problems.

Likewise, a gregarious person living with a partner or family members who takes part in a range of social activities will seek help at an early stage. A more solitary person, living alone, may leave such a consultation until they become concerned that they are unable to hear people on the telephone, at the door or when their neighbours complain of the loudness of their television.

It has been argued that there is a passive acceptance of hearing problems by older people, (Van den Brink, 1995; Van den Brink *et al.*, 1996), which Maurer and Rupp (1979) had earlier referred to as 'geriapathy'. In particular, this is reflected in the agreement with Van den Brink's (1995) statements 'Hearing problems are so much a part of growing old that there is no reason to see a doctor about it' and 'When you grow old it gets less important to hear anything'. However, in the absence of clear data covering a broad age span, we would prefer to follow Merluzzi and Hinchcliffe's (1973) concept of a gradual loss of sensitivity to the consequences of hearing impairment occurring through the individual's life.

Furthermore, there is also the tendency to attribute their hearing difficulties to external factors along the lines of 'others do not speak clearly'. Holding this attitude will again further reduce the individual's likelihood of help-seeking. The question of stigma is more complicated. This has been discussed at some length by Hétu (1996), among others. From interviews with workers with hearing impairment and their spouses, he identified elements of:

▨ Denial
▨ Minimisation of the problem
▨ Reluctance to talk about the problem and its consequences
▨ Attempts at normalisation of the problem.

The process of stigmatisation is shown in Figure 2.3.

The problems arise as hearing impairment itself is stigmatising, being still associated in popular reactions with mental slowness and with old age. On top of that is the fact that hearing aids themselves may be stigmatising, making it more apparent to those around the individual that they have a hearing difficulty with the hearing aid/s again being associated popularly with old age and progressive cognitive impairment. Thus, while having hearing difficulties is stigmatising and might make the individual more likely to seek help, the thought of then having to use a hearing aid, the most common treatment for such a condition, will deter them.

Some effort has been made to change such attitudes, such as with the Siemens poster from the late 1970s: 'Hearing aids are less conspicuous than poor hearing', and the introduction of brightly coloured and bejewelled hearing aids by Phonak in the early 1980s. Unfortunately, however, while some other hearing aid companies have followed suit in producing coloured hearing aids, use of these has generally been restricted to hearing impaired children and both audiologists and patients need to change their attitudes towards such an approach. Furthermore, most hearing aid advertising still focuses on small, inconspicuous hearing aids, which does nothing to change ingrained attitudes in this respect.

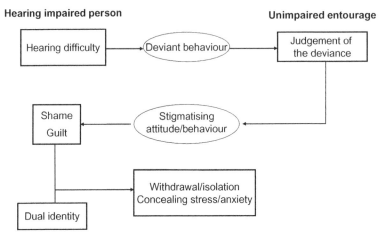

Figure 2.3 The process of stigmatisation. (*Source:* reproduced from Hétu, 1996, with permission.)

Both Van den Brink's (1995) study and that by Duijvestijn *et al.* (2003) highlighted the role that significant others have on the likelihood of the individual seeking help. This reflects the finding from a number of clinical studies (e.g. O Mahoney *et al.*, 1996) that, in older patients attending audiology clinics, the predominant motivation for referral comes from significant others. Consequently, it is to be expected that having a family member who is keen that the individual seek help is a strong motivating factor.

There is little information on the effect of demographic factors, such as age, gender and social class, on such help-seeking. Humphrey *et al.* (1981) and a number of subsequent authors report that, as might be expected, the more severe the hearing impairment, the more likely the individual is to have sought help. They also found that 62% of those who had not sought help were female compared with 54% of those who had done so. There was no significant age difference in those seeking and not seeking help in their sample of older people and no information on social class effects. Similarly, Van den Brink (1995) found no significant effect of age and gender in help-seeking behaviour, after hearing level had been controlled for.

However, those seeking help are more likely to have had hearing problems prior to their retirement (58% versus 16%) and to have tinnitus (55% versus 47%) (Humphrey *et al.*, 1981). Further, Swan and Gatehouse (1990) found that patients going to an audiology clinic were more likely to have an asymmetrical hearing impairment than those not seeking help, even after controlling for better ear hearing level and a number of demographic factors.

Within the data from the MRC–ENT study (Davis *et al.*, 2007), it is not easy to separate the results for those having sought help from those who had but had not been referred on. However, as may be seen from Figure 2.4, there were no major gender effects when we look at those with a hearing aid as a proportion of those with reported hearing difficulty. However, there is a marked increase in the percentage who had obtained hearing aids in the older age bands. This cannot be explained by the fact that reported hearing problems are less in older patients than in younger patients with the same hearing level (Merluzzi and Hinchcliffe, 1973; Gatehouse, 1994).

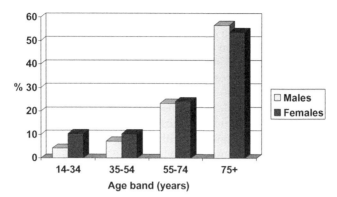

Figure 2.4 Proportion of those reporting hearing difficulty who had been fitted with hearing aid/s in the MRC–ENT study. (*Source:* derived from Davis *et al.*, 2007.)

Within the individual's work environment there will be conflicting influences on help-seeking. People with hearing aids may need help in order to manage within that environment, but may be worried about having a hearing aid in case that compromises their job prospects and promotion within their existing jobs. These will influenced by the nature of the work, how auditorily demanding it is, whether they are interacting with the general public and the attitudes of those around them in their workplace.

The accessibility of the system may be considered in different ways: organisational accessibility, financial accessibility and geographical accessibility. Organisational accessibility concerns how complex the individual's health care system is and how many stages they must pass through in order to obtain appropriate rehabilitative help. Thus, in the traditional UK health system, the individual would consult their primary physician (GP), who might then refer them to an ENT surgeon, who in turn might refer them on to the audiology service. For older patients, without complications, this has been largely simplified so that the primary physician may refer the patient directly to audiological services. Elsewhere, this has been even further simplified by the patient being able to refer themselves directly to an audiology clinic, although there are potentially a number of problems with such an approach, which requires highly trained audiology personnel performing a triage of the patients. In any case, it may be assumed that many patients would be more likely to attend an audiology clinic were their access to it simple and straightforward.

Financial accessibility concerns the direct monetary costs of help-seeking to the individual in relation to their income or wealth. In many European countries, there is no or minimal direct cost to the individual when they seek rehabilitative help. In other countries, such help entails direct expenditure for all or part of the cost of the service, depending perhaps on whether they have private health insurance This has always been a deterrent to help-seeking, even in wealthy Western countries, and makes the situation almost impossible for most of the population of developing counties, where the cost of a hearing aid may exceed the individual's annual income. Thus, it is not surprising that hearing aid possession is directly related to a country's gross domestic product (GDP), and to whether the country has a health care system free at the point of delivery (Stephens, 1983b).

Finally, geographical accessibility concerns how far the individual may have to travel in order to obtain rehabilitative help. This will be regardless of the health care system, so that those people living in remote rural communities will be less likely to seek help unless it is provided on a domiciliary or seriously decentralised basis. This factor is particularly important in older people who may also have related mobility problems. Thus, studies in the United States have indicated that hearing impaired people living in rural areas are less likely to have hearing aids than those in metropolitan areas (e.g. Johnson, 2004a). The same author found that such lack of intervention also applied for visual problems (Johnson, 2004b).

Other factors concern the attitudes of those around the patient, particularly health care professionals and other individuals with hearing difficulties. They may be aware that such professionals have limited knowledge and enthusiasm regarding hearing problems and are consequently unlikely to be sympathetic to the individual's difficulties. On the other hand, one or more of the health professionals may have a particular interest in hearing problems and so the patient will be, consequently, more likely to consult them.

Similarly, if the patient has acquaintances with hearing problems, much will depend upon how these individuals were managed. If they were considerably helped by an audiology department, the patient will be more likely to seek help. If their experience was disappointing, the patient may regard help-seeking as worthless until their own problems become more severe.

Referral for hearing help

In most countries, the first stage of help-seeking takes the individual to a primary physician (GP). Such professionals often act as the gatekeepers of health service provision but, unfortunately, many patients do not get beyond the gatekeeper. Thus, in their population studies on people aged over 70 years with hearing levels of 35 dB or worse, Gilhome Herbst et al. (1991) found that, in both London and Wales, 56% of those consulting their GP were not referred on. Both GP practices were staffed by highly motivated doctors, concerned for their patients, so the general figure could be even worse. Within the Netherlands, Van den Brink (1995) found a smaller proportion coming within this category (35–40%, depending on the audiometric criterion used).

In an unpublished study on the older Welsh population sampled by Stephens and Meredith (1991c) enquiries were made of both patients and doctors as to why they were not referred, and it appeared that, in the majority of cases, this was because of low motivation on the part of the patient, who merely sought reassurance that they did not have a sinister condition. In other cases, the doctor judged them unlikely to persist with the rehabilitative process. In considering the range of possible explanations for this, a number of other factors also needed to be taken into account (e.g. Stephens, 1983a). These are shown in a modified form in Box 2.2.

The attitude of primary physicians covers a number of factors, coloured by their training, experience and personality. The most extreme example will be negative attitudes towards hearing impairment in older people, represented by the comment 'What do you expect at your age?' resulting in a failure to take the individual's symptoms seriously. They may also regard hearing impairment as a fairly trivial symptom and have little interest or motivation to arrange appropriate rehabilitative intervention. On the other hand, some GPs will be concerned to improve the individual's hearing activity as far as possible, realising that their communication with the patient will be facilitated and that better hearing may attenuate the impact of other health problems on the individual.

Box 2.2 Factors influencing the GP as to whether to refer the patient to an audiology clinic.

GP attitude
GP audiology knowledge
Aetiology of hearing loss
GP local knowledge
GP knowledge of patient
Hearing aid stigma reported by patient and significant other
Geographical considerations

The aetiology of the individual's hearing impairment will also have an influence on the GP's attitude. Thus, for example, if the patient complains of a discharging ear, the GP is more likely to be concerned with that than with the associated hearing loss. Similarly, in patients with Menière's disorder, all intervention may well be concentrated on treating the patient's vertigo when, often, the associated hearing impairment may be a bigger problem for the patient (Stephens *et al.*, 2009a). Again, in asymmetrical or unilateral hearing impairment, the primary physician may be concerned to exclude a vestibular Schwannoma, so is likely to refer the patient to an ENT surgeon, who, on eliminating that possibility, may arrange subsequent referral to audiology. Indeed, this may be the main factor behind Swan and Gatehouse's (1990) finding that patients referred on to audiology are more likely to have asymmetrical hearing impairment compared with those not consulting.

The local knowledge of the GP is important, given the fact that, inevitably, not all audiology departments provide a high-class service. Thus, for example, if the GP is aware that the local provisions are of relatively poor quality, they may refer only patients who they consider to have a serious disability, encouraging others to either come to terms with their hearing impairment or consider referral to a more distant facility. On the other hand, if the GP is aware that local facilities are of a high standard, they may be happy to refer patients with relatively mild problems.

Related to this is the GP's knowledge of their patients' attitudes towards, motivation concerning and likely compliance with rehabilitative intervention. As mentioned earlier, this factor seems to have played a large part in the 56% of older patients not referred on in our study in Wales (Gilhome Herbst *et al.*, 1991). Indeed, many patients seek only reassurance that their problem is not life-threatening or serious and, while they are happy to have such reassurance, they feel that there is no real need for further intervention. This is equally true of early intervention or population screening studies, such as the Leiden 85-Plus study in the Netherlands, which found that three-quarters of their older subjects with significant hearing impairment declined participation in a rehabilitation programme (Gussekloo *et al.*, 2003).

A part of this is related to the stigma felt by the patients and those around them regarding hearing aids. Van den Brink (1995) found this a major factor separating those who consulted their GP and were not referred for hearing aids from those who took up the offer of a hearing aid. The statements with which respondents were to agree/disagree included 'I think people will behave quite differently when they see you wearing a hearing aid' and 'I think people will no longer regard you as fully fledged, when you are wearing a hearing aid'. This comes on top of the elements of stigma relating to hearing impairment as a whole, which influence the process of help-seeking, and which may be perceived by the individual's GP.

Finally, we come to the question of geographical considerations, also considered in the context of help-seeking, which will influence whether the patient accepts being referred to a distant centre for a symptom that may seem relatively minor. This can also have some bearing on the GP's decision and advice, given that they may take into account the patient's mobility and general health.

Before concluding this section, it must be remembered that many patients bypass the orthodox health care system to make their first, and often only, port of call a hearing aid dispenser. Indeed, in many parts of the world this is the predominant approach.

In that context a number of the same considerations, and some different, ones will apply. This will depend to some extent on the regulations in the country concerned specifying what patients should be referred on by the dispenser for medical and other professional help, the training and ethical approach of the dispenser and the facilities which they are able to offer. Frequently, dispensers will overcome geographical considerations by being more prepared to visit patients in their homes, although sometimes the facilities they have for evaluating and fitting patients under these circumstances may be limited. In addition, dispensers are often more attuned to the question of stigma and will be more likely to fit smaller and less conspicuous hearing aids. However, such aids may not always be appropriate for the patient concerned.

Furthermore, it is important not to forget socio-economic considerations. People from poorer families are, in general, less likely to seek rehabilitative help than those from wealthier backgrounds, even when such facilities are provided free of charge to the patient. This will be accentuated when the patient is required to purchase their hearing aids, and a number of studies (e.g. Stephens, 1983b) have indicated a higher level of hearing aid possession in countries in which hearing aids are provided via state health care systems.

Ethics/philosophy of adult screening

Should we be concerned that only a small proportion of individuals with significant hearing impairment have hearing aids? Even a simple question like this is problematic. First, what is a significant hearing impairment? Second, is it impairment or disability that we should be considering? Third, do hearing aids comprise the approach of choice for all individuals with hearing impairment, and should the proportion fitted be regarded as a criterion for the effectiveness of a health care system?

These various problems will be addressed below but, at this stage, it must be admitted that, by any criterion, there are many people within the community who could benefit from audiological enablement but who have neither sought it nor received it. We would argue here that we should not be concerned by those individuals who are unaware of the fact that they have a significant hearing impairment, as highlighting such an impairment could result in more emotional stress than could be relieved by relevant intervention. Our concern should be with those individuals who are aware that they have a problem but who are discouraged from acting to reduce this problem in one way or another. As may be seen from previous sections, factors resulting in such discouragement may be stigma, limited expectations, difficulty in accessing the system, attitudes of both professionals and significant others and concomitant disabilities.

In the short term, three approaches may be considered: first, publicising the benefits of early intervention through the media; second, improving local services and making them more accessible; third, by introducing some form of national screening programme. While the last has a number of problems, some of which have been discussed elsewhere (Gianopoulos and Stephens, 2005), such an approach has been the subject of a number of detailed studies (e.g. Davis *et al.*, 2007). However, any evidence for media-based approaches and the impact of improving local services is, at best, anecdotal. The possible impact of such services, together with a long-term approach to reduce the stigma of hearing impairment and hearing aids, is shown in Figures 2.5a and 2.5b.

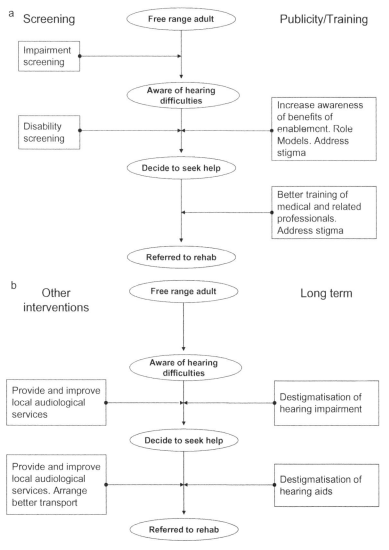

Figure 2.5 a Possible stages of intervention in screening and publicity. **b** Other approaches to intervention in the short and long term.

If we consider first screening, which stands out from the other three approaches as an intrusive intervention, we would argue strongly that the first stage must be to determine whether the individual experiences hearing problems (i.e. has one or more disabilities). This approach was adopted in some of our earlier studies in Wales (e.g. Stephens *et al.*, 1990a; Davis *et al.*, 1992) and then extended in the recent Health Technology Assessment study (Davis *et al.*, 2007). Thus, subjects were formally included within the intervention only if they responded positively to the question 'Do you have any difficulty with your hearing? Yes No' (Stephens *et al.*, 1990a). Measures of impairment (pure tone audiogram) in those indicating difficulties were then applied, to help determine what might be the most effective intervention for that particular individual.

In the Health Technology Assessment study, such a two-stage approach with one or two simple questions followed by an audiometric screen proved the most efficient way of identifying those prepared to accept intervention compared with the use of more sophisticated techniques including speech audiometry, otoacoustic emissions and so on (Davis *et al.*, 2007).

In a study using just audiometric screening in older patients, Gussekloo *et al.* (2003) found that, even with a criterion of >35 dB better ear hearing level across the frequencies 1–4 kHz, 77% declined to take part in a rehabilitation programme. Apart from any direct considerations of cost-effectiveness, this study raises two important questions. First, should we be looking for an impairment measure as the first line of approach in adults who are capable of making their own decisions when screening for a non-life-threatening condition? Second, at what age should we be performing the screening?

The first of these points raises the issue as to whether we are justified in proposing intervention for a condition which apparently results in no activity limitation or participation restriction and which is not of great importance to the individual. In newborn hearing screening, where a baby cannot articulate its feelings, it is certainly arguable that an impairment-based measure provides the optimal approach. In addition, in the context of a child who has not developed speech and language, not intervening has a far greater deleterious effect on the subsequent development and later life than it might in an older person with a moderate hearing difficulty. We would strongly argue that if the individual were unaware of any hearing problems it would be ethically unacceptable to intervene, or even to indicate to them that they did, in fact, have a hearing impairment. This has been discussed further elsewhere by Gianopoulos and Stephens (2005). Thus, in the UK National Screening Committee's (NSC) recommendations (2003) point 15 states, 'The benefit from the screening programme should outweigh the physical and psychological harm (caused by the test, diagnostic procedures and treatment).'

Second, there is the question of the age at which any screening should be performed. Again, the NSC recommends that the 'condition should be an important health problem'. This implies that it should be either common or have serious implications for the health of the individual. Few would strongly argue that late-onset hearing impairment comes in the latter category, therefore screening for it can be justified only when the condition becomes common. Earlier studies (Stephens *et al.*, 1990a; Davis *et al.*, 1992) concentrated on the 50–65 years of age group on the basis that it is in this age band that the prevalence of hearing impairment begins to increase markedly (Davis, 1995). The more recent Health Technology Assessment study (Davis *et al.*, 2007) took a wider band of 55–74 years, based in part on the results of the earlier investigations.

An extension of the earlier studies in Wales included a sub-study which also targeted patients aged over 65 years (Stephens and Meredith, 1991c). This indicated that the proportion of patients over the age of 80 years who were aided as a result of the screening was smaller than the proportion already aided. Again, in the 50–55 years age group, the newly aided group was small, owing to the relative scarcity of significant impairment in that group. Hence, the approach of 55–75 years seems appropriate in view of the reduced cost-effectiveness of aiding individuals for the first time both below and above this age band.

Returning to less intrusive interventions, there are a number of broad areas in which relevant interventions could be made, covering attitude changes, information provision, training of professionals and improved accessibility of the services. Attitude changes and information provision can be achieved via health education programmes in the media aimed at the general and, in particular, the older population. The approach adopted by Brooks (e.g. Brooks, 1989), of pre-clinic visits to the patients who had been referred, can be helpful in terms of hearing aid use by that group, but fails to address the problem of those who do not consult their GPs or who are not referred on by their GPs.

Approaches via the media, making clear to individuals what is available and attempting to reduce stigma, can be considerably helped by role models among famous people. The late Ronald Reagan, president of the United States, was a good example of this, but less was made of the hearing impairment of Bill Clinton, another president, or of that of many media stars, such as Joan Collins. However, some individuals in the spotlight, such as Tony Benn and the artist David Hockney, have been much more open about their hearing difficulties and possible benefits of intervention, but have not been effectively used in health promotion in this respect. There is a much greater need for the health promotion arms of governments and NGOs to be forward-looking and promote healthy hearing in the same way as they are devoting attention to healthy eating. As well as a structured campaign through programmes and adverts on television, the Internet, newspapers and magazines, such as those targeted at retired or pre-retirement age groups (e.g. SAGA), there is a need for audiology professionals, aware of the problem, to use their contacts in the media to promote such healthy hearing.

The informational aspect of such a media-based approach would need to target the hearing society around those with impaired hearing. This would emphasise the particular communication difficulties experienced in noisy places, aspects of hearing tactics and improved access for people with hearing difficulties, including loop systems and communication facilities, which are actually implemented and activated as well as merely being installed. The cost-effectiveness of such a media-based approach will need to be assessed and the process refined.

Linked with this is the question of better audiological training of health care professionals in contact with middle-aged and older people. At the present time, the audiological training of most doctors is minimal and a greater effort is needed to remedy this, particularly in the training of GPs and geriatricians. Even many ENT doctors have little training in the communication needs and rehabilitation of people with hearing difficulties. This is even truer of nurses and other staff based in health centres, pre-retirement clinics and day centres for older people.

Tolson and Stephens (1997), in their audiological care model for nursing, had considered possible roles of nurses in the hearing health care of older patients. However, as long ago as 2000, both Hines and Fooks et al. highlighted the inadequate training of medical and nursing staff in deaf awareness, and little has been done to address this deficit since that time.

Finally, there is the question of accessibility. Even in the countries of northern Europe and the Antipodes, where hearing health provision for older people is essentially free of charge at the point of delivery, uptake of hearing help, as discussed above, has been poor. Part of this problem stems from the limited mobility of many in this age group, and from a tendency for audiology centres to be based at large centralised hospitals. There is a considerable need for this to be more decentralised, even if it entails staff from the audiology centres providing a regular service in local hospitals or health centres, with only those found to have severe problems being referred to the main, centralised, department. There have been discussions about involving private hearing aid dispensers in such a provision, but this may entail a significant conflict of interest. In addition, health care models in advanced countries but without a universal health care provision need to be reconsidered by the lobbying of relevant politicians.

Conclusion

The process of help-seeking by an individual with a hearing impairment passes through several stages: becoming aware of hearing difficulties, deciding to seek help for these difficulties and achieving referral to an audiology centre. Each of these steps acts as a hurdle to be overcome and is influenced by a number of factors, psychological, demographic and physical, which have been highlighted in the chapter. However, in most advanced societies, it is generally agreed that barely one person in four with a significant hearing impairment has received help for their hearing problems. In an attempt to improve this situation, various programmes of screening for middle-aged and older adults have been proposed. It is stressed that these should be based on the difficulties experienced by people within society rather than on a particular level of impairment.

3 Types of hearing impairment and their consequences

Introduction

The basic approach of this chapter is a pragmatic one. It aims to introduce the reader both to the implications of activity limitations, which are caused by the onset of lesions in the auditory pathway, and to approaches which can be taken to reduce these. As such, we make no attempt to provide a detailed review of the anatomy, physiology and pathology involved, and merely highlight elements which can have important implications for the enablement process. Readers wanting more information on these domains, basic to the experience of hearing, are advised to consult Gelfand (2004) and Chermak and Musiek (2007) for various aspects of the central auditory system.

Basic anatomy and physiology and their implications

The auditory pathway stretches from the auricle to the auditory cortex, and different aspects of auditory processing occur at each stage. Indeed, much remains to be learnt about the roles of different parts of the auditory system and, for example, the importance of the insula of the cortex in temporal processing has only recently been highlighted (e.g. Bamiou *et al.*, 2003). Overall, however, it may be stated that the more peripheral the lesion, the more severe its impact on hearing level, and the more central the lesion, the more subtle its impact. In this context, Jerger (1964) coined the term *the subtlety principle*, which stated that the more central the lesion, the more subtle the test required for its diagnosis.

A schematic representation of the overall layout of the auditory system is shown in Figure 3.1, which indicates a crossed system with bilateral representation of the input from both ears from the level of the superior olivary complex in the brainstem rostrally (upwards). In general, however, the majority of the input from the left ear passes to the right auditory cortex and from the right ear to the left auditory cortex. This has the implication that, as speech processing takes place predominantly in the left auditory cortex, input from the left ear has to pass from the right temporal lobe via the corpus callosum for integrated processing.

The external ear

The outer, or external, ear comprises the auricle and the external acoustic meatus. These are responsible for collecting and transmitting sound to the middle ear.

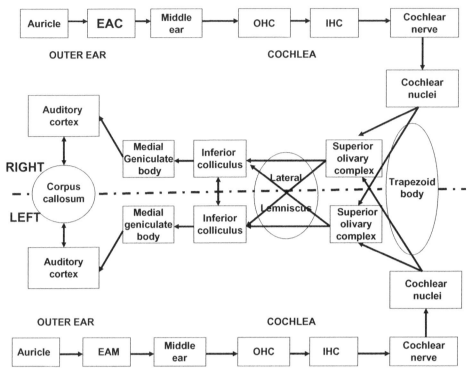

Figure 3.1 Schematic diagram of the main pathways in the afferent auditory system. EAM = external acoustic meatus; OHC = outer hair cells; IHC = inner hair cells; EAC = external auditory canal.

Sound arrives at the auricle, or pinna, in which some transformations occur with sound from different locations being reflected into the external acoustic meatus with different delays. This process provides important clues for the directionalisation of sound in the vertical plane and, to a lesser extent, in the horizontal plane (Batteau, 1967; Blauert, 1983), although the latter is predominantly based on differences between the inputs from the two ears.

The external acoustic meatus, or ear canal, is basically a tube, about 2.5 cm long, connecting the auricle and the tympanic membrane. The outer third is surrounded by cartilage and the inner two-thirds by bone. From a functional standpoint, the main effect of this is in terms of the sound resonances which occur here, leading to some amplification of the mid-frequencies, particularly frequencies in the 2–3 kHz range, important in the recognition of speech (Shaw, 1974). Cerumen, or earwax, is produced by a combination of the ceruminous and sebaceous glands in the skin lining the outer one-third, and has antiseptic and moisture-retaining characteristics, important for the health of the tympanic membrane and related structures.

The middle ear

The middle ear, or tympanic cavity, is an air-filled space between the outer ear and the cochlea, or inner ear. Air reaches it from the nasopharynx via the auditory, or Eustachian, tube. Functionally, it is bounded by the tympanic membrane and the oval window. It contains three ossicles and two muscles: the tensor tympani and the stapedius.

The tympanic membrane and the three ossicles (the malleus, the incus and the stapes) may be considered together from a functional standpoint. Their main role is to overcome the air–fluid impedance mismatch between the sound travelling through air to the fluid vibrations which it sets up in the cochlea, or inner ear. Without this effect, the auditory system would be functioning at a level some 30–40 dB less sensitive than it does in practice (Nedzelnitsky, 1980). This is achieved mainly by the ratio of the areas of the tympanic membrane and the oval window, partly by the lever function of the ossicular chain and partly by the buckling effect of the tympanic membrane. The effect of this transfer function is greatest at about 1 kHz, adding to the resonance effects from the outer ear.

The cochlea

The cochlea (the auditory section of the inner ear) is the key part of the auditory system in which the acoustical signal arriving at the ear is converted into electrical discharges which pass up the cochlear nerve to the brain. It is a complex mechanism, beyond the remit of this book, and readers are referred to Møller (2006) and Moore (2007) for up-to-date information of the mechanisms involved. Essentially, the three key areas are the stria vascularis, the outer hair cells and the inner hair cells. The stria vascularis, a vascular organ, is responsible for the production of the endolymph, a fluid high in potassium and low in sodium and with a high electrical potential (+80 mV) which powers the electrical transduction in the hair cells. The outer hair cells (ca 12 000) have a largely motor function, increasing the sensitivity and the sharpness of the frequency tuning of the inner ear. The inner hair cells (ca 4000) are the main transducers and link with and stimulate the dendrites of the cochlear nerve fibres. Dysfunction of any part of this system will have a major impact on hearing, affecting the sensitivity, frequency and temporal selectivity to different extents up to and including total deafness on the affected side.

The cochlear nerve

The cochlear nerve (auditory nerve), with its cell bodies constituting the spiral ganglion of the inner ear, connects the inner hair cells with the cochlear nuclei. The 20 000 fibres of each cochlear nerve connect with the three main sections of the cochlear nuclei, the dorsal cochlear nucleus and the anterior and posterior ventral nuclei. Damage or disease of the cochlear nerves leads to distortion of sound to a varying degree, with total unilateral hearing impairment resulting from severe lesions.

The brainstem

The cochlear nuclei are located in the pons around the cerebellar peduncle. The neurones vary in complexity from the anteroventral to the dorsal cochlear nucleus and this is reflected in the complexity of their neurophysiological responses to acoustical stimulation. However, their precise function in terms of sound perception has not been clearly defined. More detailed descriptions of this and other aspects of central auditory function are given by Musiek and Baran (2007).

Nerve fibres from the cochlear nuclei pass to the superior olivary complex of both sides as well as directly to the inferior colliculus. Some pass via the trapezoid body and via the lateral lemniscus, but, again, the role of these structures is not clear.

The superior olivary complex is the most caudal part of the auditory system to receive inputs from both ears and is known to be involved in the lateralisation and localisation of sound. Most of the input comes from the anteroventral and posteroventral sections of the cochlear nucleus via the trapezoid body. The superior olivary complex, situated in the medulla, in turn comprises three sections, the lateral and medial superior olive and the medial nucleus of the trapezoid body. The medial superior olive is an important relay centre for the acoustic stapedial reflex, which can modify the transmission of sound through the middle ear.

The lateral lemniscus is the main ascending auditory pathway through the brainstem to the inferior colliculus. It receives inputs from the cochlear nuclei and the superior olives from both sides with some of the neurones ending in the nuclei of the lateral lemniscus and some continuing directly to the inferior colliculus. The function of the nuclei of the lateral lemniscus is not clear.

Higher centres

The next major auditory centre is the inferior colliculus, located in the dorsal part of the midbrain. It receives its main inputs from both superior olivary complexes and from the contralateral dorsal cochlear nucleus. This implies a role in localisation of sound and in the complex processing of sounds. Noback (1985) refers to the inferior colliculus as 'the obligatory relay nuclear complex transmitting auditory information to higher levels'.

The medial geniculate body is an eminence on the inferior surface of the thalamus, lateral to the midbrain. Its main inputs are fibres from the ipsilateral inferior colliculus, and fibres project from it to the primary and association auditory cortical areas AI and AII, with some projecting to the insula. Beyond being a relay station, its precise function is unclear.

The cortex

The auditory cortex comprises several sections with the primary auditory cortex (AI) and the association auditory cortex located on the superior surface of the temporal lobe. It is thought that the primary auditory cortex is essentially associated with frequency and intensity analysis, and non-primary areas are involved in computation and integration of sounds (Hall *et al.*, 2003). There is lateralisation of many aspects of auditory function, with basic speech and language processing taking place in the left cortex but tonality and intonation recognition on the right side. These are connected via the corpus callosum and the anterior commissure. The insula is linked to both the medial geniculate body and the auditory cortex and is now considered responsible for temporal resolution (Bamiou *et al.*, 2003).

In parallel to this reasonably well-defined afferent system, there is an equivalent efferent system from the cortex to the cochlea, which can modify the input passing up the afferent system. The best studied part of this is the olivocochlear system with the crossed olivocochlear bundle projecting onto the outer hair cells and the uncrossed system onto the cochlear nerve dendrites connecting with the inner hair cells. More detailed information on the efferent system may be found in Berlin (1999).

Purposes and process of assessment

Traditionally, audiometric testing has been concerned with defining the site of the lesion responsible for the hearing difficulties described by a patient. However, with the development of imaging and electrophysiological techniques, this role has been largely usurped. Formerly, auditory assessment preceding enablement would comprise at best a pure tone audiogram, speech audiometry and uncomfortable loudness level measures, but subsequently a range of other psychoacoustical measures has been used to help define the impairments experienced by the individual. In the present section, we shall briefly consider the most important of these measures mainly from the standpoint of the enablement process, while also mentioning their role in diagnostic audiology.

Much basic testing to determine both hearing levels and site of peripheral hearing lesions can be done on the basis of clinical tests, such as whispered voice and a wide range of tuning fork tests. While these are invaluable in many circumstances, including as a check of the validity of more sophisticated audiometric tests, they will not be considered further at this stage, where we are concerned with defining the specific auditory impairments experienced by those individuals with hearing difficulties.

The most widely performed hearing test is manual pure tone audiometry (PTA). This is a test in which pure tones, generally at octave frequencies from 250 to 8000 Hz are presented at various intensities to define the lowest level at which the testee can hear the sound 50% of the time. These are usually presented through air-conduction supra-aural headphones, but also by bone-conduction transducers placed on the mastoid, for which testing is usually limited to the range 500–4000 Hz. A comparison of the, adequately masked, thresholds obtained by the two techniques can indicate whether the individual has a 'conductive' element to their hearing impairment, arising from the outer or middle ear with a difference in the two thresholds of 15 dB or greater. Beyond that, which indicates an attenuation, or softening, effect of the incoming sound, the value of PTA is that it provides information of the severity of the loss of sensitivity experienced by the individual. In addition, the frequency configuration of any hearing loss will provide information as to what type of sounds the individual is most likely to have difficulty hearing. Thus, the common high-frequency impairment will result in the person having difficulties, particularly with fricatives in speech.

More detailed information as to the frequency configuration of the hearing loss can be obtained from sweep-frequency Békésy audiometry, in which the individual tracks their hearing threshold over a predetermined frequency range (Békésy, 1947). A more recent sweep-frequency technique is the Audioscan (Meyer-Bisch, 1990, 1996), which can demonstrate notches or small irregularities in the hearing of individuals who otherwise appear to have normal hearing, such as those with King-Kopetzky syndrome (Zhao and Stephens, 1999a, 1999b).

The first basic perceptual abnormality arising from cochlear damage to be extensively studied was that of an abnormal growth of loudness to suprathreshold sounds, commonly known as *recruitment*. This was studied by binaural loudness balance techniques dating back to the 1930s and later by monaural loudness balance and testing for the detectability of small increments in the sound level. The tests relevant to enablement are measures of the uncomfortable loudness level (ULL) and the most comfortable loudness level (MCL) first used systematically by Watson (1944). In the former, the listener is asked to indicate as soon a sound, increasing in steps, becomes uncomfortably loud. This is then repeated across the range of frequencies and can be performed using sweep-frequency Békésy audiometry. In the MCL, the listener is asked to indicate the most comfortable listening level for the test signal and, again, tracking techniques can be used to define it.

In terms of the value of these measures, the ULL can be used to define the maximum output of any hearing aid and is currently incorporated into several hearing aid fitting programs. The MCL can be used to define the hearing aid gain needed, but has the drawback that both intrasubject and intersubject variability are high for this measure (e.g. Stephens *et al.*, 1977). However, it can be extrapolated from the PTA and ULL measures, coming (in dB) about two-thirds of the way between the threshold and the ULL (Keller, 1971; Lundborg *et al.*, 1973). The ULL itself has high intersubject variance, owing in part to personality factors (Stephens and Anderson, 1971), but this can be regarded as a bonus in achieving patient-appropriate hearing aid fitting.

Recruitment is, in part, a reflection of impaired frequency resolution in the cochlea and Moore (2007) discusses this and other psychoacoustical aspects of damage in detail. Frequency resolution can be measured by critical band tests, psychophysical tuning curves, notched noise tests and a range of other measures. The impact of such poor frequency resolution is that extraneous noises have a much greater masking effect on the signal that the listener is trying to hear. The classical example of this is the difficulty that most people with cochlear damage have hearing speech in the presence of any background noise.

The other significant distortion which is experienced in the presence of cochlear damage is impaired temporal processing. This has been demonstrated using measures of temporal summation, which have been used in the clinical domain, and by measures of forward and backward masking and of gap detection. Abnormal temporal summation, in which there is less difference between the loudness and detectability of long (e.g. 200 ms) and short (e.g. 20 ms) sounds results in people with such cochlear damage being more sensitive to impulsive noises. The question of temporal resolution, reflected in the other tests, means that soft components of speech, such as fricatives, may be masked by the loud vowels which precede or follow them.

Unfortunately, there is relatively little that can be currently done, by even the current digital signal processing hearing aids, to directly overcome these distortions in the frequency and temporal domains and their subsequent impact on speech recognition.

Speech recognition tests of one type or another have been used at least since the inception of audiology and were undoubtedly among the earliest tests of hearing to be used. They range from speech components through to running speech, and the various types are listed in Table 3.1.

Simple speech component tests such /aba/ or /ata/ for testing consonant recognition or /hid/ or /had/ for testing vowel recognition may be used in the analysis of a particular speech or speechreading deficit and to evaluate the effectiveness of specific interventions aimed at overcoming this. In addition, a range of synthetic speech component tests for more detailed testing of the recognition of voice-onset times or the harmonic separation of the components of vowels have been used in this context (e.g. Fourcin, 1980).

Word tests are probably the most commonly used speech tests in general audiological practice with both diagnostic and rehabilitative applications. There is a wide range of such tests across and within different languages. In many countries, for example the United Kingdom, monosyllabic words are used for both speech threshold and speech recognition measures, whereas in other countries, for example the United States, spondees (bisyllabic words with equal stress on each syllable) are used for

Table 3.1 Types of speech recognition tests in increasing complexity.

Category	Types	Example	Use
Phoneme recognition	Vowel–consonant–vowel	/aba/	Defining consonant confusions
	Consonant–vowel–consonant	/hid/	Defining vowel confusions
Word tests	Phonetically balanced; isophonemic	ship; rake	Defining basic speech recognition ability in diagnostic and rehabilitative audiology
	Spondees	blackbird; teapot	Determining speech reception thresholds
Sentence tests	Balanced	John saw the brown dog	Defining speech recognition before and after interventions
	High and low semantic redundancy	The boy kicked the ball; Anne found the red house	Separating auditory from cognitive influences
Continuous discourse tracking	Any relevant written material		Monitoring progress after rehabilitative interventions
Low-redundancy speech	Monaural (e.g. filtered, interrupted)		Testing central auditory function
	Monaural or binaural masked		Measuring overall function and effectiveness of interventions; Testing central auditory function
	Bilateral competing	Rt cowboy Lt doorbell	Testing central auditory function
	Bilateral integration	Segments alternating between the two ears	Testing brainstem function

speech threshold determination. Other languages, for example Finnish, have few if any monosyllables, so use bisyllabic words for the same purposes. All may be scored using either whole words or the constituent phonemes.

Sentence tests are generally used in an enablement context to determine the need for a particular type of intervention and subsequently the effectiveness of such an intervention. These may be scored using either whole sentences or the component words. Some sentence tests may be deliberately based on a combination of sentences with high and low redundancy. In the former, different components will give cues as to the likely nature of others. Thus, in the example in Table 3.1, if the listener recognises 'The boy kicked', there is a strong likelihood that the final word will be 'ball'. In the second example, there is little to suggest what 'Anne' might have found. This approach to separating the auditory and cognitive components of speech recognition was introduced to audiology in the SPIN test (Kalikow *et al.*, 1977).

In the SPIN test, the material is presented in a background of noise. Such speech-in-noise tests, which may use words or sentences as their basis, have been used to make the test more difficult than presenting speech in quiet and to provide a more realistic test of the difficulties which an individual patient may be experiencing. In addition, they may be used to monitor the patient's progress after intervention. Tests of this nature are insufficiently specific to be used further as diagnostic tests as speech recognition in noise may be affected by lesions in many parts of the auditory pathway from the cochlea to the cortex. However, monaural speech tests have been used in patients with normal hearing thresholds to compare the two ears and test for possible unilateral cortical lesion (e.g. Olsen *et al.*, 1975).

Continuous discourse tracking is an approach developed by DeFilippo and Scott (1978) as a means of monitoring improvements in speech recognition during and following therapy. In it, the tester reads from a book or other text appropriate to the listener's language skills and interests. If the listener fails to repeat what is said, the tester increases stress patterns and provides other cues until the listener is able to correctly repeat the phrase. This is done over several minutes and the scoring is on the basis of the number of words correctly repeated per minute. Other sections of the same text may be used on subsequent visits.

A range of speech tests have been used, dating back to Bocca's work in the 1950s (e.g. Bocca, 1958), to test different aspects of central auditory function. These range from monaural tests, in which the redundancy of the speech is reduced by filtering or interruption, through to a range of binaural tests with competing messages or integration of the information from the inputs from the two ears. The diagnostic value of the various types of tests involved has recently been discussed by Baran and Musiek (2003) but, at the present time, their role in the monitoring of therapy for central auditory processing disorders remains unclear.

Those authors also discuss a range of non-speech tests of central auditory function, such as masking level difference and temporal patterning, to which may be added a range of lateralisation/localisation tests and temporal summation, which provide diagnostic indicators. However, the role of such tests in rehabilitative assessment and outcome measures has yet to be established.

In addition to such tests of auditory perception, a wide range of electrophysiological tests of auditory function ranging from admittance testing with stapedial reflex measures, otoacoustic emission testing and auditory evoked potentials extending from the cochlea to the frontal association areas, have been described and have an important role in diagnostic testing. Their role in the enablement process is more problematic (Stephens, 1979), although the use of middle latency responses in evaluating possible improvements in central auditory processing disorders has been advocated (Baran, 2007). In addition, electrical brainstem responses are frequently used to assess aspects of the function of cochlear implants.

Types of hearing impairment and their consequences

The external ear

The most common external ear condition resulting in hearing difficulties is excessive production of cerumen, or wax. This causes a significant hearing impairment only if it completely occludes the ear canal, and it can be easily removed by appropriately trained professionals.

Permanent hearing impairment can be caused by a complete congenital atresia or lack of formation of the external acoustic meatus and attempts to surgically construct a canal are rarely permanently effective. This will result in a permanent conductive hearing impairment, which may be overcome using direct stimulation of the cochlea with a bone-conduction technique. Finally, severe otitis externa, inflammation of the external canal, may block the meatus and similarly result in a conductive hearing impairment. This may respond to topical treatment but, in the most severe cases, may necessitate direct bone-conduction stimulation.

The middle ear

Middle ear disorders, resulting predominantly in a conductive hearing impairment, predominantly have an attenuation effect on the auditory input with relatively little distortion of the input signal. Because of this, sounds seem softer but not less clear, and are therefore very amenable to amplification. It has been suggested that there is a 'conductive recruitment', with a reduced dynamic range in the case of middle ear disorders, but the evidence for this remains controversial and, in any case, the effect is far smaller than in cochlear disorders. Consequently, the individual's ability to recognise speech in noise is not significantly impaired.

Despite the lack of distortion, patients with moderate to severe conductive hearing impairments (45–75 dB) appear to report a greater disability than those with cochlear hearing impairments of the same levels (Lutman et al., 1987). Those authors found that speech-hearing activity limitation and general participation restriction were most affected. Noble (1998) reports similar results with poor speech-hearing activity limitation and a non-significant difference in localisation difficulties.

The two most common conditions resulting in middle ear disorders in adults are chronic otitis media and otosclerosis. Both can involve the inner ear as well as the middle ear, although their predominant effects are on the middle ear. Chronic otitis media is a possible consequence of an acute infection of the middle ear. This may result in scarring of the tympanic membrane with fibrosis of the middle ear and possible erosion of the ossicles or can result in an ongoing purulent infection. The former is relatively easy to manage but chronic suppurative otitis media can cause a range of problems from the standpoint of instrumental rehabilitation, and is discussed further in the next chapter.

Otosclerosis is predominantly an autosomal dominant condition of incomplete penetrance, with a possible trigger effect of certain viral infections such as measles. It usually manifests itself in the mid-20s in women and mid-30s in men and shows a progressive course with spongy bony growth affecting particularly the stapes footplate. Some eight gene loci have been proposed but no specific genes have been identified and a complex genetic mechanism may be involved (Declau and Van de Heyning, 2007a).

The cochlea

Within the cochlea, a variety of disorders may occur stemming in particular from damage to the hair cells and from disorders of the metabolic function of the inner ear, particularly the stria vascularis. Apart from a range of genetic disorders, caused by more than 100 different genes, damage to the cochlea can be caused by infection, trauma (including noise effects), damage by a range of chemicals and drugs, as well as a number of vascular and metabolic conditions. Here so-called presbyacusis, or age-related hearing impairment, is caused principally by a combination of these factors (Lim and Stephens, 1991), and so is not considered as a separate entity.

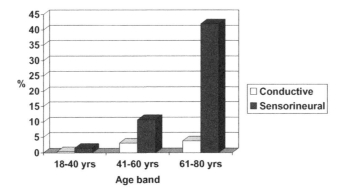

Figure 3.2 Percentages of better ear hearing levels (averaged 500–4000 Hz) greater than 25 dB HL in the population by middle ear and cochlear hearing impairment. (*Source:* derived from Davis, 1997.)

Different genes are expressed in different parts of the cochlea (Snoeckx and Van Camp, 2007), but the perceptual implications of this have not been related clearly to the specific parts affected.

From an enablement standpoint, the most important effects of cochlear lesions are in speech recognition and, in particular, speech recognition in the presence of background noise. Such impaired speech recognition in noise can occur even in the presence of essentially normal pure tone audiograms, although with abnormalities in sensitised measures such as Audioscan tests and Distortion Product Otoacoustic emissions (Zhao and Stephens, 2000).

More severe cochlear impairments affecting, for example, the high frequencies can result in difficulties hearing specific sounds, such as high-frequency bells or other warning signals, as well as the inability to hear the calls of certain birds and other animals such as cicadas. This can impact on the individual's ability to hear speech clearly, even in the quiet, and in particular speech, as from the radio, for which the listener receives no visual cues.

Severe to profound hearing impairment is most commonly the result of cochlear lesions with the consequence that the individual can hear little or nothing from the affected ear or ears. In such individuals, hearing aids can usually offer only a very distorted input, alerting the individual to environmental sounds and perhaps facilitating speechreading, and better speech recognition can generally be obtained only with the use of cochlear implants.

The common impacts of these and other aspects, particularly of cochlear lesions, are discussed further in Chapter 5, in which the effects of the individual being in what to them is a 'dead' environment are also considered. Furthermore, at this stage, it must be emphasised that the great majority of bilateral hearing impairments in adults, particularly with increasing age, stem from disorders affecting the cochlea (Figure 3.2). However, the differences are smaller when based on worse ear measures, and that will be considered further in the context of unilateral/asymmetrical hearing loss later in this chapter.

Cochlear nerve

Disorders affecting primarily the cochlear nerve are much less common and essentially result in a range of distortions of speech and other auditory signals. The most extreme version of this is *auditory neuropathy*, which is found in some children in whom otoacoustic emissions are normal but auditory brainstem responses are abnormal, acoustic stapedial reflexes are missing and speech recognition is very poor. Unfortunately, this is a poor term, implying that such a lesion is restricted to the cochlear nerve, whereas one of the most common causes, a mutation of the otoferlin gene, affects the junction between the inner hair cells and the cochlear nerve. The condition may also be caused by conditions affecting the cochlear nucleus, such as hyperbilirubinaemia.

While secondary degeneration of the cochlear neurones following cochlear damage is relatively common, primary lesions of the vestibulocochlear nerve, for example from a vestibular Schwannoma, are rare. They will usually result in disproportionately poor speech recognition and abnormal adaptation, in which the individual has difficulty listening to a sustained tone, which fades away or becomes distorted.

Central auditory pathways

Disorders arising in the auditory pathways are generally very subtle and may not be immediately obvious. This stems from the fact that there is considerable redundancy of neurones within the central pathways and a lesion would have to affect both sides before it results in a major auditory deficit. Such deficits have been defined in an American consensus conference (Jerger and Musiek, 2000) as being 'associated with difficulties in listening, speech understanding, language development and learning'.

The most recent consensus definition from the American Speech-Language-Hearing Association (ASHA; 2005) specifies that it may be demonstrated by poor performance in one or more of sound localisation and lateralisation, auditory discrimination, auditory pattern recognition, temporal aspects of audition or auditory performance in the presence of competing signals and with degraded acoustic signals.

Baran and Musiek (2003) sub-classify the deficits according to whether the lesion is affecting the low brainstem, the high brainstem, the auditory cortex or the interhemispheric pathways, and indicate the specific deficits which may be associated with these. One of the problems is that the lesions affecting the central auditory nervous system may be diffuse (e.g. multiple sclerosis, strokes, tumours, trauma) and affect several different parts of the auditory pathway. It is only in such cases that pronounced auditory deficits may be experienced (Fourcin *et al.*, 1985; Musiek *et al.*, 2007).

King-Kopetzky syndrome

This is a condition, also known as *obscure auditory function* (Saunders and Haggard, 1989), in which an individual will report a particular difficulty hearing speech in background noise while, at the same time, having a normal pure tone audiogram. The individual complains specifically of difficulties recognising speech, particularly in background noise, and a range of psychological consequences (Zhao and Stephens, 1996a).

While in most cases the lesion involved may stem from a minor deficit in the cochlea and or psychological disturbances, a subset of some 10% may have only a central auditory disorder and so may be considered with other cases in that group (Zhao and Stephens, 2000). The aetiological factors are not clear, although in a significant proportion the condition may represent the early stages of a late-onset dominant genetic disorder (Stephens and Zhao, 2000). Pryce and Wainwright (2008) argue that the condition comes within the spectrum of 'medically unexplained symptoms', with the patient responding disproportionately to their perceived hearing difficulties.

Severity of hearing impairment

The severity of the hearing impairment has a major effect on the disabilities experienced by the individual. In cases of middle ear (conductive lesions), the maximum loss which will be experienced in a purely conductive disorder will be of the order of 60 dB. However, many cases of both chronic otitis media and otosclerosis also have a sensorineural (cochlear) element, with the cochlea in part affected by the disease processes.

In 'pure' conductive disorders, the only significant effect is one of attenuation. Thus, while the condition is mild, sounds will appear a little soft or distant, and as it becomes more severe these effects will be more pronounced, so that the individual has problems hearing speech at normal levels, some warning signals and most environmental noises apart from loud impulsive noises such as doors slamming. In association with this is the phenomenon of Paracusis (Willisii) in which such individuals may report hearing better in the presence of background noise. The best examples of this still seems to be from the description by William Holder (1669), who reported a case of someone hearing speech better when a drum was playing continually in the background, and another of someone arranging for important conversations to take place in a stagecoach driven fast. In such circumstances, the speakers, by the Lombard effect, would speak loudly and the listener would hear what they were saying without distortion.

Such behaviour would be disastrous for an individual with a cochlear lesion, because they would have considerable difficulty hearing in such background noise, even when they had only a mild hearing impairment. This stems primarily from the loss of frequency resolution in the cochlea, particularly as a result of damage to the outer hair cells, which provide by their mechanical action much of the basis of fine tuning in the inner ear. Such distortion also results in the phenomenon of recruitment, or abnormal growth of loudness, so that they would be able to hear speech at a relatively normal level until more severe distortions of the mechanism become established.

The other complication with cochlear hearing impairments lies in the configuration of the impairment. Most disorders affecting the cochlea due to acquired and genetic causes affect initially the high frequencies, progressing to the mid- and low frequencies as they become more severe. When only the high frequencies are affected, providing that the listener can also see the face of the speaker, complementing their auditory reception of speech with speechreading, they will be able to communicate well. However, as the mid- and low frequencies become affected, this benefit will be much less and, at the same time, there is increased distortion of the sounds.

More severe hearing impairment, up to the total deafness which can arise from cochlear lesions, will lead to increased communication difficulties, with very little auditory recognition of speech, even in the quiet, together with more problems hearing warning signals and a total lack of awareness of environmental sounds. Such a severe impairment of hearing and speech recognition will generally have a major impact on the individual and may result in severe psychological problems (e.g. Thomas and Gilhome Herbst, 1980; Zhao *et al.*, 1997; Kramer, 2005). See also Chapters 5 and 6.

Lesions affecting the cochlear nerve will generally result in increasing distortion with progression of the disorder, leading to a total hearing impairment. However, even mild lesions here can result in quite severe distortion.

Within the central auditory nervous system, the effects of lesion progression on the auditory effects has not been examined systematically, although in general the more extensive the lesion the greater the effects. This is particularly true when both sides of the ascending auditory pathways are affected.

Unilateral/asymmetrical hearing impairment

The preceding discussions have focused particularly on bilateral hearing impairments, largely on the grounds that they are the most frequently experienced and have the greatest impact on the affected individuals. However, while their impact is generally less than in more severe hearing impairments, a number of recent studies have indicated significant disabilities stemming from unilateral impairments (e.g. Reeve, 2003). While most of this work has concentrated on children, some similar effects have been reported in adults.

Davis (1997) indicates that in asymmetrical hearing impairment there is often a conductive element to the impairment in the poorer ear. Unilateral impairments may be conductive, generally from chronic otitis media, or sensorineural (predominantly cochlear). Such impairments have effects on the bilateral integration of sounds, resulting in difficulties particularly in localisation of sounds in the horizontal plane and on the recognition of speech in noise.

Localisation effects for louder sounds will be less in cochlear impairments as the recruitment effect may compensate for the threshold impairment in the poorer hearing ear. However, a number of studies have found that poor localisation in such individuals may impact on participation restriction and emotional effects (e.g. Noble and Gatehouse, 2004).

That study was based on individuals with asymmetrical hearing impairments who had been shown earlier to be more likely to use bilateral hearing aids, suggesting that they experienced greater problems (Chung and Stephens, 1986). Swan and Gatehouse (1990) report that individuals with asymmetry of their hearing are more likely to consult, seeking a hearing aid fitting than those with a matched symmetrical hearing impairment. They are also more likely to have participation restriction and emotional effects consequential to their hearing impairment.

Age of onset

Within this context, the most important question is concerned with differences between those with a congenital, or pre-lingual, hearing impairment and those whose hearing impairment is acquired at a later age. However, Gilhome Herbst (1983) suggests a greater impact in terms of psychosocial consequences between those people who develop a hearing impairment during their working age and those in whom it becomes apparent after retirement.

One important question which has to be answered with regards to people with a congenital hearing impairment is: 'If you have never heard anything, can you be aware of an impact of hearing impairment?' Indeed, when Deaf school leavers or Deaf adults are questioned as to their hearing problems, they will generally deny having such problems, and this is a very genuine response. However, if one questions the parents or significant others of such individuals, a range of difficulties emerges (Meehan *et al.*, 2002). Nevertheless, the question arises as to whether it is ethical to propose interventions for an individual not experiencing or reporting problems. In any case, it is debateable as to whether the offer would be taken up and implemented.

The same is true of those with a congenital unilateral hearing impairment, who may often be unaware of their impairment until a chance remark when they are in their teens or later.

However, this does not imply that those with pre-lingual hearing impairment have no problems. Griggs (1998), in a 20-year follow-up of deaf school leavers, found a high level of psychological illness, more pronounced in those with deafness of unknown aetiology. Werngren-Elgström *et al.* (2003) found older pre-lingually Deaf people to have higher depression scores and insomnia than hearing older people, but did not compare them with older people with late-onset hearing impairment. They also found no difference in *well-being* and Griggs (1998) highlights the different concept of *Deaf wellness* found among people in the Deaf community.

One study that reviewed the literature on suicide among Deaf people (Turner *et al.*, 2007) concluded that, while there was an increased level of depression in such individuals, the risk factors for suicide were much as in the general population, but any increased risk of suicide was not clear.

Unpublished data from a study by Middleton *et al.* (in press) offer the opportunity to compare some views of members of Hearing Concern and the British Deaf Association. Respondents were separated according to whether they lost their hearing as a child after they had developed language, as an adult between the ages of 18 and 49 or as an older adult. Table 3.2 indicates whether they regarded themselves as Deaf (culturally deaf), deaf, hard of hearing, deafened or hearing impaired, and which community they identified with. The groups were not controlled for severity of hearing impairment as those data were not available.

Table 3.2 Views of people with acquired hearing impairment by age of onset (%).

Self-descriptor	Age at which hearing was lost		
	3–17 years	18–49 years	>50 years
Deaf	16	6	4
deaf	22	16	9
Hard of hearing	41	48	69
Deafened	11	13	4
Hearing impaired	10	16	13
Community they identify with			
Deaf	11	0	0
Hard of hearing	23	20	30
Mainstream hearing	42	66	54
All communities	24	13	16

The most notable aspects of this table are the fact that appreciable numbers of all groups regarded themselves as culturally Deaf, but only in the childhood-onset group did any identify with the Deaf community. The majority of the two adult-onset groups identified with the mainstream hearing community, but a significant minority of all groups identified with the hard of hearing community, which is a rather nebulous concept.

As might be expected, the majority of the pre-lingually Deaf respondents, derived from a different source, identified with the Deaf community, but with over 20% reporting that they identified with all communities. In addition, the vast majority there regarded themselves as Deaf or deaf.

Genetic issues

The influence of genetic factors on the psychosocial aspects of hearing impairment has been the subject of a number of studies (e.g. Stephens and Jones, 2006; Stephens, 2007). However, in general, it has proved difficult to differentiate between the impact of genetic conditions per se and the impact of role models, within the family, who also have hearing impairment related to a variety of causes.

A clear impact of genetic hearing impairment can be found in small isolated communities in which a mutation resulting in recessive hearing impairment has entered the gene pool. This was true of nineteenth-century Martha's Vinyard in the United States (Groce, 1985) and in the current situation in the village of Bengkala in Bali (Branson, 1996). In both communities, when the prevalence of profound hearing impairment reached a certain level within the population, hearing villagers came to use sign language as a natural form of communication, and the Deaf people were accepted as full members of society.

In more general investigations, there seems to be a difference between the results of epidemiological studies (Stephens et al., 2003a, 2006; Sindhusake et al., 2006), which suggest that the impact of hearing impairment may be greater in those with a family history than in those without, and clinic-based studies. The latter appear to highlight the positive effects of a role model (Coulson, 2006; Kramer et al., 2006a). However, in all large-scale studies, the impact of having a family history seems to be less than that of the severity of the hearing impairment or its age of onset. Jones et al. (1987) report that adults with hearing impairment who had direct experience of their parents' hearing impairment while they were children found this helpful and a positive experience.

The epidemiological studies (e.g. Stephens, 2007) indicate that those with a family history are more likely to have worse hearing than those without, but also that they are more sensitive to such a hearing loss and annoyed by it. Furthermore, a family history of hearing impairment may affect the impact of associated tinnitus and hyperacusis.

Within clinical studies, positive effects of the family history were reported 2–3 times more frequently than negative effects were (Stephens and Kramer, 2005), although this is apparent only where the individual is aware of having such a family history and sees their antecedents as role models from whom they can learn (Coulson, 2006; Kramer et al., 2006b). This can be in terms of benefiting from positive experiences of family members or by taking action (e.g. early fitting of hearing aids) to avoid their negative experiences.

In pre-lingually deaf adolescents, both Vernon and Koh (1970) and Conrad (1979) found that having role models in their Deaf parents resulted in better academic achievement than in those who had a genetic disorder but hearing parents. Griggs (1998) in her long-term follow-up of Conrad's subjects also found that those with genetic disorders were less likely to have psychiatric problems as adults than those with unknown or acquired causes for their hearing impairment.

A more recent study by Fortnum et al. (2006) found a benefit on educational achievement in those with 'totally deaf' parents, but little impact on their quality of life. It also notes that such effects of a family history were small compared with those resulting from a range of demographic factors.

Otosclerosis is a genetic disorder (or group of disorders) with a complex mechanism of inheritance in which about half of affected patients have a family history (Declau and Van de Heyning, 2007a). Middleton et al. (2006) examined a series of patients with and without a family history and found no difference in the psychosocial impact of the condition in the two groups. However, Stephens and Lemkens (2006) asked those with such a family history whether that had influenced their reaction to the condition and how, and two-thirds indicated that having a family history had a positive effect on their reaction. The overall results were very similar to those found with non-specific genetic disorders.

Progressive/sudden onset

In general, the onset of adult hearing impairment is a gradual process to which the individuals may adapt as the impairment worsens. In some, however, it is a sudden change which can have a severe impact on those affected. Fortunately, in most cases, such an acute change is often unilateral and, when bilateral, is either generally not severe or is followed by some degree of recovery (Booth, 1997).

Lehmann (1954) describes sudden hearing loss as 'one of life's most terrifying experiences'. However, unfortunately, there has been little systematic work on the condition since those words were written. In most studies (e.g. Hallam et al., 2006), while sizeable proportions of the patients with profound acquired hearing impairment studied had a sudden onset, the results from these are not presented separately from those with a more gradual onset.

Sato-Minako et al. (2005) report that a combination of hearing loss and severe tinnitus contributed to the difficulties experienced by those with sudden deafness. They also report that, unlike those with a gradual onset, there was no correlation between their scores on the Hearing Handicap Inventory in Adults (HHIA) and their hearing level. Earlier, in sudden unilateral hearing loss, Chiossoine-Kerdel et al. (2000) had reported similar results with no relationship between hearing loss and HHIA scores. Interestingly, they similarly failed to find a relationship between such scores and the time lapse since onset of the hearing loss.

Conclusion

Within this chapter, the different types of hearing impairment, their severity and onset, are considered in relation to how they may affect the patient and influence the enablement process. First, the basic anatomy and physiology of the auditory system is briefly presented with a consideration of tests which can localise the patient's disorder within the auditory pathway. The impact that lesions at different levels of the auditory pathway may have on the patient is emphasised and the influence of the severity, age of onset, rate of onset of the hearing impairment and whether it affects one ear or two is discussed. Some 50% of hearing impairment is genetically deter-mined and the specific impact of such an aetiology is beginning to be unravelled. This is further considered in Chapter 7.

4 The influence of other factors on assessment and goals of enablement

Introduction

Some younger patients with hearing impairment have such a loss in the absence of any other related symptoms. However, the majority of individuals have hearing impairment associated with other symptoms, either in the auditory system, more generalised aural symptoms or symptoms of disorders elsewhere in the body. Any of these may interfere with their auditory function and its management. Such a proportion will, inevitably, increase with increasing age, and so will impact more and more on patients with hearing impairments, which become more common with increasing age.

Within this chapter, we discuss how some of these conditions influence the impact of hearing impairment on the individual, as well as their implications for the process of enablement.

Auditory symptoms

Tinnitus

Tinnitus occurs in some 60% of people with hearing impairment either some or most of the time (Coles *et al.*, 1990). In addition, over 80% of people with tinnitus can be shown to have some degree of hearing impairment and many of those with normal audiograms have a significant hearing impairment on sensitised testing (Sirimanna *et al.*, 1996). Some recordings and simulations of different types of tinnitus are available via the web site accompanying this book (http://www.wiley.com/go/stephens).

Tinnitus itself may be associated with a range of psychosocial impacts on the patient, many of which will be dependent on the underlying personality of the individual and the stressors to which they are submitted. These effects can range from mild insomnia or anxiety through to severe depression and even suicide, although the last is exceptional without a number of other contemporaneous precipitating factors (Lewis *et al.*, 1994). In population studies, while some 12% of the adult population report significant tinnitus, only 0.4% report it as having a severe effect on their quality of life (Davis, 1995).

Many patients with tinnitus attribute their hearing difficulties to their tinnitus and deny any actual hearing impairment per se. This was observed by Itard (1821), almost two centuries ago, who suggested testing for it using sustained pressure on the carotid artery, with the hearing improving if the apparent impairment was related to the tinnitus! However, a real impairment of hearing can generally be demonstrated using carefully performed audiometry, and most patients will accept the results of this. The degree to which tinnitus can actually interfere with the hearing has been the subject of some debate and the consensus is that its impact is more one of distraction rather than of masking.

In many such patients, the fitting of a hearing aid or aids, with open moulds, can provide considerable relief to both their hearing and their tinnitus. In directly helping their hearing, the patient does not have to strain to hear, so making them less aware of their tinnitus.

Approaches to more general psychosocial aspects of the tinnitus have been the subject of much controversy. For many patients, counselling and reassurance is sufficient, particularly when coupled with investigations to exclude sinister causes. For those who are more disturbed, the most effective approaches at the present time would appear to be based on cognitive behavioural therapy and relaxation techniques (Tyler, 2000; Andersson et al., 2005). However, even these approaches frequently leave some residual problems, and a range of other approaches is currently being investigated (Stephens and McKenna, 2008). In that context, Goebel and Floezinger (2008) found a greater psychological disturbance when the tinnitus was associated with hyperacusis.

Among the psychosocial effects reported by patients with tinnitus are impaired concentration, sleep difficulties, anxiety and depression (Tyler and Baker, 1983; Sanchez and Stephens, 1997). Impaired concentration and lack of sleep will interfere with people's hearing problems in difficult listening situations and so need to be taken into account in the planning of any enablement programme. In addition, particularly in patients with severe hearing impairment, any anxiety and depression may stem from a combination of the effects of the tinnitus and of any coexistent vertigo, and needs to be addressed seriously.

As mentioned earlier, appropriate amplification can help both hearing difficulties and tinnitus, but needs to be addressed carefully, avoiding any occlusion effect, which, in many patients with tinnitus, may aggravate that symptom. This emphasises the need for careful follow-up, and Stephens and Meredith (1991b), using an open-ended approach to hearing aid shortcomings, found that 8% of patients reported aggravation of their tinnitus by the hearing aid fitting. Other benefits for tinnitus of appropriate audiological management, including environmental aids, will be that they find themselves in a noisier environment, less distracted by their tinnitus and better able to concentrate.

Thinking in terms of positive impacts of both the tinnitus and hearing impairment, one area frequently reported is the lack of disturbance by extraneous noises at night, with a consequent facilitation of sleep (Kerr and Stephens, 2000). Other positive aspects reported of tinnitus experience overlap with those of hearing impairment, and include 'personal development' and 'empathy with others' with tinnitus, hearing problems and other disabilities (Kentala et al., 2008).

Pressure sensation

A feeling of pressure or blockage in the ear is traditionally associated with otitis media with effusion (OME), often known as *glue ear*. While this is generally true for children, among adults the sensation is often associated with inner ear disorders. In the latter context, it is best known as being one of the characteristics of Menière's disorder, but may also occur in a number of other conditions, being particularly associated with a sudden change in hearing. Whether this is related to the development of endolymphatic hydrops remains unclear.

A study of patients with sudden deterioration in their inner ear hearing found it in 83% of those studied, but unrelated to the tinnitus, often found in such individuals, both in terms of its onset and of its recovery (Sakata *et al.*, 2008). Its recovery did seem to relate to a recovery of hearing for the lower frequencies.

From the standpoint of auditory enablement, the main implication of this symptom, which many individuals find disturbing and may refer to as *pain*, is on any hearing aid fitting. In severe cases, the affected individual may find it too uncomfortable to be able to tolerate a hearing aid or earmould in their external meatus, necessitating medical/pharmacological treatment of the symptom before such a fitting can proceed.

More commonly, it will be essential to avoid a tightly fitting earmould, which could aggravate the patient's discomfort and cause them to reject their hearing aid. It is thus essential to have as open an earmould as possible for any hearing aid fitting to an ear affected by such a pressure sensation. With improvements in hearing aid feedback suppression techniques, this is now generally feasible. In patients with severe hearing impairment, it may still be achieved by the use of a vented earmould with a sintered filter in the vent (French St George and Barr-Hamilton, 1975).

Hyperacusis

Hyperacusis refers to the intolerance of sounds and is sometimes used as a synonym for *phonophobia*, the aural equivalent of *photophobia*. Hyperacusis is defined in *Dorland's Pocket Medical Dictionary* as 'an exceptionally acute sense of hearing' and phonophobia as 'a morbid dread of sounds or of speaking aloud' (Anon, 1982).

Subsequently, particularly with regard to tinnitus, a condition with which hyperacusis is commonly associated, the use of the term has been restricted to those people with essentially normal hearing, in order to distinguish it from the phenomenon of recruitment. Thus, Andersson *et al.* (2002) and Goebel and Floezinger (2008) use the term hyperacusis to denote 'increased sensitivity to ordinary environmental sounds' and phonophobia as 'a discomfort to special environmental sounds, and the patients express fear of specific sounds'. Goebel and Floezinger further comment that 'hyperacusis and phonophobia are often found together, but both of these phenomena can also be diagnosed separately'. Interestingly, they argue that hyperacusis is the result of a psychological disorder rather than the cause of it.

Andersson *et al.* (2002), in a postal survey of a random sample of the population aged 16–79 years, found a prevalence of hyperacusis for the total population of 8%, dropping to 5.9% when those with reported hearing problems were excluded. There was no significant relationship with age or gender but, in the normally hearing group, there was an association with hypersensitivity to light or colours. Elsewhere, in a UK population survey, Stephens *et al.* (2006) found that among individuals over the age of 60 years who reported themselves as having normal hearing some 65% reported being at least slightly annoyed by loud sounds. This proportion was even higher in those with a family history of hearing problems.

Aetiological factors and approaches to the measurement of hyperacusis are discussed extensively by Andersson *et al.* (2005). They propose that it comprises three components: 'noise sensitivity', 'annoyance/irritation' and 'fear of injury or of the symptom becoming worse', which interact to result in the patient's symptoms.

The relevance of hyperacusis to audiological enablement is related to its effects on any possible amplification and its impact on the patient's response to certain sounds in his or her environment. With regard to the former, Goebel and Floezinger (2008) found a good relationship between the results of uncomfortable loudness levels (ULLs) and those obtained with a questionnaire on the subjective stress related to hypersensitivity to loud sounds. Thus, arguably, incorporating ULL measures in the patient assessment protocol should address that problem. Further, they argue that hyperacusis is amenable to either cognitive behavioural therapy or counselling accompanied by maskers/noise generators. In addition, Saglier *et al.* (2004) found that appropriate hearing aid fitting can reduce hyperacusis. This emphasises also that patients entering an enablement programme should always be asked about this symptom.

General aural symptoms

Otorrhoea

Otorrhoea is the term which describes discharge from the ear. This may arise in the outer ear or, after a perforation of the tympanic membrane, in the middle ear. It generally consists of the purulent consequences of an infection, although on occasions it may take the form of a clear discharge.

The main implications of otorrhoea for auditory enablement concern hearing aid fitting. In this context, the otorrhoea can block the acoustical pathway from the output transducer of the hearing aid to the middle/inner ears and, in addition, the occlusion of the ear canal by the earmould or hearing aid can lead to an accentuation of the infection. Furthermore, in certain cases, owing to poor hygiene or, more rarely, to an allergy to the earmould material, the presence of the earmould/hearing aid in the ear can provoke discharge.

Otorrhoea stemming from an outer ear infection or allergic reaction can generally be controlled by appropriate aural toilet and antibiotic/anti-inflammatory eardrops. The main problem is not to exacerbate it by provoking further irritation or allergy, and well-made earmoulds of a hypoallergenic material are important in this respect. Where earmoulds made of silicone and related materials fail, silver-coated or even porcelain moulds may be considered. In addition, it is essential that any earmould/hearing aid fitting should be as open as possible, avoiding complete occlusion of the external meatus.

There are some individuals whose otorrhoea stemming from the external canal (chronic otitis externa) resists all treatment. In such cases, if the opposite ear is unaidable, alternative instrumental approaches must be tried. If the cochlear component of the hearing impairment is not severe, the patient may be fitted with a bone-anchored hearing aid (BAHA). An alternative approach would be to consider a middle ear implantable hearing aid such as the Vibrant Soundbridge, comprising a transducer with a coil and magnet, which is fixed to the long process of the incus. Unfortunately, long-term evaluations of such devices are sparse, and a study by Schmuziger *et al.* (2006), involving a two-year follow-up, indicated a significant deterioration in the hearing of the aided ear and suggested, interestingly, that its use should be limited to patients with chronic otitis externa.

Chronic suppurative otitis media (CSOM) occurs after there has been a perforation of the tympanic membrane following acute otitis media or trauma. It involves a chronic infection of the middle ear which may lead to erosion of the ossicles and, in severe cases, can go on to involve the cochlea or even cause bony erosion and lead to meningitis. Most commonly, however, it causes an unpleasant smelly discharge from the ear. This can interfere with sound transmission from a fitted hearing aid, and can be exacerbated by the occlusive effect of the hearing aid fitting.

The condition can often be controlled by antiseptic or antibiotic eardrops, although the potential of aminoglycoside eardrops causing hair cell ototoxicity via the round window remains controversial. As with otitis externa, as far as possible, non-occluding earmould fittings should be used, although this is made more difficult by the conductive element to any hearing loss, which generally accompanies this condition. Surgical intervention with a radical mastoidectomy to eradicate the infection may be effective, but otherwise BAHAs are the most useful answer for patients with persistent CSOM.

Vertigo

Many conditions which affect hearing can result in vertigo or other balance abnormalities. *Vertigo* can be defined as an abnormal sensation of movement in which either the environment of the individual appears to be moving or the person feels that they are moving themselves. Such sensations can be of either spinning or swaying, with the most common being a feeling that the individual is swaying (subjective swaying vertigo) or that the room is spinning (objective rotatory vertigo). Such sensations arise from lesions in the vestibular labyrinth, the vestibular nerve or in the central balance pathways.

From the perspective of audiological enablement, the most relevant condition is that of the Tullio phenomenon (Tullio, 1929). In this condition, loud sounds can result in the patient experiencing vertigo, which potentially interferes with any hearing aid fitting. The patient may complain of such a problem when a lorry passes them while they walk along the road, or the balance difficulties can be triggered by a range of other sounds. If the maximum output of the person's hearing aid is too high, this can trigger such a sensation. It can be tested for clinically using the sono-ocular test (Kacker and Hinchcliffe, 1970; Stephens and Ballam, 1974), which is broadly analogous to the test for uncomfortable loudness levels, but with any nystagmus being observed or recorded. Other techniques have entailed the use of posturography (e.g. Pyykkö et al., 1992) and vestibular-evoked myogenic potentials (e.g. Brantberg and Verrecchia, 2008).

Many of the early cases of the Tullio phenomenon were associated with fenestration surgery for otosclerosis but, subsequently, it was found to be associated with a range of conditions including Menière's disorder, perilymph fistula and superior canal dehiscence. While the occurrence of the condition after hearing aid fitting has not been systematically recorded, Lesinski et al. (1998) report its occurrence following cochlear implantation.

A range of balance disorders have a psychosocial impact interacting with the effects of hearing problems, limiting the individual's activities and affecting them psychologically. Indeed, vestibular problems are amongst the most common causes of severe falls in older people.

There is a complex interaction between balance and psychological symptoms entailing both psychosomatic and somatopsychic effects (Jakes, 1997; Jacob et al., 2003) and these can be presumed to interact with the primary effects of any auditory disorder.

The main effects of balance disorders are anxiety and depression. However, while these can increase the psychological impact on tinnitus (Hallam and Stephens, 1985), the interaction with the effects of hearing problems is less clear. The specific psychological impact of hearing problems is discussed in Chapter 6.

Atresia

Atresia is defined as 'a congenital absence or closure of a normal body opening or tubular structure' and *aural atresia* as an 'absence or closure of the auditory canal' (Anon, 1982). While this is generally taken to refer to congenital developmental abnormalities, from a hearing standpoint, acquired atresia due to chronic otitis externa can be a significant problem. Both result in a conductive hearing impairment.

Congenital atresia is often associated with abnormalities of the auricle (pinna) and of the middle ear (Declau and Van de Heyning, 2007b). The condition may affect either one ear, as in hemifacial microsomia, or both, as in Treacher Collins syndrome. A wide range of reconstructive surgical techniques have been described for congenital atresias, with the aim of constructing a patent external ear canal. Such surgical treatment is often unsuccessful, and Jahrsdoerfer *et al.* (1992) suggest that only some 50% of individuals with this condition are candidates for such surgery. In particular, few surgeons would seriously consider such repair in patients with a unilateral atresia and a normal canal on the other side.

In the past, the enablement process normally entailed the use of bone-conduction hearing aids and, more recently, the use of BAHAs has become the approach of choice in such affected individuals. These are discussed further in Chapter 11, but basically consist of a hearing aid producing a vibratory output connecting with and fixed into the mastoid bone in a surgical intervention. They provide better quality sound than a traditional bone-conduction vibrator, provided that the individual has reasonably normal cochlear function (Snik *et al.*, 2008). Such surgery can be performed at any age when the mastoid bone is sufficiently well developed, generally from the age of 3–5 years.

Chronic otitis externa, an infectious or allergic inflammation of the external ear canal, generally occurs in later life, and in severe cases can result in a complete obstruction of the ear canal. Most cases will be treatable with appropriate eardrops and aural toilet and will represent only a short-term problem from the standpoint of the individual's hearing. However, in hearing aid users, this problem can sometimes be exacerbated by a reaction to the earmoulds. In addition, in many cases, only one ear is affected.

However, in a small minority of cases, it may result in chronic bilateral acquired atresia, which is resistant to medical interventions. In such patients, BAHAs should be considered. providing that there is sufficient cochlear function. In people with associated inner ear problems, implantable hearing aids such as the Vibrant Soundbridge can be considered, although the maximum output of such devices is somewhat limited, and there is a possibility that they can result in a further deterioration of cochlear function.

Pinna abnormalities

Abnormalities of the pinna, or auricle, may often be associated with atresia or middle ear abnormalities, when congenital, but may occur in isolation. In addition, acquired abnormalities may result from trauma, such as boxing, or from surgical interventions to treat skin tumours. Isolated abnormalities with normal ear canals and middle ears will result in only relatively minor effects on directionalisation, but will cause problems for the fitting of hearing aids if the individual has other, generally unrelated, hearing problems.

Surgical reconstruction of the pinna has long been attempted, but has rarely had good cosmetic success. More recently, artificial pinnas have improved in quality and appearance and may be fixed to the side of the head using a similar type of titanium screw as used for BAHAs. In addition, a fitting for such BAHAs may be inserted at the same time in those with related ear canal or middle ear abnormalities.

From the standpoint of hearing aid fittings, either in-the-canal or in-the-ear fittings may be used in most patients, provided the ear canal form and size are appropriate. In addition, it is possible to use postaural aids, sitting in a normal position on an artificial pinna.

Vision

Visual information is essential for normal communication, and many people with hearing problems have visual impairments. Such impairments may range from mild abnormalities in the lens through to complete blindness. Those with more severe visual and auditory impairments are categorised as *deafblind*, although the degree of such impairments may vary considerably. In addition, the age of onset of these impairments will have a considerable influence on their impact on the individual concerned (Möller, 2005).

By far the largest proportion of people with dual impairments are older people, who have mild to moderate refractory impairments which may be largely corrected by the use of spectacles and hearing aids. The main impact that this will have will be on the individual's ability to speechread and to detect cues of non-verbal communication. The former can be particularly important in those with high-frequency hearing losses, which can compromise the auditory detection of fricatives. These, in turn, are relatively easy to speechread, so that people with good vision can compensate, at least in part, for the auditory impairment, provided that they can see the face of the speaker (Sumby and Pollack, 1954; Ewertsen, 1974). Hardick *et al.* (1970), in normally hearing subjects, found a significant relationship between their visual acuity and their speechreading ability. It is thus important that people with hearing difficulties and visual problems should have the latter checked to ensure that their visual impairment is corrected as far as possible, and this should be considered in enablement programmes (see Chapter 10).

The psychosocial aspects of deafblindness have been extensively reviewed by Möller (2005), with further findings presented by Möller and Danermark (2007). Essentially, Möller considers those affected in three categories: those born deafblind, those with early onset of deafblindness and those with late onset. The first may be due to rubella syndrome and a number of congenital disorders, the second often to Usher syndrome, particularly Usher type 1, and the third to a range of acquired disorders.

Inevitably, people in all three groups have restricted participation in all situations and are very dependent on the support which they receive from their families, significant others and from state provisions. For example, Möller and Danermark (2007) show that, in a group of young people with Usher syndrome, the considerateness of those around them was a key factor in determining the impact of their condition.

In the psychological domain there appears to be a difference in the impact of the condition dependent on the age of onset. Möller (2005) argues that in young people with a pre-lingual condition, behavioural disorders such as head-banging, self-injury and other repetitive habits are common. These can be reduced by a range of approaches, including the use of alternative sensory stimulation using smells and tastes. Interventions in this group will include the learning of an appropriate tactile or symbolic language, a consideration of appropriate instrumentation according to the severity and nature of their hearing impairment, but primarily an approach tailored to their specific needs and orientation. The different tactile sign systems, particularly the Tadoma system, are discussed by Rönnberg and Borg (2001).

In post-lingually developed deafblindness, there are reports of depression, psychosis and suicidal tendencies perhaps related to the loss of independence and identity. Thus, for example, young people with Usher type 1 syndrome, who have congenital deafness but onset of retinitis pigmentosa (RP) in their teens, will often have identified with and involved themselves in the Deaf community, but begin to experience major problems as their RP expresses itself in deteriorating vision. Thus, for example, having previously been opposed to the concept of cochlear implants, they now feel they would like to have them to maintain contact with their environment, even if, at this stage, such a device is unlikely to provide them with adequate speech recognition. It could be argued that such individuals should receive bilateral implants in infancy so that they will be able to develop reasonable speech and language and have auditory localisation abilities when their visual impairment later becomes severe. Furthermore, Rönnberg et al. (2002) suggest that the use of any residual vision is critical in the enablement process and Danermark and Möller (2008) emphasise the importance of the development of trust by the patients in those around them during any such process.

Late-onset deafblindness can result in the development of depressive conditions and the exacerbation or enhancement of dementia (Vernon and Duncan, 1990). Little has been written about this condition and it would appear that it should be addressed like any other enablement process, involving problem-solving and the use of any residual hearing and vision to an optimal extent. Saeed et al. (1998) emphasise that such patients, where appropriate, may benefit considerably from cochlear implantation.

Cognitive and intellectual factors

Influences on hearing in this domain can range from severe intellectual disability (learning difficulty) and dementia to minor short-term memory problems. The influence of the latter and other aspects of cognitive function on speech recognition are discussed in the next chapter. It is of note that one review (Akeroyd, 2008) suggests that, while measures of working memory, particularly reading span, may influence speech recognition, more general measures of intellectual ability were rarely shown to have a significant effect.

It must be noted, however, that while Akeroyd found general verbal and non-verbal IQ measures to have no effect in this context, the studies reviewed used subjects essentially within the 'normal' range of intelligence. Here we shall consider briefly the problems posed by those outside such norms.

A range of conditions resulting in intellectual disability, such as Down syndrome, are frequently associated with middle ear and occasionally inner ear problems (Toriello *et al.*, 2004). Indeed, otitis media is almost invariably present in people with Down syndrome and, in addition, a progressive premature ageing effect on the cochlea occurs in adulthood. These both have an impact on the individual's ability to communicate and, indeed, to develop meaningful speech in the first instance.

Attempts to treat the middle ear problems surgically have generally been unsuccessful and there has been more emphasis on early hearing aid fitting. This can be problematic in terms of the individual's tolerance of an aid in their ear, but can generally be achieved with care and persistence, together with a sympathetic approach. Where such an approach fails, and, indeed, in conjunction with such an approach, there will be a need to consider alternative methods, including the use of Makaton, a simplified sign language, environmental aids and communication tactics for the carers. The need for help for such people with intellectual disabilities is becoming a more common problem with the increase of life expectancy during the past half-century (Fisher and Kettl, 2005). The importance of providing any information in as comprehensible a way as possible to such individuals cannot be overemphasised.

The other area which is assuming greater importance with increased longevity in the general population is that of dementia. While many studies (e.g. Gilhome Herbst and Humphrey, 1980) have found a co-occurrence of hearing impairment and dementia in older people, there is no evidence for poor hearing being the cause of the condition, although any concomitant hearing impairment can accentuate the symptoms associated with it. Indeed, a range of studies have found no clear relationship between cognitive and hearing impairments (e.g. Gussekloo *et al.*, 2005). However, Gates *et al.* (2008) emphasise that central auditory function will be impaired in a range of cognitive impairments including Alzheimer dementia.

The importance of appropriate communication between professionals and both patients with dementia and their carers is paramount in order to provide support in ameliorating the impact of the condition. A broad approach to enablement is essential, and one which considers all aspects of intervention that can be appropriate. Given such an approach, a number of studies have shown that hearing aids can be beneficial to such individuals (e.g. Allen *et al.*, 2003; Petitot *et al.*, 2007).

Neuromusculoskeletal problems

While neuromusculoskeletal problems may occur congenitally as a result of genetic disorders (Toriello *et al.*, 2004) or pre- and perinatal insults, the most common problem in the context of hearing problems are the later-onset conditions. The main concern here is not generally the direct effect on hearing but rather on the implications for any instrumentation, particularly hearing aid fitting.

In terms of any direct effect on hearing, there is debateable evidence of the impact of conditions such as rheumatoid arthritis or the muscular dystrophies on hearing (e.g. Rogers *et al.*, 2002). However, the impact of neurological disorders such as stroke or multiple sclerosis is clearer, but not inevitable. The consequences of any of these conditions on the individual's motor control and sensation in their fingers can have a critical impact.

The most extreme condition in this context is, obviously, either a total loss of the upper limbs or a loss of their function. An example of this is a patient who had lost both arms and had been fitted with bilateral behind-the-ear hearing aids which he

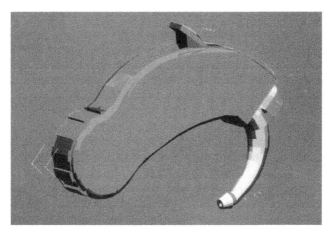

Figure 4.1 A design for an ergonomic hearing aid. (*Source:* reproduced with permission from Roberts, 1992.)

could not control once his partner had put them in his ears. A much more reasonable approach was subsequently achieved by the use of an adapted body-worn aid with large controls that he could manipulate with his legs, and so make appropriate adjustments for particular environments.

More commonly found conditions are those in which patients with severe arthritis or who have had strokes lack the manipulative skills to be able to fit a hearing aid appropriately or adjust its controls. The same will be true of individuals with severe tremors, as in Parkinson's disease or hyperthyroidism. Finally, a range of neurodegenerative conditions such as multiple sclerosis can result in an impairment of the individual's ability to feel the small controls. In fact, in practice, the most common problem occurs in older people with a combination of mild tremor, manipulative and sensory difficulties and some confusion, possibly related to early dementia.

While some of these problems may be overcome by a hearing aid with a remote control system, this is not always practicable or acceptable. Alternatively, many of the problems may be overcome by simple modifications of the earmould (Meredith *et al.*, 1989), making it easier to fit to the ear, and by ergonomically designed hearing aids.

An attempt to design such an aid was made by Roberts (1992), see Figure 4.1, following a survey of the problems experienced by older hearing aid users.

In this hearing aid, the volume control was built into the battery compartment and hence easy to access and manipulate. The on/off switch is a simple toggle switch, again easily controlled by the patient. Patients who had difficulties with standard hearing aids found this easy to manipulate and were enthusiastic about the design. Unfortunately, there has been little interest among hearing aid manufacturers in the development of such ergonomic aids.

Conclusion

A range of other factors and disabilities may influence the patient's hearing problems and the approaches needed to address such difficulties. These factors may be auditory, but can also be aural, visual, cognitive or related to the neuromusculoskel-etal system. Auditory factors include tinnitus, hyperacusis and pressure sensations, all of which need to be addressed at the same time as the hearing difficulties. Among other aural problems are vertigo, ear discharge and malformations of the outer ear. These can have a major impact on the choice of any instrumentation in the process of enablement.

Visual problems may range from short-sightedness to deafblindness, and all levels of severity can affect the individual's communication skills and deficits. Each needs to be addressed in a way that is relevant to the patient's needs. Mild cognitive differences may affect speech communication, and are discussed further in the next chapter. However, more severe impairments such as dementia or intellectual disabilities can have a major impact as to how the enablement process is structured to make it relevant to the needs of the individuals concerned and those around them. Finally, disorders of the nervous system and of the musculoskeletal system may affect how the individual can cope with any instrumental assistance and the choice of such interventions.

5 Communication

Introduction

Communication is a broad concept. It is a process by which information is exchanged between or among individuals. That includes conversing, speaking, listening, hearing, writing and expressing feelings. Communication can occur both verbally and non-verbally and it involves spoken language, signs, signals and behaviour.

While communicating, humans interact with their surroundings. Hearing and communication may therefore be seen as interactive processes between individuals who are also interacting with their social and physical environments. The science that studies the interactions between individuals and their interactions with the environment is called *ecology*. Ecological approaches towards disabilities arising from hearing impairment are advocated by Noble and Hétu (1994) and by Borg (2003) and their perspectives will be described in the next section. In addition, on the accompanying website (http://www.wiley.com/go/stephens), we refer to websites demonstrating as to how speech may sound to individuals with different hearing impairments.

Ecological audiology

In their ecological approach towards auditory disability and handicap, Noble (1983) and Noble and Hétu (1994) focus on the system of interactions among people, environments and interfaces. They emphasise the relevance of such an interactive approach when defining a person's limitations and restrictions resulting from hearing impairment and when considering rehabilitative interventions. For example, when an individual experiences communication difficulties owing to hearing impairment and seeks help, adjustments are required not only at the level of the individual (e.g. hearing aid prescription, speechreading lessons, emotional counselling), but also in other domains. Thus, adjustments of environmental conditions (i.e. reducing background noise, changing attitudes of significant others) are equally important and may even be more effective in certain circumstances than adjustments at the individual level. It means that the assessment of difficulties and any means of reducing those difficulties can only be made with reference to specific situations and interactions. Taking into account all interactions, disabling or enabling, offers a wider range of enablement possibilities than does focusing on the individual alone.

An ecological approach differs from an individualistic and a collectivist approach in that the latter focuses on the environment only while neglecting the adaptations an individual needs to make to overcome hearing difficulties. An individualistic

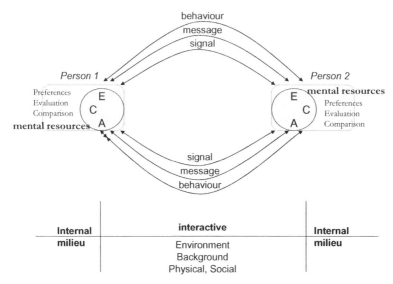

Figure 5.1 Representation of Borg's (2003) ecological conceptual framework.

approach focuses on the individual while neglecting any possible intervention at the level of the environment of the person. A consequence of an ecological approach is that audiological enablement can be considered successful only if both partners in the communication process (e.g. the person with the hearing impairment and the significant other) are satisfied with the outcome.

The conceptual ecological framework for auditory communication, as elaborated by Borg (2003), differs from that of Noble and Hétu (1994) in that it mainly focuses on communication. In doing so, it identifies different levels and additional concepts and components. The framework is illustrated in Figure 5.1. The interaction with another person is conceptualised into three levels: signal (acoustics of the speech sound), message and behaviour. The environmental factors comprise the acoustical, physical, social, psychological and attitudinal environment in which people live and conduct their lives, similar to the environmental factors in the *International Classification of Functioning, Disability and Health* (ICF) model (WHO, 2001).

The framework then distinguishes between different components comprising the so-called *internal environment*, which, together, determine a person's auditory communicative ability. Those components reflect pathways with different directions and are referred to as *ACE*:

1. The first component is defined as the *afferent* (A), or bottom-up, *signal-related component*. It involves the physiology, anatomy and pathology of the hearing organ and reflects the quality of the system at the receptor or input level. Analogous to the ICF model (see Chapter 1), an abnormality in the anatomical structure or physiological function of the hearing organ is defined as *hearing impairment*.
2. The second component is the *central language-processing-related factor* (C). This factor is influenced by the person's cognitive capacities (mental resources) that reflect that person's knowledge, interests, vocabulary, attention, memory and speed of information processing. This factor is often identified as the top-down

processing component in speech perception and will be further discussed in the following paragraphs.

3. The third component is the *efferent speech/language-related component* (E), which involves the production of sounds including speech and vocalisation. Poor expressive language and speech (poor articulation, a vocabulary that is not well understood) and poor talking behaviour (disregard of turn-taking, talking while moving away) may have a negative effect on the communication.

According to this framework, a person continuously perceives and evaluates the communication process and relates it to his or her communicative self-image (also referred to as *preference, preferendum, internal reference* or *ecological optimum*). The internal reference is influenced by various factors such as individual needs, societal norms and the personality of the individual.

When there is a mismatch between the internal preference and the actual communication situation, an error signal (emotional reaction) may be produced, reflecting the misbalance in the system. Examples of such error signals are feelings of failure, loss of confidence, irritation or anger, creating a release of mental energy. To reconstruct the communication situation again, either the internal preferendum may be modified or an external coping strategy (feedback), such as asking for repetition or a change of the environment, may be applied.

The conceptual ecological framework of Borg provides a broad holistic perspective. It not only includes the interaction between the individual and the environment, but it also recognises (the interaction with) the internal preferendum (self-image), which, if not in balance with the actual communication situation, may lead to emotional reactions and inappropriate coping behaviour.

The framework has been proven a useful and valid tool for diagnostic and rehabilitative purposes (Borg and Stephens, 2003; Borg *et al.*, 2008). Even more interesting is its perspective of generating new questions for the analysis and understanding of patients with many different types of hearing impairment.

Ramsdell's classification

A rather different classification to describe communication and hearing is that proposed by Ramsdell (1947). Whereas Borg's (2003) model only deals with the communicative ecological system, Ramsdell's (1947) classification goes beyond communication and focuses on hearing in general. Ramsdell argues that to understand the psychological changes which accompany the loss of hearing it is first necessary to comprehend how normal hearing operates. Ramsdell discusses normal hearing as though it occurs at three hierarchical psychological levels: the symbolic level, the signal level and the primitive level (Table 5.1). He emphasises that each of those levels is essential for a human being.

The following sections provide an overview of the different levels, showing that Ramsdell's classification is still up to date and relevant. In particular, the distinction of the different levels substantiates what it means to live with hearing difficulties.

The symbolic level

The first level of hearing as described by Ramsdell is the *symbolic level*, which refers to language. As mentioned in the previous section, it is the level that most people

Table 5.1 Ramsdell's (1947) classification of hearing into three basic levels according to the level of meaning and relatedness to the environment provided by each.

Level	Type
Symbolic	Speech, Language
Signal	Warning signals
Primitive	Connectedness to the world

associate with hearing impairment. The majority of people with hearing problems would indeed confirm that difficulties in following conversations are notorious and common, as are difficulties following the radio and television (Stephens *et al.*, 1990b; Kramer *et al.*, 1998). The vast majority of studies on the impact of hearing impairment using self-report outcome measures rely heavily on the self-reported ability to understand speech (Bentler and Kramer, 2000). Similarly, performance measures focusing on the intelligibility of speech are increasingly common in the laboratory and clinical practice, even though the pure tone audiogram still serves as the gold standard. Tests measuring the intelligibility of speech have been developed over the years to ensure that performance tests would represent the daily life situation.

Sentence tests
Well-known performance tests assessing the comprehension of sentences that are auditorily presented in quiet or against a background of noise are the Speech Perception in Noise (SPIN) test (Kalikow *et al.*, 1977; Bilger *et al.*, 1984), the Connected Speech Test (CST) (Cox *et al.*, 1987), the Bamford–Kowal–Bench (BKB) sentence test (Bench and Bamford, 1979), the Hearing in Noise test (HINT) (Nilsson *et al.*, 1994) and the Speech Reception Threshold (SRT) test (Plomp and Mimpen, 1979a). The last forms the basis of a National Hearing Screening test by telephone and over the Internet (Smits *et al.*, 2004) which is now implemented in a number of European countries.

Earlier in this chapter, we described the conceptual ecological framework of Borg (2003), which identifies the internal preferendum, referring to a person's auditory communicative ability. As portrayed, two of the factors in that preferendum determining a person's auditory communicative ability were (a) the quality of the peripheral bottom-up auditory processing and (b) the individual's top-down cognitive capacities (mental resources).

Bottom-up versus top-down processing
Bottom-up peripheral auditory processes refers to the coding of the acoustical signal in the peripheral auditory system and the subsequent transfer and processing through the central auditory system to the auditory cortex. The quality of bottom-up peripheral auditory processes depends on the accuracy in the coding and transfer of the acoustic signals and is based on elementary perceptual features, such as loudness, pitch and timbre.

Borg's (2003) assumption that both bottom-up peripheral auditory and top-down cognitive processes are involved in speech comprehension is in line with a rapidly increasing number of studies on the involvement of top-down cognitive processes in speech comprehension (Humes and Christopherson, 1991; Pichora-Fuller *et al.*, 1995;

Wingfield, 1996; Rönnberg, 2003; Pichora-Fuller and Singh, 2006; Houtgast and Festen, 2008). The relevance of cognitive processes depends on the listening demands. When listening conditions are adverse because of interfering noise or reverberation, or a reduced quality of the auditory signal owing to hearing impairment, the need for effortful top-down processes during speech comprehension increases (Pichora-Fuller *et al.*, 1995; Schneider *et al.*, 2002; Rönnberg, 2003; Rönnberg *et al.*, 2008).

The most relevant cognitive functions associated with speech communication are:

- the speed of information processing
- working memory
- attention
- the ability to use linguistic context.

The speed of information processing has been extensively studied by presenting time-compressed recorded speech to young and older listeners (Wingfield, 1996). The speed of processing declines with increasing age, which has an adverse effect on speech comprehension in difficult conditions, especially when there is little contextual support (Pichora-Fuller and Souza, 2003).

Working memory comprises a system for the temporary storage and manipulation of information (Baddeley, 1998). It is the ability to simultaneously process and manipulate information in memory. There is ample evidence that working memory is associated with speech comprehension, in particular in adverse listening conditions (Daneman and Carpenter, 1980; Daneman and Merikle, 1996; Rönnberg, 2003; Rönnberg *et al.*, 2008). In order to integrate successively heard words, phrases and sentences into a coherent representation, listeners must have access to the results of earlier processes (Pichora-Fuller *et al.*, 1995). Working memory during speech comprehension is such that when resources are allocated to improve the comprehension of the speech information fewer resources are available for manipulating the auditory information and storing it in long-term memory (Pichora-Fuller *et al.*, 1995, Pichora-Fuller, 2003b).

The working memory framework for the Ease of Language Understanding (ELU) model, as developed by Rönnberg (2003), demonstrates that speech understanding requires more mental effort (or explicit cognitive resources) when speech input cannot be easily matched to memory representations of language (Rönnberg *et al.*, 2008). That may be the case when the speech signal is masked by background noise (George *et al.*, 2007; Rudner *et al.*, 2008). In an optimum listening situation, the speech signal is processed effortlessly and automatically. It means that the cognitive processing involved is largely unconscious and thus implicit.

A range of working memory tests is available. For an overview of tests often used in the field of audiology, we refer the reader to Akeroyd (2008), who concludes that the Reading Span test is probably the most effective in explaining interindividual differences in speech comprehension ability.

The role of attention in speech communication is important. Three types of attention are distinguished (Pichora-Fuller and Singh, 2006):

1. Vigilance and *sustained attention* are required when maintaining awareness during listening over a longer period.
2. *Selective attention* is required when listening to a person in a noisy environment. While listening to the speaker, attention needs to be directed to the speaking person, whereas attention to the surrounding noises needs to be inhibited.

3. The third type is *divided attention*. This is illustrated by the example of having a conversation while engaged in another task, such as walking or driving a car. Rakerd *et al.* (1996) found that when people with hearing impairment performed two tasks simultaneously speech listening was extraordinarily effortful.

Finally, speech comprehension is influenced by the ability to make use of linguistic context. For example, if the last word of the sentence 'Yesterday, I drove my own *car*' is incomprehensible because of background noise or a hearing loss, most people will be able to guess the correct word based on the first part of the sentence and the topic of the conversation. Individuals who are better able to use the linguistic context to fill in the gaps in the auditory information will be better able to communicate with others despite a hearing loss or the presence of background noise (Wingfield, 1996; Schneider *et al.*, 2002; Rönnberg, 2003). Usually, high- and low-context sentences are used to manipulate the availability of context in the speech and to investigate its influence on speech comprehension. Evidence suggests that older individuals are better able to use linguistic context when available than younger individuals are (Speranza *et al.*, 2000).

Unravelling auditory and non-auditory influences in speech communication

The examination of the separate contribution of auditory-specific (bottom-up) and cognitive (top-down) factors in speech comprehension, and their interaction (Rönnberg *et al.*, 2008), is relevant for both research and clinical purposes.

One means of unravelling the auditory and cognitive processes in speech communication or hearing in general is to perform parallel testing. That is to apply similar tests in different sensory domains, such as the auditory domain (listening) and the visual domain (reading text) (McFarland and Cacace, 1995). One could then search for non-auditory central factors in hearing and speech comprehension by investigating the correlations between the parallel tests. If performance on both the visual and the auditory test is totally dependent on peripheral bottom-up sensory processing, then no associations between the two should be expected. But, if similar modality-specific processes are involved in both tasks, then an overlap, and thus a certain share in variance in scores of listeners, would be expected. For both speech and text comprehension, top-down functions improving the comprehension of verbal information become more relevant when the amount or quality of the information is reduced (Grant *et al.*, 1998). It is likely that the cognitive abilities relevant for compensating difficulties in speech and text comprehension partly overlap (e.g., Humes *et al.*, 2007; Zekveld *et al.*, 2007a; Kramer *et al.*, 2009).

Watson *et al.* (1996) explored parallel testing in speech comprehension. They found evidence for the existence of a non-specific cognitive source of variance in speech recognition among normally hearing college students. Using a visual Fragmented Sentences Test (FST; sentences with portions erased) and auditory parallel tests, the correlation coefficients between the composite auditory scores and the non-auditory visual FST test were significant and varied from 0.30 to 0.44. These results imply a modality-aspecific, cognitive source of variance in speech recognition among college students with normal hearing.

Humes *et al.* (2007) also applied parallel tests in the visual and auditory domains. The objective of their study was to discern whether presumed central auditory processing deficits are not simply consequences of deficits in the auditory periphery, cognitive processing or both. Young and older people with normal hearing as well as older people with hearing impairment participated in their study. Auditory and visual versions of the SPIN test and the auditory speeded-spelling test using word lists were presented. When baseline levels of performance were taken into account, any significant group differences in the comprehension of high-context sentences disappeared. In other words, group differences in the ability to use linguistic context were not found. However, even when controlling for auditory and visual peripheral functioning, the older people groups (normally hearing and hearing impaired) performed worse than the young participants did on the auditory speeded-spelling task and the auditory speech recognition test for time-compressed syllables. Furthermore, significant associations of performance on similar tasks across modalities (visual and auditory) and within modalities were found. Humes *et al.* (2007) conclude that performance on the speech tasks was mediated by common underlying modality-aspecific abilities (e.g. the ability to reconstruct the whole from its degraded fragments) as well as modality-specific abilities.

The widely used Reading and Listening Span tests as described by Daneman and Carpenter (1980) are also parallel visual and auditory tests. These complex verbal working-memory tests examine the ability to process and store linguistic information. Pichora-Fuller *et al.* (1995) used those tests in groups of young and older listeners. Their results seemed to give evidence for a processing model in which resources that can be reallocated can be used to improve auditory processing when listening becomes difficult either because of noise or because of age-related degradation of the auditory system. Because of this reallocation, these resources are unavailable to more top-down cognitive processes such as the storage and retrieval functions of working memory, so that the bottom-up processing of auditory information is adversely affected.

Further research on analogous tests in the auditory and visual domain was conducted by Zekveld *et al.* (2007a). They developed a visual analogue of the auditory SRT in noise test (Plomp and Mimpen, 1979a, 1979b). The visual analogue of the auditory test uses everyday short Dutch sentences similar to those of the SRT test. The sentences, masked by a bar pattern, are presented on a computer screen (Figure 5.2).

The procedure of the test is identical to that of the SRT test and the percentage of unmasked text is varied according to an adaptive procedure. The sentences are presented word by word and the presentation rate is equal to the presentation rate of the words in the auditory SRT test. The score on the visual equivalent is defined as the Text Reception Threshold (TRT) (i.e. the threshold at which 50% of the sentences can be read and reproduced correctly).

Using the TRT test, two experiments were run, the first among listeners with normal hearing (Zekveld *et al.*, 2007a) and the second among listeners, some of whom had normal hearing and some with hearing impairment (George *et al.*, 2007). Both studies demonstrated significant associations between the auditorily presented SRT test and the visually presented parallel task. This finding was confirmed in a secondary data analysis (Kramer *et al.*, 2009). About 30% of the interindividual variance in SRT scores was shared with variance in TRT performances. Furthermore, the visual parallel test appeared to contribute significantly in the equation developed to predict SRT scores among listeners with hearing impairment. Thus, again, evidence was found for a non-auditory modality-aspecific component involved in listening to speech in noise.

Clinical relevance

The disentanglement of the auditory and non-auditory cognitive or linguistic processes and the relationship of each to speech comprehension may be relevant for both

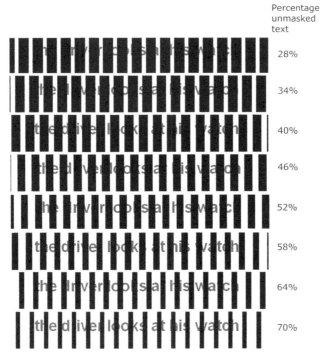

Percentage
unmasked
text

28%

34%

40%

46%

52%

58%

64%

70%

Figure 5.2 The visual analogue of the Speech Reception Threshold in noise test. (*Source:* from Zekveld *et al.*, 2007a. Reproduced by permission of the American Speech-Language-Hearing Association (ASHA).)

research and clinical purposes. Patients with hearing impairment may want and need to know the origin of their communication difficulties. Once the contribution of the different factors to an individual's hearing problem can be unravelled, the tailoring of audiological enablement programmes becomes possible.

Some examples of interesting studies in this respect are those of Gatehouse *et al.* (2006a, 2006b). In a group of 50 clinic patients using hearing aids, listening effort, satisfaction and reported speech intelligibility in two different conditions were investigated. The two conditions differed in the fitting strategies used in the hearing aids. The first profile was a slow-acting automatic volume control; the second strategy was a fast-acting wide dynamic range compression. As well as assessing benefit on each of the three outcomes measured, the investigators also related the benefit to other variables such as lifestyle and the individual's cognitive capacities. The results showed that listeners with greater cognitive capacity derived greater benefit from the fast-acting compression than the slow-acting volume control. The reverse was observed for those with lesser cognitive capacities.

Additionally, reports of auditory lifestyles and measures of the acoustical variability of listeners' environments showed that greater benefits from the slow-acting (linear) fittings were associated with less varied lifestyles and environments, whereas the opposite was the case for fast-acting wide dynamic range compression fittings. The study revealed that patterns of candidature for hearing aids include measures beyond auditory function in the domain of cognitive capacity and auditory ecology. Similar findings are also reported by Lunner (2003).

The results of these studies clearly indicate that an appreciation of the diverse dimensions of hearing aid benefit, and the importance of auditory, ecological and cognitive influences on outcome, is required for the comprehensive assessment of technological and fitting features. This finding will apply to both research and clinical practice settings and needs to be implemented in audiological enablement programmes.

Consequences of impaired speech communication

Alterations in the ability to communicate on the symbolic level owing to acquired hearing impairment inevitably affects life in an encompassing way. Frequently observed psychosocial effects of impaired communication are isolation, withdrawal, loneliness and depression. These effects are described by Ramsdell (1947). Extensive reviews of the consequences for different populations, such as children, working-age adults and older people are given in Stephens and Jones (2005). The consequences vary from changes in interpersonal interactions and relationships, including family life and social relationships to changes in leisure activities, working and community life as well as education. These issues are further elaborated on throughout the following chapters. A consideration of strategies to 'repair' communication breakdowns is included in Chapter 12.

The signal level

The second level of hearing as distinguished by Ramsdell (1947) is that of *signs or warning signals* requiring conscious awareness, serving to alert the individual. There is growing interest in this level of hearing despite the fact that speech and verbal communication have long been considered the most important domains in hearing and hearing impairment.

Eriksson-Mangold and Erlandsson (1984) were among the first to describe the psychological importance attached to categories of sounds other than speech. In the early 1980s, they performed a study on how hearing impairment would affect sound perception. A hearing deficiency was induced by means of occlusion of the ears of 28 normally hearing subjects. The authors observed that the misinterpretation of movements of other people and the inability to hear produced tension and stress, leading to feelings of insecurity and loss of control of the situation.

More recently, the work of Bregman (2004) has contributed uniquely to the rapidly expanding field of hearing complex auditory environments. Bregman investigated how the human auditory system analyses mixtures of overlapping sounds in order to extract descriptions of the individual sound components and to hear the individual sound sources. This process is called *auditory scene analysis*. Such analysis is used continuously by listeners to keep connected to what is happening in the world around them.

Other terminology that refers to the same phenomenon, and which is frequently used within this context is *auditory streaming, segregation of sounds* or *spatial segregation*. The capacity to separate and group sound components into auditory objects enables an individual to focus attention on a single sound source. People with hearing impairment have difficulty performing auditory scene analysis, which consequently affects their ability to focus attention on a warning signal in a noisy environment, a talker in a crowded restaurant or the sound of an approaching car in a busy street (Edwards, 2007).

Gatehouse and Noble (2004) were inspired by the work of Bregman and developed the Speech, Spatial and Qualities of Hearing Scale (SSQ). The SSQ focuses on the reality of hearing in the everyday dynamic and demanding world. It measures a range of hearing abilities across several domains, such as hearing in competing contexts, the ability to segregate sounds and to attend to simultaneous speech streams, spatial hearing (directionality, distance, movement) and qualities of hearing (ease of listening and naturalness, clarity and identifiability of speech and sounds). In their study, they compared SSQ scores of 153 clinic patients with an independent measure of 'handicap' covering distress and related emotional effects. It was found that the disability–handicap relationship was mainly governed by 'identification of sounds', 'attention' and 'effort problems'. The authors emphasise that 'in real contexts, listeners must continuously locate, identify, attend to and switch attention between signals, so as to maintain communicative competence and a sense of connection with their surroundings' (Gatehouse and Noble, 2004).

It may be argued that some of the aspects highlighted by the SSQ have received attention in earlier studies and in audiological enablement in the past. For example, the issue of localising sounds and the adverse effects of asymmetrical hearing losses on this ability have long been studied (e.g. Noble and Atherley, 1970a, 1970b; Noble et al., 1994; Stephens et al., 2001). However, Gatehouse and Noble (2004) justifiably argue that, with a few exceptions (e.g. Hétu et al., 1994), traditional research in audiology predominantly focused on speech hearing alone, whereas the other functions of hearing as served by the auditory system have not always been regarded as equally important.

Similar conclusions were drawn by Kramer et al. (2006c). In their study, the occupational performance of a group of 151 employees with hearing loss was compared to that of a matched group of 60 workers with normal hearing. Workers with hearing impairment reported experiencing mental distress, fatigue and strain leading to sick leave significantly more often than those with normal hearing. The need to continuously distinguish between and identify sounds at work rather than the need to converse in a noisy environment appeared to be the most important factor in the regression model predicting sick leave due to mental distress.

Focus groups among workers with self-reported hearing loss and occupational noise exposure conducted by Morata et al. (2005) revealed similar findings. The employees' primary concerns were about job safety as the result of a reduced ability to hear environmental sounds and warning signals in a noisy environment. Also, their inability to monitor essential equipment sounds was a concern.

Besides speech communication, the importance of the ability to hear and interpret non-verbal contextual sounds in life and its relationship with distress among those with limited hearing has been demonstrated. To live with hearing loss, the second level of hearing, as distinguished by Ramsdell (1947), is more important than has long been assumed. Fortunately, awareness of these aspects of hearing is emerging (Edwards, 2007). There is no longer a consensus that the consequences of hearing impairment should be assessed solely in terms of the effects of hearing impairment on speech communication, rather than on the hearing of non-speech sounds.

The primitive level

The third level described by Ramsdell (1947) is the *primitive* level. It involves the unconscious awareness of background sounds, which gives individuals a sense of self and of being part of their environment. Thus, environmental sounds provide contextual cues that enable individuals to recognise important aspects of their surroundings and stay connected with the world around them. Examples are the tick of a clock, the distant roar of traffic or vague echoes of people moving about in other rooms of the house.

In particular, research in the domain of cochlear implantation shows that the awareness of environmental sounds is of great importance for a person's well-being, both in children and in adults. In studies focusing on the benefits of cochlear implantation, environmental awareness is consistently one of the most frequently reported positive consequences (Tyler and Kelsay, 1990; Kelsay and Tyler, 1996; Zhao *et al.*, 1997; Stephens *et al.*, 2008). In particular, among pre-lingually hearing impaired individuals, the increased awareness of sounds and improved perceptual skills seem to be the main benefits of cochlear implantation, rather than significant improvements in speech recognition abilities (Zwolan *et al.*, 1996).

Among adults in work situations, the enhanced awareness of environmental sounds as a result of cochlear implantation appears to lead to an increased feeling of safety and confidence (Chee *et al.*, 2004).

Qualitative studies revealed that being aware of background sounds is an existential value. Karlsson-Espmark and Hansson-Scherman (2003) conducted open-ended interviews among a group of older people with hearing impairment. Describing their experience of living with hearing loss, the respondents reported that hearing is not only important for verbal communication and spatial orientation, but that it also affirms their existence as a human being. The interviewees reported that 'not until they experienced the lack of sound as a lack of contact with life was there any interest in help in the form of hearing technology'.

Adults who have heard normally and then have lost their hearing not only complain about the loss of hearing but also report that the world around them appears to be quite dead and that life seems to have lost its on-going character. Loss of the primitive level of hearing results in a loss of a very basic and reassuring relatedness to their environment. Smith and Kampfe (1997) point out that misunderstanding environmental sounds generally leads to embarrassment, fear, anxiety and some form of withdrawal and isolation. Moreover, it takes away the ability to enjoy sounds such as music, voices of children, birds, a stream.

In contrast to the results above, Barcham and Stephens (1980) report that the majority of 500 consecutive clinic patients with hearing impairment in their study did not attach much importance to hearing environmental sounds, whereas understanding speech was rated as very important by almost all patients. Apparently, the primitive level of hearing is not perceived as very important, unless this function is restored. People then become more conscious of its importance.

Attitudes of the Deaf

At the end of this chapter, a note must be made about the values of the Deaf world which conflict with the values of the hearing world on the issue of communication and audiological enablement. The Deaf world is a culture with its own (sign) language, customs, values and organisations. Those identifying with Deaf culture regard themselves as being Deaf (Lane and Bahan, 1998). They communicate with sign language, which is a language in its own right. It has a distinct syntax and structure that are different from spoken language. Examples are British Sign Language (BSL) and

American Sign Language (ASL), which are dissimilar from Sign Supported Languages. Deaf people obtain information primarily through vision and they rely on vision rather than on hearing. As a consequence, Deaf people reject the suggestion that they have an impairment or a disability and they strongly criticise any means to restore levels of hearing. More extreme members of the Deaf community see all oralism, mainstreaming, cochlear implants and genetic counselling as potential threats to their community (Austin and Coleman, 2004). Whereas people with disabilities may seek medical care or audiological enablement services, culturally Deaf people rarely attach any importance to those services (Lane and Bahan, 1998; Middleton *et al.*, 1998).

An exception to this generalisation may occur when Deaf people find themselves in a situation in which they want to use and enhance any aural skills that they may have. Examples of this are when a Deaf couple have hearing children whose speech development they want to encourage, or if a Deaf person has a change in their job which necessitates the use of some speech communication.

A different situation may occur in some people with Usher I syndrome, who have a profound pre-lingual hearing loss and identify with the Deaf community. However, when their vision deteriorates markedly with the development of retinitis pigmentosa, they may seek help in the form of a cochlear implant. They are generally aware that implantation at such a late stage (teens to twenties) will not give them speech recognition, but are keen to have help in order to have environmental awareness and alerting to warning sounds. Implants must be considered seriously in such circumstances.

Conclusion

Communication is a key area that is affected by hearing impairment. Both bottom-up peripheral auditory and top-down cognitive processes are involved in speech comprehension. Examples of top-down processes are the speed of information processing, working memory, attention and the ability to use linguistic context. One means of unravelling the auditory and cognitive processes in speech communication or hearing in general is to perform parallel testing, that is to apply similar tests in different sensory domains, such as the auditory domain (listening) and the visual domain (reading text). An example of a visual analogue of the auditory Speech Reception Threshold (SRT) in noise test is the Text Reception Threshold (TRT) test. Whereas communication is often regarded as the most important area that is affected by hearing impairment, Ramsdell (1947) argues that the loss of hearing at any of the three hierarchical levels of hearing he identifies may have a considerable impact on human functioning. These levels are: the symbolic level (speech, language), the signal level (warning signals) and the primitive level (connectedness to the world). Several studies demonstrated the specific consequences of hearing impairment at any of these levels and these have been described in this chapter.

6 Social and emotional aspects of hearing impairment

Introduction

Hearing impairment may have a wide range of consequences for an individual and his or her personal surroundings. A large body of studies on the psychosocial effects of hearing impairment is available. Mainly negative effects have been found, but positive consequences have also been reported. This chapter provides definitions of the various concepts and gives an overview of the possible effects of hearing impairment.

Participation in life

When defining a person's involvement in life situations, the World Health Organization (WHO) distinguishes nine areas of participation:

a. learning and applying knowledge
b. general tasks and demands
c. communication
d. mobility
e. self-care
f. domestic life
g. interpersonal interactions and relationships
h. major life areas
i. community, social and civic life.

Participation restriction is defined as the problems a person may experience in involvement in life situations (WHO, 2001).

Hearing impairment may impact on people's lives in profound and all-encompassing ways. It means that any of the areas as defined by the WHO may be affected to a certain degree.

Domains that are most likely to be influenced are those mentioned under (c) communication, (g) interpersonal interactions and relationships, (h) major life areas and community and (i) social and civic life. Nonetheless, aspects of physical or behavioural functioning (e.g. mobility, body care and movement) have also been found to be influenced by hearing impairment (Bess *et al.*, 1989; Chia *et al.*, 2007), in particular among those with severe levels of hearing impairment. To illustrate this, a number of population-based studies have shown that individuals with severe levels of hearing impairment were more likely than individuals without hearing impairment to have reduced performance of activities of daily living (ADL), such as maintaining body position, personal grooming, dressing, eating and getting in and out of bed. Similarly, controlling for age, gender, educational level and comorbidity, greater difficulties with instrumental activities of daily living (IADL; pulling or pushing large objects, lifting or carrying weights, preparing meals, doing light and heavy housework and doing laundry) were found to be related to hearing impairment (Carabellese et al., 1993; Cacciatore et al., 1999; Strawbridge et al., 2000; Dalton et al., 2003). Likewise, using the results of the Cardiff Health Survey among 3129 people over 60 years of age, Stephens et al. (1991d) observed that the older (70+) female participants with hearing impairment were more physically disabled than the non-hearing disabled population.

In addition, the increased risk for falling among frail elderly people with hearing impairment has also been reported (Bumin et al., 2002), and is most probably due to balance problems arising from the same pathology as the hearing problems.

There is thus some evidence that even the domains (4) mobility, (5) self-care and (6) domestic life may be influenced by auditory difficulties. It remains to be investigated whether the relationship between these two is direct or indirect. For example, a mood disorder such as depression may act as a go-between for hearing impairment and reduced physical performance. Also, it must be added that conflicting results have been reported. Using generic measures of quality of life, including physical performance scales, Mulrow et al. (1990), Parving et al. (1997) and Bess (2000) were not able to demonstrate significant associations.

Nevertheless, there is little doubt that areas in which psychosocial problems are most likely experienced are those requiring communication in interaction with other people. In addition, as described in Chapter 5, misunderstanding environmental sounds may also lead to psychosocial disturbances or dysfunction.

Psychosocial dysfunction

A review of the audiological literature reveals that *psychosocial* is a multidimensional concept, covering a broad range of reactions towards hearing impairment. The variety of reactions may be the reason why the definitions ascribed to 'psychosocial health' differ widely in the literature (Kramer, 2005; Preminger, 2007). This diversity is, in particular, reflected in the outcome measures used to assess 'psychosocial health'. A comprehensive table listing questionnaires dealing with the assessment of psychosocial aspects is provided in a review by Kramer (2005).

In an attempt to classify the different categories of reactions towards hearing impairment, one may distinguish between emotional, cognitive, interpersonal, physiological and behavioural responses (Trychin, 2002; Preminger, 2007). It is assumed that a combination of the various responses determine a person's overall psychosocial health status. The category *behavioural reactions* includes limitations of daily activities or reduced physical performance, such as those described in the previous section, and the relationship between these and hearing impairment has been described there. Each of the remaining categories will be considered separately in the following sections.

Emotional reactions

Losing your hearing as an adult is, in most cases, a gradual process that pervasively impacts on a person's emotions (Jones *et al.*, 1987). Patients' reactions to hearing impairment consistently include feelings of frustration, anger, annoyance, fear, anxiety, loss of control, mood changes, low self-worth and embarrassment (Heine and Browning, 2002). Distrust may occur when it is felt that people talk about the person with hearing impairment rather than with him or her (Smith and Kampfe, 1997). Some people blame themselves for having a hearing impairment and experience feelings of inferiority, guilt and shame. This may happen in situations where the wrong answer is given as a result of having misunderstood the question. The fear of being stigmatised as deviant from normal is strong and frequently felt (Hétu, 1996).

Persistent negative emotional reactions and lack of confidence generally go along with downhearted feelings and may finally result in isolation and depression. An essential feature of depression is the loss of interest in life activities. Self-report outcome tools measuring depression include questions like 'During the past week, did you feel that everything was meaningless?' Most studies report significant associations between hearing impairment and depression (Carabellese *et al.*, 1993; Cacciatore *et al.*, 1999; Tambs, 2004; Fellinger *et al.*, 2007, Nachtegaal *et al.*, 2009a), although Mulrow *et al.* (1990) failed to find such a relationship. It should be noted that, while there is a significant association, one cannot consider every person with hearing impairment as being depressed. Group mean scores in those studies often fall within the normal range, despite a wide distribution of scores, with many participants in the normal range and many with clinically deviant scores. A significant association means that with every step in the reduction of hearing (the definition of a step differs per study), the risk for developing depression increases to a certain extent.

Positive emotional reactions towards hearing impairment may also occur. Kerr and Stephens (1997) administered an open-ended questionnaire to consecutive patients of an audiological rehabilitation clinic. In the initial sample of 125 consecutive patients, 27 (21.6%) reported one or more positive experiences. The authors finally created a sample of 79 subjects who reported positive aspects to their hearing impairment and analysed their comments. Even though most of the reactions fell into the category 'reduced disturbance from unwanted sounds', a number of reactions emphasised self-appraisal and the use of individual resources to cope with the hearing impairment as potentially beneficial. Examples of such reactions are self-development, self-reliance, positive self-image and affinity to other Deaf people or other people with hearing impairment.

Cognitive reactions

In general, the term *cognition* refers to the processing of information by a human being. It is a dynamic process which comprises implementing new approaches, developing new problem-solving skills, gaining information, changing and adding routines and making adjustments. Each of those elements seems to play an important role in the process of adjusting to acquired hearing impairment. Herth (1998) interviewed 32 adults with acquired hearing impairment and found that integrating hearing loss into one's life requires constant learning of how to adapt to changes. Adjusting to acquired hearing impairment is a cognitively demanding process, in particular for those people with limited hearing who are actively involved in life.

While the degree of hearing impairment increases with age, cognitive functioning (i.e. working memory and processing speed) evidently decreases with age (Wingfield, 1996; Pichora-Fuller, 2003a, 2003b). Controlling for age, various quantitative studies have found a relationship between hearing impairment and reduced cognitive functioning. Thus, using the Mini-Mental State Examination (MMSE) as a measure of cognitive status, Cacciatore *et al.* (1999) found an adverse relationship between hearing impairment and cognitive functioning. Other studies using the same outcome measure have confirmed those findings (Naramura *et al.*, 1999; Bazargan *et al.*, 2001). Lindenberger and Baltes (1994) measured five cognitive abilities (speed, reasoning, knowledge, memory and fluency) in a group of 156 (very) old individuals (mean age = 84 years). They found strong associations between sensory functioning (vision and hearing) and cognitive functioning. Van Boxtel *et al.* (2000) report a relationship between mild-to-moderate levels of hearing impairment and verbal memory performance. In a study group of 1191 older people (70–75 years), Carabellese *et al.* (1993) found an independent association between hearing and cognition only among those with double sensory dysfunction (vision and hearing), but not among those with hearing impairment alone.

The tests of cognitive functioning applied in the studies above were all verbally administered. The question arises as to whether the individuals with hearing impairment performed less well on the cognitive tasks because they did not hear the questions adequately. For example, Thomas *et al.* (1983) found a significant relationship between hearing acuity and cognitive functioning when analysing the scores on the verbally administered Jacobs' Cognitive Screening Exam (Jacobs *et al.*, 1977) in a group of 259 older individuals. This association was not seen for the Halstead Category test, a non-verbal test of cognition, which was administered to the same group of people. In agreement with these findings, Zekveld *et al.* (2007b) failed to find a significant association between hearing impairment and cognitive functioning when using non-verbal visually presented cognitive tasks. Furthermore, participants with severe levels of hearing impairment even performed better on a spatial working memory subtest than those with milder levels of hearing impairment did.

In contrast to the argument above, Lindenberger and colleagues, in their later study (2001), explicitly examined the possibility of assessment-related sensory acuity accounting for the age-related increase in the association between sensory and cognitive functioning. They manipulated hearing and visual acuity in middle-aged adults and administered cognitive tests. The performance of this group in the simulated conditions was compared to a control group tested under normal circumstances. The results did not support an assessment-related age effect and the authors claim that the often reported independent relationship between sensory decline and reduced cognitive functioning holds and should be ascribed to the general brain ageing processes.

The role of cognition in hearing, in particular in the comprehension of speech, is further explored in Chapter 5 of this book.

Interpersonal interactions and relationships

Maintaining interpersonal and social relationships is about carrying out the actions and tasks required for basic and complex interactions with people (strangers, friends, relatives, family members and lovers) in a contextually and socially appropriate manner (WHO, 2001). Even though communication may occur non-verbally (as in a virtual community), verbal communication is still the essential basis for maintaining interpersonal and social relationships.

Hearing impairment inevitably hinders communication with others and thereby affects the quality and frequency of interpersonal and social relationships. Even when a certain level of interpersonal and social interaction is maintained, the type and quality of the conversation may be altered owing to strategies on the part of the person with hearing impairment (Jones et al., 1987). For example, one may interrupt, take over and dominate the conversation in order not to need to listen.

Such alterations in interpersonal interactions may carry over into every human relationship. For example, intimate contacts within couples may change owing to irritation (Hallberg, 1996) or less frequent intimate and personal talks (Jones et al., 1987). Within the family, the dynamics may change as a result of misunderstandings, misconception, the need to repeat, changes in family roles and independent functioning (the spouse becoming the caregiver) (Smith and Kampfe, 1997). The impact of hearing impairment on significant others is further elaborated on in Chapter 7.

Number of friends

The number of friends a person with hearing impairment has may be reduced as well. In a study by Gilhome Herbst (1983), older people with hearing impairment reported having fewer friends than in the past, whereas the normally hearing controls in that study did not report such a situation. Similarly, the social network size, defined as the number of people with whom an important and regular relationship is maintained, has been found to be smaller among people with hearing impairment compared to that of their normally hearing peers (Kramer et al., 2002).

Withdrawal

Withdrawal from social life is a regularly observed, notorious phenomenon among people with hearing impairment. Various studies have reported on this issue. Compared with normally hearing adults of the same age, individuals with hearing difficulties seem to be less active in exploring their free time and enjoying it (Strawbridge et al., 2000; Wallhagen et al., 1996). Owing to embarrassment and fear, they may not feel competent to engage in social and civic life (Aguayo and Cody, 2001) and are less likely to go out without being accompanied by another person (Gilhome Herbst, 1983). Using the Hearing Handicap Inventory for the Elderly (HHIE) as an outcome measure, Newman et al. (1997), as well as Mulrow et al. (1990), found that people with auditory difficulties are less active when it comes to 'shopping', 'attending services' and 'meeting new people'. In other words, hearing impairment results in an impoverished social life. A participant in a study reported by Rutman and Boisseau (1995) gave a succinct illustration: 'Noisy places become hostile zones and social withdrawal seems to be the ultimate choice.'

Loneliness

Social withdrawal, a reduced number of friends and alterations in the interpersonal contacts easily turn into loneliness. Loneliness is defined as the discrepancy between what one desires in terms of interpersonal affection and intimacy and what one actually experiences; the greater the discrepancy, the greater the loneliness (de Jong Gierveld, 1987). The most common factors predicting loneliness are gender, living arrangement and marital status. In general, females have a higher risk of developing loneliness than males do. Those living alone suffer more from loneliness than those living with others and being separated, divorced or widowed enhances the risk of loneliness (Savikko *et al.*, 2005; De Jong Gierveld, 1987). Controlling for those factors, hearing impairment consistently emerges as a predictor in studies focusing on the determinants of social isolation and loneliness in the general population (Strawbridge *et al.*, 2000; Kramer *et al.*, 2002; Hawthorne, 2008). Knutson and Lansing (1990) observed extreme levels of loneliness among people with profound hearing impairment who were candidates for cochlear implantation.

Physiological reactions

Examples of physiological reactions towards hearing disabilities are distress, anxiety and somatisation. *Distress* refers to the 'direct manifestation of the effort people must exert to maintain their psychosocial homeostasis and social functioning when confronted with stress' (Terluin *et al.*, 2006). Symptoms are worry, tension and poor concentration. Mild distress can be considered part of normal life. However, severe distress forces a person to give up major social roles, such as their occupation.

Distress is closely related to *anxiety*. Symptoms of anxiety are irrational fear, muscle tension, sleep disturbance and avoidance behaviour.

Increased effort, tension, anxiety and distress are common phenomena among individuals with hearing impairment (Tambs, 2004; Hallam *et al.*, 2006) and they may be assumed to be among the most disturbing complaints. Communication in challenging listening situations, such as in background noise or in reverberation, but also the inability to identify contextual sounds and insecurity in social settings often lead to distress and auditory fatigue (Knutson and Lansing, 1990; Eriksson-Mangold and Carlsson, 1991; Kramer *et al.*, 2006c). Symptoms such as insomnia and muscle tension in the neck have also been found to be related to hearing impairment, in particular among those with high-stress work (Werngren-Elgström *et al.*, 2003; Danermark and Coniavitis Gellerstedt, 2004). It must, however, be noted here that the majority of studies in audiology dealing with symptoms such as stress, insomnia and other types of physiological reactions primarily focus on tinnitus.

Distress and strain are due to the cost of adapting to the auditory disability and arise when trying to cope with the hearing impairment. Demorest and Erdman (1986) express it accurately: 'the individual's attempts to compensate and to communicate optimally require vigilance: a constant effort to hear, to pay attention and to respond properly.'

As auditory fatigue and distress mostly result from compensatory efforts, they ought to be considered as *indirect* consequences of hearing impairment rather than as *direct* effects. Hétu *et al.* (1988) introduced the term *secondary handicap* to describe that phenomenon in his framework for understanding the psychosocial effects of hearing impairment. Subsequently, Stephens and Hétu (1991) proposed an extension of the WHO *International Classification of Impairments, Disabilities and Handicaps* (ICIDH) classification (WHO, 1980) to include these levels of participation restriction. This concept was further elaborated on by Stephens and Kerr (1996), but was ultimately superseded by the WHO developments of ICIDH at that time, which led to the publication of *International Classification of Functioning, Disability and Health* (ICF; WHO, 2001). However, although the model included in ICF has two-way interactions and the role of contextual factors, the concept of primary and secondary handicap is not clearly spelt out.

It is assumed that when explicit cognitive processing, as discussed in Chapter 5, is required to understand speech, listening requires more effort. Several studies have indeed shown that individuals with hearing impairment rate adverse listening situations as more effortful than their normally hearing peers (Hällgren *et al.*, 2005; Larsby *et al.*, 2005) and that effort features prominently in the experience of participation restriction (Gatehouse and Noble, 2004).

Physiological and behavioural measures

Most of the research on effort, distress and anxiety in relation to hearing impairment has used self-report outcomes to measure the effort allocated to listening tasks. Only a few studies attempted to measure listening effort directly and objectively by means of physiological measures. An example is a study by Kramer *et al.* (1997). They used pupil dilatation as a measure of processing load. The diameter of the pupil directly reflects the activity of the autonomous nervous system. As such, it can be used to measure the arousal level in an individual. Changes in pupillary diameter have been shown to reflect the level of arousal in response to task demands (Janisse, 1977). Pupillary dilatation increases systematically with processing load in multiple domains of cognitive functioning including hearing (Kahneman and Beatty, 1966; Hoeks, 1995). Kramer *et al.* (1997) demonstrate the relationship between pupil dilatation and speech comprehension difficulties using sentences. They observed that hearing impaired individuals have a smaller reduction in the allocated effort in easier listening conditions compared with normally hearing participants. The poorer the ability to comprehend speech in noise, the less benefit was obtained from more favourable listening conditions. The authors concluded that pupillometry offers the opportunity to measure consequences of hearing impairment that are not easily assessed with traditional audiometric or psychoacoustical measures. Their findings encourage further study in the domain of physiological consequences of hearing impairment. Much can be learnt from the literature on the physiological stress response (stress hormones) in patients with Menière's disorder (Van Cruijsen *et al.*, 2005).

Another index of effort required to understand a message is the *response time*. It is the time elapse between the occurrence of a message and the initiation of a response to it by a listener. Gatehouse and Gordon (1990) applied response times to assess the benefit of amplification in adults with hearing impairment. Single words and sentences were presented to 44 experienced hearing aid users, both in aided and in unaided conditions. Participants showed equal performance, in terms of the percentage of correct identification of speech stimuli, in both the aided and unaided condition, but a reduction in response time in the aided condition. Gatehouse and Gordon concluded that the response time as an outcome offers advantages over the traditional performance index (i.e. percentage of correct identification), in particular in conditions where the traditional measures show ceiling effects. However, while they regard the response time as a promising index, they argue that a more controlled paradigm would be desirable. Their work relied upon detecting the verbal response from the participant via the microphone and this is subject to external influences that are difficult to control.

Somatisation

Somatisation is the tendency to experience somatic symptoms in response to psychological stress, to attribute them to physical illness and to seek medical help for them (Lipowski, 1988). Experiencing one or just a few somatic symptoms in the absence of a disease can be considered normal under stressful circumstances. However, the more somatic symptoms a person experiences, the less likely it is that these symptoms reflect the presence of a physical illness and the more likely that they imply somatisation as described above (Mayou and Farmer, 2002). Symptoms of somatisation are nausea, an upset stomach area, headaches and tingling in the fingers. A few studies have addressed the association between hearing problems and somatisation. Controlling for confounding variables, Nachtegaal *et al.* (2009a) found higher levels of somatisation among adults with hearing impairment compared with normally hearing people. Coniavitis Gellerstedt and Danermark (2003) observed more symptoms of somatisation (back pain, stomach problems and headache) among workers with hearing impairment and high-stress jobs compared with hearing impaired workers with less stressful working conditions.

Psychosocial consequences of Deafness

Only a few studies have addressed the psychosocial consequences of Deafness while comparing the health status of Deaf people with those of hearing people. An example is a study by Werngren-Elgström *et al.* (2003), who found a higher prevalence of depressive symptoms and insomnia among pre-lingually Deaf older adults using sign language, compared with their hearing peers. However, no differences were found in their subjective well-being (as measured with the Gothenburg Profile). De Graaf and Bijl (2002) observed a higher prevalence of mental distress (as measured with the General Health Questionnaire) in Deaf people (pre-lingual and post-lingual Deaf people included) compared with the prevalence in the general population. Moreover, the prevalence of distress among Deaf women was significantly higher than among their male peers.

It may be argued that the differences in psychosocial health status between Deaf and hearing people in studies such as those mentioned above were due to inappropriate measurement methods being used. Paper-and-pencil questionnaires were administered, whereas it is known that the average reading level of pre-lingually Deaf people is far below that of the general population (Conrad, 1979; Holt, 1994). This inappropriate method may have resulted in biased findings. Similarly, interviewing techniques may result in biased outcomes owing to the intervening role of a signing interpreter. To avoid any of those inadequacies, an interactive computer-based assessment package for full self-administration was used in a study by Fellinger *et al.* (2005). The program allowed Deaf participants to read test items and to see the items demonstrated to them in sign language simultaneously. The package included three standardised questionnaires: the World Health Organization's Brief Quality of Life questionnaire (WHOQOL-BREF; 26 items), the 12-item General Health Questionnaire (GHQ-12) and five subscales of the Brief Symptom Inventory (BSI). It was administered to 236 adults who identified with the Deaf community. Their scores were compared to those of the general German population. A significantly poorer (general) quality of life and higher levels of emotional distress were observed among the Deaf adults, despite the absence of any difference in the social relationships domain of the WHOQOL-BREF questionnaire. These results support the findings of earlier studies and it seems as if the different methodologies did not have a significant influence on the outcome.

An issue that needs discussion within the context of describing the psychosocial effects of Deafness among pre-lingually Deaf people is the comparison of Deaf people with hearing people. For Deaf people living in a Deaf community, the most meaningful point of reference for mental health is other Deaf people, not hearing people (Griggs, 2004).

This brings us to the difference in psychosocial health of those with congenital or pre-lingual Deafness as opposed to those who became deafened at a later age (post-lingual deafness). For the latter group, deafness may be a much more devastating experience with much more severe psychosocial consequences than those with pre-lingual Deafness. The study of Barlow *et al.* (2007) revealed that adults with post-lingual deafness no longer felt they belonged in the hearing world. Their social network decreased and their isolation increased. Furthermore, they did not belong to the Deaf world either. Thus, late-onset deafness had left them in a twilight zone between worlds and had robbed them of their identity. Barlow *et al.* (2007) emphasise the need for enablement courses providing the opportunity for sharing with others similarly affected, giving post-lingually deafened people a sense of belonging.

Demographic factors

Various factors may influence the way and extent to which hearing impairment is associated with a person's psychosocial health and well-being and their reaction towards hearing impairment. We have mentioned some of these variables briefly in previous sections. The best known are demographic factors such as age, gender and socioeconomic status, but also environmental variables (room acoustics, support) may affect that relationship. Some of the variables and their impact will be addressed below.

Age

People of different age groups are likely to emphasise psychosocial issues differently as their lifestyles, occupational obligations and circumstances, communication needs and listening conditions may differ. However, the vast majority of studies on the relationship between hearing impairment and psychosocial health have included samples of older people, most likely because of a higher prevalence of hearing impairment among older adults. Only a small number of quantitative studies in the international literature have focused on younger age groups. Table 6.1 gives an overview.

Tambs (2004) studied a large cohort comprising more than 50 000 subjects aged 20 years and over and found younger (20–44 years) and middle-aged participants (44–65 years) reporting higher levels of anxiety and depression, lower self-esteem and sub-jective well-being compared to normally hearing peers. Moreover, among young and middle-aged adults with hearing impairment, the impact on psychosocial health was larger than among the oldest adults (>65 years of age) with a hearing impairment (Hallam *et al.*, 2006).

In particular, loneliness seems to be an issue in younger age groups. Knutson and Lansing (1990) observed extreme levels of loneliness among young and middle-aged adults with severe hearing impairment, most likely due to limited communication with family and friends. In a study on health and well-being across the lifespan, Hawthorne (2008) showed younger adults to have a higher probability of suffering from loneliness and social isolation than older people. Similar findings are reported by Nachtegaal *et al.* (2009a).

Table 6.1 Overview of the different age groups included in studies on the relationship between hearing impairment and psychosocial health.

Age mean (range)	Psychosocial outcome	Reference
80 (65–94)	Depression	Naramura *et al.* (1999)
77 (70+)	Overall functioning	Lee *et al.* (1999)
74 (65–96)	Depression	Cacciatore *et al.* (1999)
72 (HI) 69 (NH)	Depression	Mulrow *et al.* (1990)
72 (65–95)	Depression	Wallhagen *et al.* (1996)
– (70–75)	Depression	Carabellese *et al.* (1993)
69 (53–97)	Social functioning, mental health	Dalton *et al.* (2003)
68 (55–74)	Depression, anxiety, somatisation	Eriksson-Mangold and Carlsson (1991)
67 (49+)	Health-related QOL	Chia *et al.* (2007)
66	Social isolation, emotional reactions	Ringdahl and Grimby (2000)
65 (50–102)	Depression, social functioning (loneliness)	Strawbridge *et al.* (2000)
– (55–85)	Depression, loneliness, self-efficacy, social network size	Kramer *et al.* (2002)
54; 51 (21–80)	Depression, anxiety, post-traumatic stress	Hallam *et al.* (2006)
50 (20–101)	Depression, anxiety, self-esteem, well-being	Tambs (2004)
49 (22–68)	Depression, loneliness, social anxiety, distress	Knutson and Lansing (1990)
46 (18–70)	Depression, distress, anxiety, somatisation, loneliness, self-efficacy	Nachtegaal *et al.*, (2009a)
– (42–52)	Physical and mental health	Pope and Sowers (2000)

(HI = hearing impaired; NH = normal hearing)

Erdman and Demorest (1998b) mention possible differences in the adjustment to hearing impairment for different age groups in their sample of adults (16–97 years), with adjustment (as measured with the Communication Profile for the Hearing Impaired; CPHI) being poorer among the youngest and oldest individuals.

Gender

Studies specifically focusing on the differences between males and females in the way they are affected psychosocially by hearing impairment are scarce. The most cited study within this respect is that of Garstecki and Erler (1999). Using the CPHI, they found that women with hearing impairment tend to assign greater importance to effective social communication, are more likely to use non-verbal communication strategies and report higher levels of anxiety and stress, greater problem awareness and less denial of hearing problems compared to men with hearing impairment. Similar findings are reported by Erdman and Demorest (1998a, 1998b). Vesterager and Salomon (1991) observed a higher incidence of adverse coping reactions (e.g. pretending to hear and withdrawal from social events) among men compared with women with hearing impairment.

Degree of hearing impairment

Whereas diminished physical function is mainly related to severe levels of hearing impairment, adverse effects on psychosocial functioning have been observed even with mild levels of impairment. Hence, the pure tone audiogram has frequently been found to be a poor predictor of the adverse psychosocial effects resulting from hearing impairment (Kramer *et al.*, 1996; Newman *et al.*, 1997; Pichora-Fuller *et al.*, 1998; Scherer and Frisina, 1998).

Although one may conclude that severe to profound impairment of hearing and speech recognition usually leads to severe psychosocial problems, psychosocial difficulties may be reported even in cases of normal pure tone audiometric thresholds (Zhao and Stephens, 1996b). People belonging to this category experience difficulties understanding speech in background noise, despite a normal audiogram. The phenomenon is called *Obscure auditory dysfunction* (Saunders and Haggard, 1989) and the clinical picture is labelled as the *King-Kopetzky syndrome* (Hinchcliffe, 1992).

Patients with King-Kopetzky syndrome have become recognised as a distinct clinical group in audiology and ENT clinics. It is assumed that about 5–10% of the patients attending those clinics have been shown to have this syndrome (Higson *et al.*, 1994; Stephens *et al.*, 2003b).

Various attempts have been made to identify the underlying cause of the condition (King and Stephens, 1992; Saunders and Haggard, 1992; Zhao and Stephens, 1996a, 2000). And the results of these studies revealed that the King-Kopetzky syndrome is a multifactorial disorder with no single cause. Among the factors contributing to the syndrome are:

1. subclinical cochlear damage (Zhao and Stephens, 1999a)
2. central auditory dysfunction (Ferman *et al.*, 1993; Zhao and Stephens, 1999a)
3. impaired speech-reading skills or audio-visual integration
4. emotional, psychological and work-related problems (e.g. irritability, nervousness and moodiness) (King and Stephens, 1992; Zhao and Stephens, 1996a)
5. difficulties in the use of a second language
6. personality; Saunders and Haggard (1992) report anxiety-related personality traits in a group of people with obscure auditory dysfunction and found that these traits were related to the seeking of medical attention in general (Saunders and Haggard, 1989, 1993)
7. family history (Stephens and Zhao, 2000).

Pryce and Wainwright (2008) argue that the condition comes within the general category of *medically unexplained symptoms* (MUS). In such conditions the patient focuses on a particular mild symptom (e.g. difficulty hearing speech in background noise), and becomes increasingly aware of and consequently exaggerates its effect on their life.

Socioeconomic status

A person's socioeconomic status (as measured by education, occupation and income) may have great influence on a person's health status (Mackenbach *et al.*, 1997). The main issue governing the relationship between low socioeconomic status (low income, substandard education) and poor health is that economic restrictions imply a limited access to health care. Across the range of health care types within the field of audiology, various studies have shown such a relationship. For example, Sixt and Rosenhall (1997) observed and compared groups of older people with hearing impairment from different social classes. Those from higher social classes had better hearing and better access to aural rehabilitation than those of a lower socioeconomic status. Lupsakko *et al.* (2005) found 'low income' to be an explanatory factor for the non-use of hearing aids in Finland. Lee *et al.* (1996) found that adult Hispanics in the United States with incomes above the poverty line were nine times more likely to be using hearing aids compared to their peers below the poverty threshold. The study of Vohr *et al.* (2002) revealed that 'no insurance' predicted no compliance with the completion of in-hospital newborn hearing screening or re-screening (if indicated).

It is thus not surprising that socioeconomic status (and access to health care) affects the way and extent to which a certain health condition affects a person *psychosocially*. For example, Gatehouse (1990) observed educational level (verbal and non-verbal IQ) to contribute to the proportion of variance explaining self-reported hearing disability, those with higher educational levels self-reporting less disability. Similarly, Erdman and Demorest (1998b) found less frequent use of maladaptive behavioural strategies among those with higher levels of education. Nevertheless, Lee *et al.* (1999) report different results. In their study on the association between hearing/vision and well-being, including 7320 older people, socioeconomic status did not emerge as a confounding variable predicting well-being. The authors argue that psychosocial difficulties exist, regardless of economic status.

Incidentally, it must be noted here that among Deaf people, it is not only the limited access to health care per se that results in inequalities in health compared to hearing people (even though higher rates of early retirement and unemployment have been reported among Deaf working age adults (Danermark, 2005)). The main problem that Deaf people face is the lack of awareness by general and mental health staff of how to communicate with them (e.g. Ubido *et al.*, 2002; Austin and Crocker, 2004; Fellinger *et al.*, 2005). Disorders (both mental and physical) that have been misdiagnosed or untreated because of the lack of adequate communication and availability of sign users among specialists and staff workers have frequently been observed in the Deaf community (Austin and Crocker, 2004).

Conclusion

Hearing impairment may impact on people's lives in profound and all-encompassing ways. Psychosocial consequences cover emotional, cognitive, interpersonal, physiological and behavioural aspects. Examples of emotional consequences are anger, frustration and a changed mood. Cognitive effects occur when integrating hearing impairment into one's life requires constant learning of how to adapt to changes. *Interpersonal consequences* refer to changes in intimate contacts and family dynamics, social withdrawal and a reduced social network size. Distress, anxiety, (muscle) tension, somatisation and fatigue are examples of physiological aspects. The category *behavioural reactions* includes limitations of daily activities or reduced physical performance.

All of the above consequences may be labelled *negative* in nature. Positive effects may also occur. Examples are: self-development, self-reliance and an affinity with other people with hearing impairment.

Various factors may influence the association between hearing impairment and psychosocial health. The best known are age, gender, socioeconomic status and the degree of hearing impairment.

The pure tone audiogram has been found to be a poor predictor of the psychosocial consequences of hearing impairment, even though severe to profound levels of impairment usually lead to severe psychosocial problems. Nevertheless, psychosocial difficulties may be reported even in cases of mild impairment or normal pure tone audiometric thresholds. People belonging to this category experience difficulties understanding speech in background noise. Their clinical picture is labelled as the *King-Kopetzky syndrome*.

7 Hearing impairment in the family

Introduction

When considering the title of this chapter, one can think of various issues covered by it. There is the fact that living with hearing difficulties concerns not only the person diagnosed but also the significant other(s) around that person (i.e. spouse, family and friends). The first section of this chapter provides an overview of what the significant other of a person with hearing difficulties may possibly experience.

Another issue relates to the fact that hearing impairment may have a familial basis and arise from genetic causes. The second section of this chapter is concerned with this matter and touches briefly on some relevant aspects.

A third issue concerns the family history of hearing impairment that, by itself, could have an effect on the emotional impact of auditory difficulties. It may also have an effect on other aspects such as help-seeking and role modelling. The final section of this chapter taps into this area and gives an overview of results of relevant studies performed so far.

In each of the three sections, we restrict ourselves to describing effects and phenomena among adults, rather than focusing on children.

Impact of hearing impairment on significant others

Whereas the role and the position of the significant other has often been observed as supportive and as encouraging towards the person with the hearing impairment, the burden of their partner's hearing impairment may certainly affect them as well. The most common complaints reported by significant others (mostly spouses) are the need to repeat, problems with the raised volume of the television and the radio, the need to respond on behalf of their partner and getting no response at all (Hétu *et al.*, 1988; Stephens *et al.*, 1995; Brooks *et al.*, 2001). A qualitative study by Scarinci and colleagues (2008) of 10 couples revealed that the effects of hearing impairment on the (normally hearing) spouse may range widely, varying from communicative difficulties and emotional consequences to having an impact on routine everyday activities. The main effects are summarised in Box 7.1 and the major elements of these are discussed below.

Communicative difficulties

Communicative difficulties often happen when the significant other feels that a conversation cannot be carried on normally, owing to the need to repeat. The outcome

Box 7.1 Main effects of hearing impairment on the spouse.

- Communicative difficulties
- Emotional consequences
- Impact on the relationship
- Impact on social life
- Impact on routine everyday activities

(*Source:* derived from Scarinci *et al.*, 2008.)

is a breakdown in communication or conversational stress (Hallberg and Carlsson, 1991) sometimes leading to communication avoidance. The spouses in Scarinci *et al.*'s (2008) study reported a significant reduction of 'chatting' episodes in their daily communication (the interactive aspects of conversation). Such an alteration seriously affects the type of conversation in a relationship. Another reported difficulty is the lack of opportunity to spontaneously start a conversation when the attention of the person with the hearing impairment has to be attracted first.

Emotional consequences

When conversations break down frequently, communication partners may become angry or frustrated. These emotions may also occur when the spouse feels incapable of fully understanding what it means to live with a hearing impairment. Embarrassment may occur when the partner is concerned with what others may think when they use strategies to support the spouse in their communication, especially in group settings. Spouses may also feel uncomfortable when observing that their partner's hearing difficulties are being made a joke of by others or when the person with the hearing impairment is regarded as 'dumb'.

Impact on the relationship

Relationships may change because of hearing impairment, and this issue is also mentioned in Chapter 6, in the section on 'interpersonal interactions and social relationship'. All spouses in Scarinci *et al.*'s study (2008) reported an increase in tension in the relationship. As Hétu and colleagues (1993) had reported, Scarinci *et al.*'s couples experienced an alteration in intimate/sexual relationships. This may happen when one finds that whispering is no longer possible. Earlier, Jones *et al.* (1987) revealed that 40% of couples with one of the spouses having hearing problems perceived their relationship as less personal, with loss of intimate talk limiting physical and emotional intimacy.

The independence of the partner with hearing impairment may be threatened when the spouses constantly feel they need to act, speak and make telephone calls on behalf of their partner.

Impact on social life

The social life of the spouse may alter considerably when their partner with hearing impairment just 'wants to stay home' or prefers to 'invite people to their home' rather than going out to noisy gatherings. Not only may the frequency of social activities be reduced, but also if they do go to a noisy meeting there is often the need to go home early. A further social consequence relates to the spouse having to attend social events alone, rather than *with* their partner, again impacting on their relationship.

Impact on everyday activities

The effects of hearing problems on the spouse's everyday activities encompass 'increased television volume', 'the person with hearing impairment never hearing the phone ringing' and 'concerns about safety issues' when the person with hearing impairment goes out and may miss relevant traffic noises.

A further issue highlighted by Scarinci *et al.* (2008) is the spouse's need to constantly adapt to their partner's hearing impairment. An imbalance is often felt. Spouses repeatedly feel that it is they who have to make the adjustments, while the partner with hearing impairment often forgets about using hearing strategies. An example is the partner with hearing impairment starting a conversation from another room.

An interesting observation of Scarinci and colleagues (2008) is the effect of acceptance of the hearing impairment and the use of coping strategies by the spouse. Similar findings are reported by Hallberg and Barrenäs (1993) and a further overview of their study is relevant.

Coping strategies

Hallberg and Barrenäs (1993) studied the consequences of noise-induced hearing loss (NIHL) of male workers as experienced by their spouses. Additionally, they investigated how the spouses managed the consequences of their husband's hearing impairment. In-depth interviews covered seven areas of interest: onset of hearing disability, perceived stressful situations, awareness of hearing disability, technical devices, changes in lifestyle, attitudes and the phenomenon of occupational injury. Ten middle-aged females who lived with males with severe NIHL participated. Interpretation of the data resulted in the identification of two core concepts:

1. The husband's reluctance to acknowledge hearing difficulties, including aspects as 'he doesn't want to talk about it', 'he denies any hearing problem', 'he has no defects'.
2. The influence of the hearing impairment on the couple's intimate relationship. This category included issues as 'mutual irritation', 'he doesn't talk about emotional things', 'our communication is reduced', 'I become more and more silent' and 'we are doing different things'.

Four qualitatively different strategies used by the spouses to manage the situation (i.e. living with a husband with severe NIHL) were derived from combining those two concepts: co-acting, minimising, mediating and distancing. The combinations are illustrated in Table 7.1.

Co-acting

Co-acting strategies indicate that the hearing impairment is not regarded as a problem or hindrance in daily life. 'You just have to adjust to each other' as a strategy is the starting point here and both partners would say that 'everything at home functions

Table 7.1 Four qualitatively different strategies used by the spouses to manage the situation (i.e. living with a husband with severe NIHL).

		The intimate relationships	
		The spouse does not admit any impact of hearing impairment	The spouse admits impact of hearing impairment
The husband's reluctance to acknowledge hearing difficulties	The spouse is playing the game	Co-acting	Minimising
	The spouse is not playing the game	Mediating ▫ controlling ▫ navigating ▫ advising	Distancing

(*Source:* adapted from Hallberg and Barrenäs, 1993.)

well'. Hallberg and Barrenäs (1993) argue that the co-acting strategy may be a functional way of mutual adjustment to a disability rather than a denial of difficulties.

Mediating

Mediating strategies involve attempts to control the situation. This happens when the spouse listens for both herself and her husband. She navigates the husband away from stressful situations and privately advises him (e.g. 'I advise him to tell others about his hearing difficulties'). The mediating strategies clearly point out the spouse's dominant role and responsibility for the husband. The risk of such an attitude is that it may create over-protection and social dependency of the husband.

Distancing and minimising

Minimising reflects the spouse's avoidance of any conflicts with her husband, while admitting the influence of her husband's hearing problems at the same time. That strategy seems to be used when the couple wants to present itself to its surroundings as a socially normal couple.

Distancing strategies occur when the spouse does not play the game of denial or rejection of the hearing problems. Communication is minimised and it seems as though the couple lives side by side. There is mutual irritability. They no longer preserve the social image of a normal couple. Hallberg and Barrenäs (1993) mention here that it is impossible to know if the hearing disability is the main cause of the disturbed marital relationship or just a facilitating factor in a relationship breakdown.

Hallberg and Barrenäs presume that spouses who are co-acting, minimising or distancing are less motivated than the mediating spouses to stimulate the husband to partake in auditory enablement programmes. They further argue, though, that the above categories are tentative theoretical constructs which require further scientific attention.

Overall, taking Scarinci *et al.*'s (2008) findings into account as well, it seems as if the effect of the limited hearing on the spouse depends greatly on the degree of acceptance of the loss by the affected partner. That is, the more the partner with hearing impairment is perceived by their spouse as accepting the loss, the less the effect on the spouse. Accepting the hearing impairment, rather than denial, results in more tolerance, more patience and less annoyance on the side of the spouse and, in turn, facilitates adaptation.

Furthermore, the impact of the hearing impairment on the spouse seems to be influenced by whether the spouse is male or female. Overall, female spouses tend to report more problems and accentuate the unpleasant implications than male spouses (Anderson and Noble, 2005; Scarinci et al., 2008). An explanation may be that women are inclined to assign greater importance to effective social communication, report greater problem awareness and show less denial associated with hearing impairment than males (Garstecki and Erler, 1999). Males may have greater difficulties with showing their emotions. Also, females tend to take greater responsibility for maintaining the conversation.

Anderson and Noble (2005) applied the attribution theory to explore the association between relationship satisfaction and attributions for behaviours modulated by hearing difficulties. The results showed that if many attributions of responsibility are made for hearing impaired behaviours, then relationship satisfaction is low, and vice versa. These authors suggest that cognitive interventions to alter attributions may be useful in audiological enablement. In accordance with Hétu et al. (1993), they propose that communication in couples can be enhanced by sharing information about the effects of hearing impairment on behaviours and facilitating the expression of feelings and needs of both partners.

Inclusion of significant others in enablement programmes

This area has particular relevance as a high proportion of older patients attend clinics as a result of pressure from significant others (O Mahoney et al., 1996). This is discussed in Chapter 2.

The importance of including the significant other in their partner's enablement process has long been emphasised (Hallberg and Barrenäs, 1993; Hétu et al., 1993; Hallberg, 1999; Kiessling et al., 2003; Schow, 2008; this book Chapter 10) as well as the inclusion of significant others in outcome measures (Brooks et al., 2001; Noble, 2002; Stark and Hickson, 2004). However, whether clinical practices in general comply with the recommendations to actively involve significant others in their standard enablement programmes is questionable. At the present time, we are not aware of standard inclusion, despite the fact that in the international literature positive effects have been demonstrated. An example is a study by Brooks and Johnson (1981), who introduced pre-fitting interviews with the patient *and* the family and home visits as parts of a hearing aid provision programme. Positive effects on the use of hearing aids, participation and the relationship of the patient with the professional were observed. Another example is a study by Kramer et al. (2005), who developed a home-education programme for those with hearing impairment and their significant others. As explained earlier in this chapter, Hallberg and Barrenäs (1993) state that it is important to consider the coping strategies of the partner during audiological enablement as they may significantly influence the outcome.

Hearing impairment arising from genetic causes or with a familial basis

Genetically determined hearing impairment may develop at any age throughout life. There have been a number of studies on the genetics of post-lingual hereditary

Table 7.2 Genes implicated in late-onset hearing impairment.

Gene	Function	Reference
KCNQ4	Potassium channel gene	Van Eyken et al., 2006
GRHL2	Role in maintenance of epithelial cells	Van Laer et al., 2008
NAT2A	Oxidative stress-related gene	Unal et al., 2005
GRM7	Glutamate controlling gene	Friedman et al., 2009
Mitochondrial genes	Metabolic mechanisms	Fischel-Ghodsian et al., 1997

(*Source:* derived from results presented by Van Laer and Van Camp, 2008.)

hearing impairment. Karlsson *et al.* (1997) found that hereditability decreased with increasing age, but the correlation coefficient was still 0.42 in those over 65 years old. Gates *et al.* (1999) estimated that 35% to 55% of the variance of the sensory presbya-cusis phenotype (i.e. high-frequency loss; 4–8 kHz) and 25–42% of the variance of the strial presbyacusis phenotype (flat loss) is attributable to the effects of genes. Subsequent studies have confirmed this figure of about 50% for hereditability.

In late-onset hearing impairment non-syndromal autosomal dominant (NSADHI) appears to predominate. This is generally progressive and is normally mild to moderate in severity, although in some conditions a severe to profound impairment may occur.

Otosclerosis, a condition predominantly resulting in a progressive conductive hearing impairment, is generally considered autosomal dominant of incomplete penetrance. There is much uncertainty as to the mechanism underlying the condition, even though eight genetic loci have been identified (Declau and Van de Heyning, 2007a). Late-onset syndromal hearing impairment is much less common, although Neurofibromatosis 2 can result in total deafness as well as cause a number of associated neurological lesions (Neary *et al.*, 2005).

In the last few years, a number of linkage and association studies have been performed in an attempt to identify genes which may contribute to age-related hearing impairment. These are shown in Table 7.2. The role of mitochondrial inheritance has been further emphasised in results from the Blue Mountains study, indicating a major role of maternal inheritance (McMahon *et al.*, 2008).

Susceptibility to environmental factors causing hearing impairment (e.g. noise, ototoxicity, dietary factors) may also be genetically determined. In other words, some people may be genetically more susceptible to hearing impairment following noise exposure, whereas others may be genetically resistant to noise. Detailed knowledge of the genes giving susceptibility to age-related hearing impairment (ARHI) is, however, largely lacking. An important reason is that hereditary factors influencing the cochlear ageing process act together with (confounding) environmental non-genetic factors (e.g. noise, ototoxic medication) and this complicates human genetic studies on ARHI (Van Laer and Van Camp, 2007).

A frequently asked question in clinical practice is whether it is possible to distinguish a non-syndromal genetically determined hearing impairment from an auditory impairment caused by other factors. There is extreme heterogeneity in the audiometric profiles of people with later onset NSADHI, which makes it difficult to distinguish the two groups. Further deterioration of hearing with age, changing the threshold profile, makes such a classification even more difficult. It is known that many forms of hereditary hearing impairment are progressive and it seems that the ascending and U-shaped audiogram profiles show the clearest replication from parents to children (Martini *et al.*, 1996, 1997). However, age-related changes of hearing thresholds may alter the typical profiles. For example, the U-shaped audiometric profile may change to a downward-sloping pattern involving the high frequencies. It seems, therefore, that the pure tone threshold profile is of relatively little value for the diagnosis of genetic hearing impairment (Prosser and Martini, 2007). An overview of the current knowledge of such genetic profiles is provided by Huygen *et al.* (2007).

Impact of having a family history of hearing impairment

Along with the advances in genomic medicine, family history is considered a useful tool for public health and preventive medicine. For various (chronic) diseases such as diabetes, heart disease, breast cancer and asthma, the family history has been shown to help predict the risk of such health conditions (Guttmacher *et al.*, 2004). In addition, increasing awareness of having a family history is considered a potential tool to promote behavioural change in the general population (Audran-McGovern *et al.*, 2003). Research on the psychosocial impact of having a family history has been conducted for various hereditary conditions, such as breast cancer and colorectal cancer (Schwartz *et al.*, 1999; Carlsson *et al.*, 2004; Kim *et al.*, 2005).

As in many other health care disciplines, the number of studies on molecular genetics in the field of hearing disorders to investigate hereditary hearing impairment has rapidly increased (Martini *et al.*, 2007). It is therefore sensible to also consider the impact on the individual of knowing they have a family history of hearing impairment. Until recently, research on this issue was largely absent, but a number of studies included in the book *The effects of genetic hearing impairment in the family* edited by Stephens and Jones (2006) shed some light on this topic. Being aware of having a family history of hearing impairment (FHHI) may influence an individual's life in many respects. The following section presents a brief overview of the various findings reported.

Even though the question was designed for general purposes, rather than to examine the typical effects of having FHHI, Stephens *et al.* (2003a) asked 34 000 participants in a household survey: 'Did any of your parents, children, brothers or sisters have great difficulty in hearing before the age of 55 years?' The response to this question was related to questions on *activity limitation* (e.g. 'Do you have difficulty with your hearing?') and questions on *participation restriction/psychosocial problems* related to the impact of the hearing (e.g. 'Nowadays, how much does any difficulty in hearing worry, annoy or upset you?'). The degree of annoyance caused by the hearing impairment was greater when there was a family history of hearing impairment, controlling for hearing activity limitation. Similarly, the degree of annoyance caused by tinnitus was greater when people reported to have FHHI. The results seem to demonstrate that people who have a family history of hearing impairment may be more conscious of hearing problems and more sensitive to them and, hence, may be more likely to report them and consider them severe. The authors called this the *psychological sensitisation* hypothesis. The fact that those with FHHI reported more annoyance caused by loud sounds than those without such a history further substantiated this hypothesis. Overall, the findings of this study suggest a largely disproportionate negative impact of having a family history of hearing impairment on those diagnosed themselves compared to those without FHHI.

The results of Stephens *et al.* (2003a) were further supported and extended by data derived from the Blue Mountains study, a population-based survey of age-related hearing impairment in a representative older Australian community (Sindhusake *et al.*, 2006). The effects of having a family history of hearing impairment on measures of impairment (audiogram), activity limitation (self-reported hearing, i.e. 'Do you feel you have a hearing loss?'), participation restriction (Hearing Handicap Inventory for the Elderly; HHIE) and tinnitus was studied in a cohort including 2846 people of 50 years and over. The question 'Do (or did) any of your close relatives have a hearing loss?' was used to define parental or sibling family history of hearing loss as this question was repeated for father, mother, any brother(s) and any sister(s). The four possible responses were 'yes', 'no', 'unsure' or 'missing'. The responses when one or both parents reported having hearing problems ($n = 1079$) were compared with those when neither had hearing problems ($n = 1767$). In addition, for the latter group, those with one or more siblings reporting hearing problems ($n = 214$) were compared to those in which no siblings were reported to have hearing problems ($n = 1550$). The results clearly demonstrated that after adjusting for hearing and sex, individuals with an FHHI had worse hearing levels, both in the mid-frequencies (average 0.5–4 kHz) and in the high frequencies (average 4, 6, 8 kHz). Similar results were obtained for self-report measures on hearing activity limitation ('Do you feel you have a hearing loss?'). Also, HHIE scores were significantly worse for the group with an FHHI. Thus, this study confirmed earlier findings by Stephens *et al.* (2003a) indicating that individuals with a history of hearing impairment in the family are more affected than individuals without such a history.

The findings of the studies above thus seem to emphasise that having a family history mainly results in a negative impact of one's own hearing impairment. This is quite intriguing, as some other small-scale studies showed practically no differences between groups with and without an FHHI, or just positive effects. In particular, qualitative studies among clinical populations on the impact of having an FHHI showed the opposite (i.e. positive) findings. These studies revealed that having a family history is mainly a positive experience.

An example of a small-scale study is that of Carlsson and Danermark (2006). They followed a cohort of 56 individuals with early-onset hearing impairment (diagnosed before the age of five years) and compared those with an FHHI to those without such a history. At the time of investigation, the participants were between 40 and 50 years of age. In all, 14 participants confirmed that they had at least one relative (mother, father, sibling, cousin, aunt) with hearing impairment and were thus considered as having FHHI. These 14 people were compared to the remaining participants without FHHI on the following variables: degree of hearing impairment (average 0.5, 1, 2, 4 kHz), tinnitus, experience of hearing problems, hearing aid use, attending senior high school/university, employment, marital status, divorced, having children. The two groups appeared to be highly similar, as they did not differ on any of these variables, except one. Those with an FHHI were more likely to attend senior high school/ university than those without an FHHI. This finding is also reflected in studies on the academic achievement of Deaf children (Stephens, 2005; Fortnum *et al.*, 2006).

Qualitative studies were conducted by Kramer *et al.* (2006a) and by Coulson (2006). The first investigation used an open-ended questionnaire asking the person about the impact of having a family history of hearing impairment. First, it was verified whether the respondent had or had previously had a relative with hearing problems. If this question was confirmed and the respondent had specified which relative had (had) a hearing impairment, the questions were as follows: 'You have mentioned that other members of your family have or have previously had hearing problems. Does your family history of hearing loss have any effect on your reaction to your own hearing problems? (*yes, no*). If yes, please list any ways this knowledge has affected you. Write down as many as you can think of.' This question was administered both in the Netherlands (Amsterdam) and in Wales (Cardiff).

In the Netherlands, the questions were posted on the web site of the Dutch Society of Hard-of-Hearing people. Here, 41 adults participated and returned their reports either by email or by regular post. In Cardiff, the questionnaire was administered to those consecutive patients seen in the audiological enablement clinics of the Welsh Hearing Institute from whom the clinician had elicited a family history of hearing problems. Responses were obtained from 100 patients. About 40% of the Cardiff patients reported that their family history had no effect on their own hearing impairment. In Amsterdam, only one respondent reported the absence of such an effect.

Data in Amsterdam were subjected to a qualitative content analysis (Graneheim and Lundman, 2004). It is a method to group all reactions reported by the interviewees and then to compare the different classifications. The procedure entails a progressive classification of the responses (raw data) from *meaning units* to *condensed meaning units* then to *sub-themes* and finally *themes*. For a more detailed overview and examples of this process of classification, we refer to Kramer *et al.* (2006a). In all, six themes were identified:

- role modelling
- expectations/anticipation
- acceptance
- help-seeking
- sharing knowledge
- offspring/the future.

The themes and examples of reactions in each category are presented in Table 7.3.

The analyses also included an examination of the direction of each of the reactions: positive, negative or neutral. The total number of reactions in each theme, divided by positive, neutral and negative responses, is shown in Figure 7.1. In all, the 'sharing knowledge' category had the largest number of reactions. Apparently, 'sharing knowledge' is the most important issue that people associate with having a family history of hearing impairment. The number of positive reactions within this theme was large as well (52%). Other themes with the largest proportion of reactions in the positive category were 'help-seeking' (64%) and 'role modelling' (54% positive). The theme 'expectation/anticipation' appeared to be mainly neutral. No positive reactions were reported here. It seems as if issues like expectation and anticipation become mainly negative when an individual's offspring is involved. The theme 'offspring' had the largest proportion of negative reactions, indicating that anxieties about their children's future prevailed.

Surprisingly, the theme 'acceptance' predominantly comprised negative reactions. One would expect that having role models in the family would facilitate the process of acceptance. Apparently, the reverse effect may also occur. A closer inspection of the reactions within this theme revealed that negative effects may be experienced both with regard to accepting the hearing impairment and with accepting devices such as hearing aids.

When merging all reactions, the overall proportion of positive, neutral and negative reactions in Amsterdam was 36%, 30% and 34% respectively. In Cardiff, these

Table 7.3 Examples of reactions in each of the six themes identified.

Themes	Positive	Neutral	Negative
Role modelling	'My parents were hearing impaired: that made life easier as I observed them, which taught me how to cope with it.'	'I did not associate my hearing problem with my father's until I was asked if members of my family suffered from hearing problems.'	'I have seen my father struggling with inadequate hearing aids. It affected my attitude towards hearing aids.'
Expectation/Anticipation	–	'Both my father and grandfather had hearing problems, so becoming hard of hearing was no surprise for me.' 'When I was 12, I realised that I had a chance to become hearing impaired.'	'I may become isolated, like my mother, and that frightens me. I am afraid that I won't be able to work until the age of 67.'
Acceptance	'Having relatives with hearing impairment helped me to accept my own hearing loss.'	'It is "normal" for me to be hearing impaired as almost everybody in my family has hearing problems. Nothing negative, nothing positive.'	'I have difficulty accepting my hearing loss as I know that it will further deteriorate and cannot be cured.'
Help-seeking	'Having a family history of hearing loss made me determined to seek help sooner.'	'I don't think my reaction and help-seeking would be different if my hearing impairment was non-familiar.'	'My mother thinks hearing aids are useless. She told me not to use them. It made me seek help too late.'
Sharing knowledge	'Having a family history of hearing loss made me stronger, as I could share important issues with my close relatives.'	'Hearing impairment is often the topic of conversation.'	'I feel the pain that my children go through.'
Offspring/future	'I am positive about my hearing impairment and I expect that my daughter will be as well.' 'I will tell my children that their lives are valuable.'	'My children are still normal hearing.' 'FHHL did not stop us having children.'	'I feel guilty that I have carried over my hearing impairment to my children.'

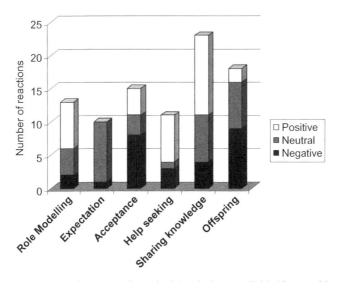

Figure 7.1 The total number of responses in each of the six themes, divided into positive, negative and neutral responses.

proportions were 57%, 19% and 24%. These data suggest that the positive effects of having a family history of hearing impairment on those diagnosed with the condition themselves prevailed.

An identification as to which themes are observed as being mainly positive, neutral or negative may yield relevant information for clinicians working with people who have a family history of hearing impairment and for those who are involved in (genetic) counselling.

It must be noted, however, that the themes identified are not necessarily mutually exclusive. A condensed meaning unit may sometimes fit into more than one theme, and overlap between themes should not be ignored. Additional quantitative research is therefore required to further support the various categories identified, and their relative importance. A first step in that direction was taken by Kramer *et al.* (2006b), who developed a structured questionnaire based on the study above. It was found that the awareness of having a family history was significantly associated with role modelling. This aspect merits further attention both in research and in clinical practices. Encouraging patients to identify and introduce suitable role models may be considered as a new and helpful elements in auditory enablement programmes.

This conclusion was also drawn by Coulson (2006).

Whereas the above study elicited six different themes comprising positive, neutral and negative effects of having a family history of hearing impairment, Coulson (2006) explored the phenomenon of FHHI from a different (qualitative) perspective. It is particularly interesting to observe that her conclusions are broadly similar to those of Kramer and Stephens, despite her completely different qualitative approach in analysing the data.

Coulson (2006) conducted semi-structured interviews among 12 adults with hearing impairment having FHHI. The focus was on the experience of adults with late-onset hearing impairment who had (had) relatives with the same condition. Data were analysed using theme-oriented discourse analysis identifying themes. The transcripts were divided into two groups:

1. Family Knowledge Group (individuals who had extensive experience and memory of affected relatives)
2. Non-Family Knowledge Group (those who were not aware of having or did not have relatives with hearing problems)

Analyses of the data resulted in a grouping of the reactions into 'relational' matters (i.e. human contacts such as relational networks, roles, self, character) and 'transactional' matters (i.e. non-human contact, everyday tasks such as television, cooking timer, everyday coping mechanisms). These relational/transactional extracts appeared to either involve the family sphere or be outside the family sphere. As such, four different categories could be created:

- Family sphere: transactional (e.g. shopping with family member)
- Family sphere: relational (roles within the family)
- Outside family sphere: transactional (everyday tasks not involving family members)
- Outside family sphere: relational (friends and other people known, embarrassment).

Overall, in the family sphere, coping mechanisms are more direct as people feel at ease. There is no reluctance in facing other family members or presenting them their good ear, for example. Outside the family sphere (in shops, dealing with customers at work) coping mechanisms are more pre-learnt and prepared. In other words, different coping strategies are applied in and out of the family environment.

Coulson's analyses revealed that those not having broad awareness of their family member(s) with the same condition (group 2) generally have limited (or different) coping mechanisms in each of the four categories above. The non-knowledge people tend to use more avoidance techniques, blame, denial and shutting off. In the public sphere (outside family) these people tend to use open gestures of asking for help, like opening their purse and asking the cashier to take the correct amount of money out. It seems as if the people in group 2 have to learn coping mechanisms from their own everyday lives and experiences. These personal experiences, however, only provide limited opportunities to learn, as they are often accidental opportunities. Also, it was found that individuals in group 2 may wonder about the cause of their hearing impairment.

Those who have had a wide exposure to and experience of family member(s) with hearing impairment, on the other hand, have had many opportunities to learn coping mechanisms from their relatives. Overall, these opportunities have enabled them to adapt more easily. The family experience seems to provide a continuous, reliable and systematic exposure to learning opportunities.

Another interesting difference between the knowledge (1) and non-knowledge (2) groups reported by Coulson (2006) is that the knowledge group predominantly talked about relational issues, whereas the non-knowledge group mainly focused on transactional and factual issues. Even when transactional issues are discussed in the knowledge group, they end up as relational issues. Also, in the non-knowledge group, family member(s) are described less positively than in the knowledge group.

Discussion

The studies of Kramer *et al.* (2006b) and of Coulson (2006) support the statement that having a family history of hearing impairment is mainly a positive experience. This is the opposite to the findings reported in population studies that predominantly show negative effects of FHHI for those with the conditions themselves. The differences in outcome may be caused by selection bias, though. As opposed to the population studies, those participating in the qualitative studies selected themselves via a web site (Amsterdam) or via the hearing clinic that they attended (Cardiff). It must be noted that only one in five of those having hearing difficulties attend clinics and seek help. It is thus possible that those who have already sought help at a clinic have a more positive attitude towards having FHHI as opposed to those with hearing impairment who did not. This issue deserves further attention in future research.

Nevertheless, the qualitative studies as presented here may be regarded as providing some basic knowledge. The effectiveness and the use of the family history in clinical care could be increased. Even though information on family history of hearing problems is routinely collected in many clinical settings, its systematic use in hearing health care is largely absent. Role models may be influential and role modelling within this context may be regarded as a strategy. Emphasising the function of role modelling could be used as a tool to facilitate appropriate intervention and to enhance the enablement process, focusing on the adjustment to hearing impairment. The concept of family history may be added to and used in advising patients about how to improve their adjustment to hearing impairment by emphasising the importance of finding appropriate role models. This should be incorporated into the enablement approach for those without having people with hearing impairment in their family by identifying and introducing the patients to suitable role models to whom they can look for advice and coping skills. This issue will be further considered in Chapter 12.

Conclusion

The first section of this chapter provides an overview of consequences that may be experienced by relatives (mostly the spouse) of the person with hearing difficulties. Areas that may be affected are: communication (less spontaneous talks, less intimate contact), emotional functioning (embarrassment, frustration), the relationship (spouse changes into caregiver), social life (partner with hearing impairment just wants to stay at home, rather than going out) and routine everyday activities (increased television volume). It is estimated that about 50% of the cases of acquired hearing impairment are attributable to genetic causes. Recently, a number of genes related to late-onset hearing impairment have been identified. Susceptibility to environmental factors causing hearing impairment (e.g. noise, ototoxicity, dietary factors) may also be genetically determined. Having a family history of hearing impairment (FHHI) may influence the lives of those diagnosed with the condition in many respects. Both negative and positive effects are reported. The question of role models, particularly within the family, can be important in terms of the patient's acceptance of their condition and in terms of early help-seeking. So far, only a small number of studies have addressed this issue. More research is needed.

8 The process of enablement at work

Introduction

Within the *International Classification of Functioning, Disability and Health* (ICF) of the World Health Organization (WHO; 2001), participation in work is acknowledged as one of the major areas in life (D8). For many people, one of the most significant determinants in their perceived status and position in society is their job (Scherich and Mowry, 1997). Difficulties that make it impossible for the person to work optimally result in participation restrictions. An increasing number of people with hearing loss are seeking help for occupational problems. Some of these problems and ways of addressing them are illustrated in a video clip on the web site associated with this book (http://www.wiley.com/go/stephens).

Statistics

In the United States, communication problems (hearing, language and speech) are estimated to have a prevalence of 5–10% in the labour force (Ruben, 2000). Ruben estimates the combined costs of communication disorders to be 2.5–3% of 'gross national product (GNP)', which means a significant loss to the US economy. The author states that modern Western economies have undergone fundamental change during the second half of the twentieth century. In the past, they were largely dependent on manual labour. In the twenty-first century, they depend on communication skills such as hearing, voice, speech and language. In the communication-age societies of this century, occupations rely more and more on communication skills. This implies a greater burden on groups of people suffering from communication disorders, such as hearing impairment or speech and language disorders.

The burden on groups of people with communication disorders may lead to a disproportionate percentage of employees taking early retirement. For example, prevalence data in Sweden show that whereas only 5.4% of the general population is reported to have a hearing impairment, approximately 12% of those taking early retirement are hard of hearing, indicating an over-representation in that group (Danermark and Coniavitis Gellerstedt, 2004).

In addition, a greater likelihood of unemployment has been found to be related to hearing impairment. Specifically, a study in Denmark revealed that about 30% of young adults with hearing impairment (aged 20–35 years) were unemployed whereas the level of unemployment was much lower (12%) in an age-matched reference group (Parving and Christensen, 1993).

The relevance of the impact of hearing impairment on work-related issues is further emphasised by the fact that in the Netherlands about 3% of the labour force (i.e. 255000 people) report that they suffer from hearing impairment (Cuijpers and Lautenbach, 2006). Owing to the ageing population and changes in retirement age, the number of older employees is increasing so leading to an increasing number of people with hearing loss seeking help for problems at work. In a large survey among Dutch Deaf and severely hearing impaired people, counselling on how to handle one's own hearing loss at the workplace was one of the most frequently reported needs (De Graaf and Bijl, 2002).

Impact of hearing impairment on occupational performance

Among the disabilities that limit a person's involvement in work, hearing impairment is clearly recognised (Colledge *et al.*, 1999). However, the vast majority of studies on the relationship between hearing and occupation are restricted to the causes of noise-induced hearing loss (NIHL), on how to protect employees from dangerous noise levels and on the development of hearing protection programmes. The relationship between work and NIHL is evident. Occupational noise exposure is a serious risk to hearing (Hétu, 1994; May, 2000; Palmer *et al.*, 2002; Nelson *et al.*, 2005). However, existing hearing impairment in employees, regardless of its origin, and even mild degrees of hearing impairment, may adversely affect occupational performance and well-being. In particular, adults with acquired hearing impairment may encounter difficulties in coping with their auditory disabilities at work. They often regard their environments and circumstances as challenging. Research on the impact of hearing impairment among those who are still active in the workforce can reveal valuable information and disclose specific rehabilitative needs (Kramer, 2008).

The impact of hearing impairment on occupational performance and well-being has barely been investigated in a systematic way. A relatively small number of studies have been published and have recently been the subject of a thorough review by Danermark (2005), who concluded that workers with hearing impairment form a vulnerable group in the labour force for whom the conditions at work are more challenging than for normally hearing colleagues.

Comparable conclusions were drawn by Kramer *et al.* (2006c), who compared the occupational performance of a group of 151 employees with hearing impairment with that of a group of 60 workers with normal hearing. The groups were matched for age, gender, educational level and type of job. The Amsterdam Checklist for Hearing and Work was used to assess the participants' self-reported environmental conditions at work, type of job, type of contract (permanent vs temporary; full-time vs part-time), general working conditions (job demand, control, support) and activities required for the performance of the job, including hearing activities. An analysis of group differences revealed that the 'self-perceived environmental noise' level was significantly higher among those with hearing loss compared with normally hearing subjects ($p < 0.01$). Similarly, the reported 'effort in hearing' needed during listening was significantly higher in the group with hearing impairment ($p < 0.001$). No differences between the two groups were found for the general working conditions, except for 'job control' (interrupting work or taking breaks when wanted). Hearing impaired participants perceived themselves to have significantly less 'control' at work compared to their normally hearing colleagues ($p < 0.01$). It is worth noting that these findings very much support the results of comparable investigations, such as a study by Danermark and Coniavitis Gellerstedt (2004) on a group of 445 employees who completed a questionnaire on the psychosocial environment at work. The scores were compared with reference data obtained from more than 8 000 people employed by local municipalities. The results showed that the psychosocial environment at work was much more demanding for the hard-of-hearing group compared with the normally hearing reference group. The most important difference appeared to be the lower self-assessed degree of control at work for those with hearing impairment.

People with hearing impairment feel a greater need to have control over their work (i.e. organising their own schedules so as to be able to take breaks; interrupt work after having had auditorily demanding activities). Providing control over their work for employees with hearing impairment enhances their well-being.

Sick-leave

The study by Kramer *et al.* (2006c) further reveals that normally hearing workers and employees with hearing impairment differ significantly in the amount of sick-leave they take. In the hearing impaired group, the proportion of employees reporting sick-leave (77%) was significantly higher than in the normally hearing group (55%) ($p < 0.01$). This appeared to be exclusively due to the higher proportion of people reporting sick-leave due to stress-related complaints (fatigue, strain and burnout) in the hearing impaired group (26%) than in the normally hearing group (7%) ($p < 0.05$). These results are illustrated in Figure 8.1. When examining the proportion of sick-leave due to 'usual' reasons, such as a fever or a cold, the proportions in both groups are equal, indicating that people with hearing impairment are not different from their normally hearing colleagues within that respect. Distress is more often experienced by those with hearing impairment than those without.

In an attempt to predict sick-leave due to distress in that same study, a logistic regression analysis was performed among hearing impaired individuals reporting sick-leave ($n = 112$). Sick-leave due to distress (yes, no) was adopted as the dependent variable and the remaining variables in the questionnaire, including demographic characteristics, were the independent variables. Two variables appeared to contribute

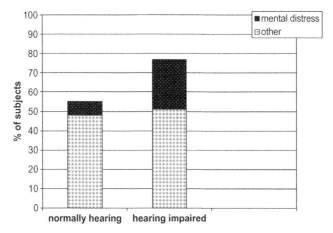

Figure 8.1 Sick-leave reported in the past 12 months by hearing impaired and normally hearing participants by reason for sick-leave (mental distress or other).

significantly in the model: job demand (a general working condition) and the necessity to continuously distinguish between and identify sounds at work. Surprisingly, the necessity to distinguish between or to identify sounds appeared to be the only hearing-specific variable dominating the relationship between sick-leave and occupational performance among those with hearing impairment. This aspect of hearing disability deserves further attention and should not be neglected. Interestingly, on the other hand, the necessity to converse in a noisy environment was not a reported factor.

Similar conclusions are drawn by Gatehouse and Noble (2004) and Morata *et al.* (2005). Gatehouse and Noble developed the Speech, Spatial and Qualities of Hearing Scale (SSQ) dealing with the reality of hearing in the everyday dynamic and demanding world. They compared SSQ scores of 153 clinic clients with an independent measure of 'handicap' covering distress and related emotional effects. They found that the disability–handicap relationship was governed by 'identification of sounds', 'attention' and 'effort problems' (see also Kramer *et al.*, 1997) rather than by 'intelligibility of speech'. Gatehouse and Noble (2004) argue that traditional research in audiology focuses on speech hearing alone, whereas other functions in hearing as served by the auditory system are equally important.

Morata *et al.* (2005) conducted focus groups among workers with self-reported hearing loss and occupational noise exposure. When reporting the difficulties they encounter when working in noise, the employees' primary concerns were about job safety as the result of a reduced ability to hear and distinguish between environmental sounds and warning signals and their inability to monitor essential equipment sounds. Misunderstanding environmental sounds generally leads to embarrassment, fear, distress, anxiety and a feeling of losing control.

A further example is a study by Grimby and Ringdahl (2000). They compared 35 hearing impaired adult full-time workers with 1256 normally hearing employed people below 65 years of age and used various measures of quality of life as outcome indicators. An important finding of that study is that hearing impaired full-time workers reported a higher degree of psychosocial distress in terms of 'lack of energy' and 'social isolation'.

Fatigue

Lack of energy or fatigue among employees is a common phenomenon. It is widely reported in the general population and frequently experienced among employees, in particular among workers with chronic diseases (Fransen *et al.*, 2003). The degree to which employees are able to recover from fatigue and distress at work is an important factor influencing their physical and mental health status. In occupational health care, this so-called 'need for recovery after work' is seen as an acute short-term reaction to work. Repeated inadequate recovery after work has been found to be an intermediate variable between exposure to stressful psychosocial working conditions and the development of psychosomatic health problems (Sluiter *et al.*, 2003).

Nachtegaal *et al.* (2009b) examined the association between hearing status and need for recovery after work in a sample of 926 normally hearing and hearing impaired workers. They used the Dutch Questionnaire on the Experience and Assessment of Work. Regression models demonstrated a significant association between hearing status and the need for recovery after work with poorer hearing leading to an increased need for recovery. The authors discuss the necessity of monitoring the 'need for recovery after work' among workers with hearing impairment, so as to be able to take preventive measures when necessary.

Lack of knowledge

Finally, Detaille *et al.* (2003) investigated what support hearing impaired people need in order to be able to cope at work. The results show that employees with hearing impairment reported a substantial lack of knowledge among colleagues, employers and even professionals about the specific limitations and needs of hearing impaired employees and about what it means to be hearing impaired. They report an urgent need for informational and training programmes to increase awareness among all stakeholders (employees, colleagues, employers, trade unions, health professionals) about how to manage hearing loss at work. Hallberg and Barrenäs (1995) and Hallberg and Jansson (1996) also report this lack of awareness among hearing impaired employees about the levels of the noise at work, the effects of noise on hearing, how to adequately protect one's hearing from hazardous noise, possibilities for financial compensation, the individual's rights at work and the possibilities of professional help.

In summary, key issues that need to be addressed in the management of employees with hearing loss are:

▪ mental distress, effortful listening
▪ job control
▪ self-reported noise levels
▪ noisy environments
▪ lack of knowledge among hearing impaired persons, other workers and professionals.

These issues are further addressed in the next section.

Impact of work-related hearing impairment on significant others

In the previous section, we addressed the issues of auditory fatigue, distress and the associated need to recover after a full day's work. Many individuals with hearing impairment who are working in acoustically demanding situations (e.g. teachers in noisy and reverberant classrooms with poorly articulating pupils) report that they need some hours of sleep or at least a period of silence when they come home from work. As a consequence, life at home may change. Social events and aurally demanding leisure activities may receive a lower priority and it may seem as though the employee with the hearing impairment shows less interest in family matters. This may impose a burden on the spouse and other family members and on a couple's relationship (Hallberg, 1996). Interpersonal relations may change when there is less intimate talking and joking (Jones *et al.*, 1987).

The impact of NIHL on the relatives of the affected individual has been extensively studied by Hallberg and Barrenäs (1993) and by Hétu and his colleagues (1987, 1988). Most of their findings, however, are commonly observed consequences of hearing impairment and do not only apply to the relatives of those who are occupationally involved. Chapter 7 further addresses the consequences of hearing impairment within the family. An outline of the social and emotional consequences of hearing impairment is presented in Chapter 6 of this book.

Vocational enablement

As outlined earlier in this chapter, various studies have identified issues that should be addressed in the enablement of employees with hearing disabilities. Unfortunately, standardised protocols delineating the components to be included in vocational enablement programmes for those people are largely lacking. Over the years, only a few examples of protocols have been described. *Vocational enablement* refers to services for maintaining, facilitating or improving the employment situation (Kramer, 2008). It seems that, in current audiological practice, the specific needs of hearing impaired adults with work-related difficulties are not dealt with in a standard manner.

Models

One example of an enablement programme developed for people affected by NIHL is that established by Hétu and Getty (1991), based on a public health model identifying different causes of the problems and several levels of intervention. They argue that an integrated (multidisciplinary) approach would be crucial for a successful management of the rather complex problems. As hearing disabilities affect not only the individual with hearing impairment but also anyone with whom they interact, Hétu and Getty argue that actions on a single level (i.e. restricting the enablement programme to the hearing impaired employee only) would have little effect. They identify different domains to be included in the rehabilitation process: the hearing impaired person, significant others (family, friends, colleagues), the workplace, health services and the society (population). An illustration is presented in Figure 8.2. The interventions applied were: psychosocial support (coping), provision of information and knowledge (types of hearing impairment, its consequences) and skill development (hearing tactics). It is obvious that in Hétu and Getty's model, these interventions were meant not only for the person with the hearing loss but also for all stakeholders involved.

Others advocating a multidisciplinary approach towards enablement are Ringdahl *et al.* (2001). They developed a multidisciplinary auditory enablement programme and describe its effectiveness. Even though the programme was designed for adults in general and not specifically for those who were occupationally involved, it includes elements focused on work, the workplace and interventions to improve well-being at work. Additional modules in their programme are hearing and speech therapy, hearing aid (re)fitting, prescription of environmental aids, counselling by social workers and group meetings.

A multidisciplinary protocol addressing the specific needs of those who are occupationally involved and who report problems at work due to their impaired hearing is described by De Jager and Goedegebure (2003). It was subsequently applied to a group of employees with hearing impairment (Sorgdrager *et al.*, 2006; Kramer, 2008).

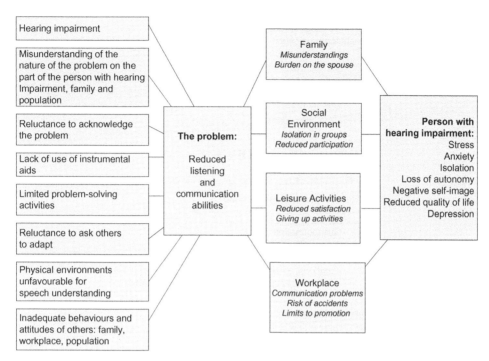

Figure 8.2 Outline of the enablement programme developed by Hétu and Getty. (*Source:* adapted from Hétu and Getty, 1991.)

Vocational Enablement Protocol (VEP)

This Vocational Enablement Protocol (VEP) comprised a half-day assessment of complex problems conducted by a team of professionals from different disciplines (audiologist, occupational physician, social worker, psychologist, speech therapist). Based on a standard procedure, the team examines the auditory functioning of the individual. It seeks to identify and clarify causes of the problems at work, evaluates the existence of additional psychosocial problems in the individual, investigates the acoustical environment at the workplace (if indicated) and finally makes recommendations for appropriate treatment. The ultimate goal is to facilitate participation in and retention of work.

Procedure

In general, employees are referred to the protocol by their occupational physician. Once an individual is referred, a set of questionnaires is sent to the patient's home. People are asked to complete the questionnaires and bring them to their consultation. The work-related questionnaire deals with various topics and provides an accurate assessment of a person's environment at work, type of job, type of contract (permanent vs temporary; full-time vs part-time), general working conditions (job demand, control, support) and activities, including hearing activities at work. Details of this Amsterdam Checklist for Hearing and Work are given in Kramer *et al.* (2006c). Also, to assess a person's ability to cope with the hearing loss and to examine further

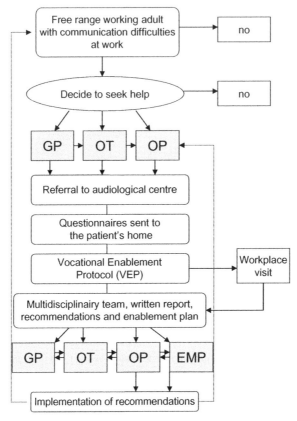

Figure 8.3 Schematic model of the Vocational Enablement Protocol. GP = general practitioner, OP = occupational physician, EMP = employer, OT = otolaryngologist.

psychosocial issues related to hearing loss, several Dutch scales of the Communication Profile for the Hearing Impaired (CPHI) (Mokkink *et al.*, 2009) are administered. A schematic model of the Vocational Enablement Protocol is presented in Figure 8.3.

In the clinic, the patient's hearing status is assessed using an extensive battery of auditory tests, including pure tone and speech audiometry, various Speech Reception Threshold (SRT) tests (in quiet, in steady state noise and in fluctuating noise) (see also Chapter 5) and a test for localisation. Loudness scaling is added if indicated. To examine aided hearing, a free-field version of the SRT in noise test is also performed.

Furthermore, a semi-structured interview is conducted by the psychologist evaluating the psychosocial history of the person, their specific needs, attitude and expectations and an evaluation of the problems at work from the patient's perspective. Referral information is taken into account. The interview is attended by the occupational physician of the team to specifically evaluate the work-related problems and to discuss the patient's view on possible solutions and legal issues.

At the end of the session, all test results are examined and considered by the psychologist, occupational physician and the audiologist and explained to the patient. Possibilities of technical, speech-therapeutic and/or psychosocial interventions are then discussed.

If indicated, the workplace itself is visited and is acoustically examined by conducting a Speech-Transmission-Index (STI) measurement. The STI provides an assessment of the intelligibility of speech in the workplace and verifies whether speech is intelligible for the employee with hearing problems (Houtgast and Steeneken, 1973). The STI measures the combined effects of background noise and reverberation.

Finally, all findings are discussed by a broad multidisciplinary team. At the end of the procedure and following the multidisciplinary team meeting, a written report is compiled, which includes the specific recommendations for the patient and the management plan. The report is then sent to the referrer. To clarify the diagnostic findings and to elucidate the reasonableness of the proposed recommendations, each referrer is telephoned by the occupational physician of the team. The duty of the occupational physician on site is to communicate with the employer and to monitor and supervise the implementation of the recommendations.

Finally, to address the enormous lack of knowledge among professionals, employers, colleagues and significant others about issues related to hearing and work, an extensive information package presented on a CD-ROM was developed (Kramer, 2006). The package provides information on a large number of matters related to hearing and work. It focuses on the understanding of difficulties of working when the individual has a hearing impairment and the various options available to reduce the occupational problems of such people.

Experiences with the protocol

Experiences with the protocol in a clinical sample of 86 patients (53% male) are described by Kramer (2008). A summary is presented below.

The 86 patients who enrolled in the Vocational Enablement Protocol had pure tone hearing losses varying from mild to severe. Their ages ranged from 19 to 64 years, with a mean of 48 years. A wide variety of jobs was encountered in the sample. The largest proportion of the employees (29%) was involved in educational settings (teaching, coaching, instructing). A slightly smaller proportion of patients (23%) was engaged in administrative jobs (office employees, secretaries, researchers, staff members). Seventeen per cent of the people were engaged in health care. The transportation sector (14%) included police officers, pilots, stewards and drivers. The section 'sales' (12%) included cashiers, shop attendants and representatives. A few people (4%) worked in a call centre, and there was one musician in the sample.

It must be noted that a job title in itself provides little information about the tasks to be performed. For example, a police officer who is conducting patrol duties by car and who assists at incidents such as criminal activities or road-related incidents is doing totally different things from a police officer who is involved with administrative procedures all day long. A detailed assessment of the tasks is therefore much more informative than the job title itself.

Reasons for referral

Most of the patients were referred by occupational physicians from all over the country. About 40% of the patients were from ENT specialists and general practitioners. Reasons for referral varied. The most common reason was a general request for advice regarding the hearing problems at work. Other referrals were more specific and included requests for the prescription of technical devices.

Recommendations

The final recommendations defined by the multidisciplinary team were essentially patient-driven. During the interview with the professionals (i.e. audiologist, psychologist, occupational physician), patients were actively encouraged to report their needs, to be involved in describing their situation at work and to bring up recommendations. Advice was given after careful evaluation of the environmental characteristics of the workplace and the conditions of the job. Recommendations were made only after having discussed these with the patients themselves and after having verified as to whether these would be most appropriate in their circumstances.

Overall, a wide range of recommendations aimed at improving the occupational conditions and facilitating participation in and retention of work were made. Table 8.1 lists the various recommendations and shows the proportion of individuals receiving the different types of advice. One of the most frequently proposed actions was a hearing aid fitting or a refitting. The latter was necessary in case of inappropriate fine-tuning earlier in the fitting process or if the hearing aids were obsolete (i.e. older than five years). In addition, environmental aids were prescribed in 20% of the cases. Those comprised FM systems, loops, infrared systems, amplified phones, tactile bleepers and visual alerting systems.

Work-related accommodations can be put into three categories: 're-delegation of assignments', 'restructuring of time schedules' and 'environmental modifications' (Scherich and Mowry, 1997). 'Re-delegation of assignment' comprises elimination of non-essential job functions or removal of highly demanding tasks (e.g. meetings, telephone work). Such a recommendation should be made with care. Some employers may interpret such advice as a declaration of the incapacity of the employee and may indicate the person to be unfit for work.

If auditorily demanding tasks cannot easily be eliminated or the individual does not wish to forego them, restructuring of time schedules is an option. Effortful listening situations, such as meetings, should be rescheduled to the morning, since lack of energy at the end of the day may worsen the listening conditions even further. As outlined in the beginning of this chapter, people with hearing impairment often experience fatigue at work owing to effortful listening and are therefore advised to

Table 8.1 Recommendations provided by the multidisciplinary team.

Hearing aid (re)fitting:	54%
Communication training (speechreading):	31%
Environmental modifications (furniture, light, removal of machines)	30%
Psychosocial counselling	21%
Environmental aids	20%
Re-delegation of assignments	18%
Restructuring of time schedules	16%
Further medical examination	8%
Occupational retraining or redeployment/ending employment	8%
Hearing protection	5%

The right-hand column shows the proportion of employees receiving the particular recommendation. (Since more than one form of advice could be given to an individual, the proportions do not add up to 100.)

reschedule such activities to the morning. Also, the insertion of breaks during the day is recommended and, if possible, a whole day off in the middle of the week is preferred above an extra day off immediately before or after the weekend. In total, 16% of the employees received this type of advice.

Environmental modifications were prescribed in 30% of the cases. Such modifications include rearrangements of the furniture in the room, the provision of lighting, the improvement of room acoustics by providing absorptive materials such as furniture, carpets and curtains. In addition, removal of machines that generate noise, such as fax machines, printers and copiers from the room is a very important recommendation within this respect.

Psychosocial counselling was suggested in 21% of the cases. This service was delivered either in individual settings or in group settings under the supervision of a social worker. Most patients who received individual counselling had it provided 'at home' by means of the Home Education Programme (Kramer *et al.*, 2005). This programme encourages the involvement of significant others (i.e. family members, colleagues).

Communication training mainly refers to training in speechreading (see also Chapter 12). Obtaining training in this skill was one of the most frequently suggested pieces of advice (31%). It could be argued that anyone with hearing impairment should receive training in speechreading. This may be particularly suitable to alternate the challenges people face in situations where understanding is difficult, with or without assistive listening devices.

In a minority of cases (8%), occupational retraining or ending employment was advised. A person was declared unfit for duty, only after both their hearing status and the conditions and circumstances under which they had to function had been considered carefully and discussed at length with the individual concerned and their employer.

In general, if the workplace does not allow any of the interventions shown in Table 8.1 to be implemented, the only way out is occupational retraining or redeployment. Few of the 86 workers were declared as unfit for work. Among those were a bath superintendent and a mechanic repairing coffee machines. The latter person had a profound symmetrical hearing impairment. He worked full-time repairing juice machines that were located in various buildings all over the country. He had to communicate with his supervisor all day long using his mobile phone, mostly while driving his car. On several occasions he had visited his occupational physician and complained about the enormous auditory demands he faced every day in the course of his job. He received neither understanding nor sympathy from his occupational physician. While he had rarely taken sick-leave over the years, this patient appeared to be totally burnt out when he visited the audiological clinic.

Hearing protection was recommended in a small minority of cases (5%). The explanation is that only a few employees in the present sample worked in places with hazardous noise levels. The advice was given after the workplace was visited where noise measurements were performed.

Overall, the majority of patients who participated in the current project were highly satisfied and reported that the vocational programme had facilitated their participation in work. A few encountered reluctant employers who were not willing to cooperate and who refused to implement the recommended interventions. Some others were not satisfied and continued to experience difficulties. Overall, it was observed that people with hearing impairment are highly motivated to work, provided that appropriate interventions are offered.

Discussion

Experience with the VEP, as described above, has yielded useful information. In agreement with Hétu and Getty (1991), it was found that an integrated approach is crucial for an accurate assessment and management of the occupational difficulties experienced by employees with hearing impairment. Neither the hearing status in itself nor the job title as such provides sufficient information to determine the extent to which the worker matches the job. A thorough evaluation of the workplace, the tasks to be performed and the conditions under which they have to work are of utmost importance.

A multidisciplinary team has added values. It provides specialised knowledge and ample experience in the various disciplines involved. Also, communication of the message to the professionals at the workplace (e.g. occupational physicians, employers) is much easier when that is done by specialists in the team who come from the same discipline.

A further important conclusion is that the requirement of the VEP is not restricted to workplaces where background noises are hazardous. The vast majority of employees in the present project were employed in places where hearing protection was not required. Despite that, barriers in the workplace had interfered with effective job performance.

Even though this programme may be regarded as a step forward in the management of people with hearing impairment who experience problems at work, there is still room for improvement. A drawback of a multidisciplinary approach is that none of the team members may feel overall responsibility for the patient. One person of the team has to fulfil the role of a case manager who monitors the process from the very beginning to the very end and who facilitates communication among professionals and with the patient.

Another limitation of the present project is that the findings to date cannot be generalised to other groups of employees with hearing impairment. The proportion of recommendations can be totally different in other groups of patients, with different types of hearing loss, different backgrounds and different types of jobs.

Furthermore, no scientific evidence is available for the effectiveness and efficiency of the recommendations proposed. Empirical research should investigate the effectiveness of the multidisciplinary approach and to what extent each of the recommendations separately significantly reduces barriers at work, enhances well-being and improves occupational performance. Also, a range of variables affecting the results (i.e. age, gender, degree of hearing loss, personality) need to be systematically examined.

The different elements of the VEP are broadly similar to those of other models of auditory enablement (see Chapter 1). An example is Stephens' (2003) updated model including 'evaluation of activity and participation', 'integration and decision-making' (goal-setting), 'short-term remediation' and 'ongoing remediation'. These elements are extensively discussed in Chapters 10 to 12. The model of Kiessling *et al.* (2003) covers the same elements and includes a section on 'outcomes measurement', an issue that needs further attention in the VEP.

The VEP may be seen as an example of a model facilitating the enablement process of a specific population: employees with hearing impairment. Even though it may be regarded as a potential model for good practice in this field, there is still room for improvement. For example, tests examining a person's cognitive and linguistic capacities have not yet been included in the protocol.

Conclusion

'Participation in work' is considered as one of the major areas in life. Hearing difficulties are estimated to have a prevalence of about 3–10% in the labour force. For many workers with hearing impairment, the conditions at work are more challenging than for normally hearing colleagues. Common problems reported are lack of energy, fatigue, job safety, lack of control and environmental noise. Hearing impairment at work has been found to be associated with early retirement, unemployment and sick-leave due to stress-related complaints. It is argued that VEPs addressing the specific needs of workers with problems due to hearing impairment are necessary to maintain, facilitate or improve the employment situation of workers with hearing problems.

This chapter presents a recently developed VEP that is characterised by an integrated approach (occupational physician, otolaryngologist, audiologist, social worker/psychologist, speech-language pathologist). Experiences with the procedure among 86 workers are described and recommendations for future practice and research are discussed.

The programme is presented in relation to other enablement programmes that also advocate a multidisciplinary approach in order to accurately assess and manage the difficulties experienced by employees with hearing impairment.

9 Leisure and the wider social environment

Introduction

Various aspects of the individual's social environment have a number of factors in common from the standpoint of an individual with hearing difficulties and these will be considered first of all. Even before that, it is important to consider how frequently patients articulate such problems.

In addition, it is important to remember that pre-lingually Deaf people may have a different approach. In particular, Dye and Kyle (2001) found that 57% of Deaf people surveyed agreed with the statement 'Deaf people seem to have fewer interests than hearing people.'

Prevalence

In the initial study using the Problem Questionnaire in 500 patients attending a clinic for audiological enablement in London, 102 (20%) reported difficulties in meetings and 48 (10%) in the theatre and cinema (Barcham and Stephens, 1980). No mention was made of church attendance in the responses to that study, whereas in response to a verbally presented version of the questionnaire in Poland, 30% reported difficulties in church, 29% at meetings and 9% with the cinema and theatre (Golabek et al., 1989). This probably reflects different attitudes to religion in the two countries, and 48% of a subgroup of older Polish patients complained of problems in church.

In a general population study in which individuals were able to list only their greatest problem, only two out of 625 individuals reporting hearing difficulties specified problems with cinemas, theatres or chapel attendance (Stephens et al., 1991c). However, several other clinical studies (e.g. Lormore and Stephens, 1994) found some 8–10% of patients reporting 'avoidance of church, theatre, cinema, meetings' with fewer such complaints listed by their significant others. Finally, when an attempt was made to split such responses to the Life Effects questionnaire into *activity limitations* and *participation restrictions*, 21 leisure-related responses from 100 patients were classified as participation restrictions and six as activity limitations. Of these, 16 concerned 'community life' and 11 'recreation and leisure' (Stephens et al., 2001).

Many studies have shown, however, that difficulties with the television and radio are amongst the most commonly reported (e.g. Stephens and Zhao, 1996), and these will be considered in more detail later. Complaints in these domains appear to be largely independent of the severity of the hearing impairment (Zhao et al., 1997).

In a quantitative study of older people, Karlsson-Espmark *et al.* (2002) included two statements in this domain: 'I avoid going to the theatre and cinema' and 'I enjoy listening to music'. They found only small differences between those with and without hearing impairments, which were significant only among their female respondents. The only significant effect which they showed was in the response to the statement 'I enjoy sounds in nature', with which over 75% of hearing impaired male respondents disagreed. The result for the females was also significant.

Ringdahl and Grimby (2000) studied patients with severe to profound hearing impairment using the Nottingham Health Profile. They found no significant difference from a hearing control group in terms of 'holidays and hobbies', although those with hearing impairments were significantly more likely to report that their 'social life' was affected. However, the impact on 'holidays and hobbies' was significantly greater in those with the most severe hearing impairment, the older respondents and those with additional impairments.

Solitary versus interactive pastimes

This raises the general question as to the type of leisure activities favoured by the individual, whether they are solitary or whether they involve interaction with other people. It is a question which covers all aspects of leisure activities from hobbies to religious practices. This includes whether they participate in such activities with family, friends or other people as opposed to something which they do by themselves.

It may be argued that those involving the least interaction with other people will be the least affected by any hearing impairment, although this is not to deny that even many solitary pastimes entail an auditory input, so may be affected by such an impairment. This will apply particularly to people whose interests are listening to music, the radio and birdwatching, where they may have problems distinguishing and localising various birdsongs and calls. It seems probable that some people with hearing difficulties specifically seek solitary activities, although there is a dearth of evidence to support such an assumption.

The role of leisure

For people of working age, leisure activities provide an opportunity to relax and 'recharge their batteries', as well as providing an opportunity to reinforce their relationships with family and friends. Various studies have shown that leisure activities help working-age people cope with stress using both challenging leisure activities and passive/recuperative activities, although the role of different activities has been shown to be complex (Trenberth and Drewe, 2002, 2005).

Among retired people, while there is a tendency to report that leisure activities decline with increasing age, much of that may depend on the definition of such activities. Indeed, most older people participate in a variety of leisure activities, both solitary and interactive.

While there has been no identifiable work on the role of leisure activities in coping with hearing difficulties, studies on the development of dementia have indicated that activities such as reading, playing board games, dancing and playing musical instruments are associated with a reduced risk of developing the condition (Verghese *et al.*, 2003). Likewise, physical leisure activities are associated with a lower mortality (Kujala *et al.*, 1998) and leisure activities as a whole facilitate coping following traumatic injuries and the onset of chronic illness (Hutchinson *et al.*, 2003). However, in terms of their influencing the quality of life, it appears that the satisfaction with such activities plays the most important role (Lloyd and Auld, 2002).

Such sources of enjoyment and their identification are particularly important for people with hearing impairment. This must always be considered as Strawbridge *et al.* (2000) and Wallhagen *et al.* (1996) found that people with moderate to severe hearing impairment and older people were less likely to enjoy their free time than their hearing peers. From the point of view of any enablement process, the important point is to find what hobbies or other pastimes the individual enjoys and to encourage them to develop those interests in the directions which will be feasible given their hearing impairment and all relevant interventions. Attempting to encourage the development of new interests, which might be feasible with their hearing impairment, in the absence of enthusiasm from the patient is likely to be counterproductive. However, that does not necessarily preclude suggesting possible activities in a non-directive manner.

In this context, the opportunities for indulging any pleasurable interests in an individual manner can be explored. Thus, for those who enjoy exercise and attend sports facilities for this, the possibility of equivalent exercise in terms of running, cycling, swimming or even the purchase of exercise machines can be considered. Music and film fans can be encouraged to think more about home entertainment in this way and other interactive interests could be focused on one-to-one activities in acoustically friendly surroundings.

Opportunities for entertainment and leisure

Such an approach does not preclude the individual's involvement with broader aspects of public entertainment in cinemas, theatres and sports stadiums. However, some of these are more conducive than others to people with hearing difficulties, offering facilities to compensate for their problems. In this respect, the availability of loop systems, infrared devices, subtitling and visual reinforcement of any acoustical stimulus through large screens can be critical in making such performances more available and enjoyable for people with such hearing difficulties.

Where such facilities do not exist, it is very much the responsibility of both hearing professionals and people with hearing difficulties to lobby for their introduction. Indeed, many countries have legislation which promotes or at least facilitates such equalities of access for people with a range of disabilities.

Even group activities such as card or board games, participation in chamber music, lifelong learning courses, council or committee meetings can be facilitated by a combination of good personal amplification combined with the use of suitably quiet, non-reverberant environments for such activities. The use of personal loop systems or FM radio systems linked to appropriately placed microphones can be invaluable in these circumstances.

Participation in certain activities such as contact sports may, however, present more problems for enthusiasts with hearing difficulties, as they generally preclude the use of personal amplification. These are, to some extent, being addressed by the formation of sporting teams of people with hearing impairments, although these mainly involve

Deaf people fluent in sign language, which provides the means of communication in such events.

Community life

Within the World Health Organization's *International Classification of Impairments, Disabilities and Handicaps* (ICF; WHO, 2001) this comprises 'engaging in all aspects of community social life, such as engaging in charitable organizations, service clubs or professional social organizations'. The three principal categories specified are 'informal associations', 'professional associations' and 'ceremonies'.

Informal associations and professional associations

These comprise groups of people with a common interest in local social activities or specific professional groups such as lawyers, ex-servicemen, doctors or teachers. Similar hearing problems will be encountered in all cases, particularly in terms of difficulties hearing in background noise and in reverberant situations, particularly when the competing noise is the speech of people other than those who the individual wants to hear.

Barcham and Stephens (1980) found that difficulties in such 'meetings' were listed spontaneously by some 20% of their clinic respondents, being the seventh most common category of response, with a moderate to severe rating. Similar overall results were found by Golabek *et al.* (1989) in a study in Poland, which, not surprisingly, showed that such difficulties were reported more than twice as commonly among working-age patients as among pensioners (38% vs 18%). An interesting, if not surprising, finding from the study by Tyler *et al.* (1983) was that while 5% of their hearing aid candidates reported problems in small meetings over 10% found large meetings difficult. The former was lower in hearing aid users, but problems in large meetings were no different between hearing aid candidates and hearing aid users.

Ways of reducing such problems can entail a combination of instrumental approaches, hearing tactics and acoustical changes to the environment. Good personal amplification with the bilateral fitting of hearing aids is the first approach in most cases. However, such bilateral fitting must be done on a case-by-case basis. Noble and Gatehouse (2006) found that, while the use of two aids gives significant benefit in terms of the ability to ignore competing sounds, it does not help in terms of separating two sounds.

To improve the signal/noise ratio in meetings, loop systems, FM radio systems or infrared systems may be used. While loop systems are relatively inexpensive and will help most hearing aid users, infrared and FM systems can provide better-quality sound and may be more applicable if a large number of the participants in such meetings experience hearing difficulties. From the standpoint of logistics, people with difficulties hearing in any meetings should discuss with the organisers the possibility of using a room or hall where such facilities are available.

Such an approach will also apply to the acoustics of the room. Thus, a room with soft, sound-absorbing furnishings with few hard surfaces, resulting in favourable reverberation times may solve many of the problems encountered by people with hearing difficulties without the expense of additional environmental aids.

Finally, the role of hearing tactics must be considered. An extraverted hearing impaired person may be prepared to inform the meeting publicly of their difficulties and how they may be mitigated. A shyer person may discuss their problems with the chairperson of the meeting, who can inform the other participants in a way not embarrassing to the person with hearing difficulties. In addition, people with hearing difficulties may position themselves with their back to the light and close to any potential key speakers at the meeting.

Ceremonies

Social ceremonies and other non-religious ceremonies such as civic marriages and award ceremonies are relatively infrequent events in most people's lives. They are subsequently unusual as a specific source of complaint, even though the difficulties experienced by people with hearing impairments at such events may be considerable. These may be addressed in ways similar to those concerning meetings, although it will be difficult in terms of any interventional hearing tactics.

It is therefore important that the person with hearing difficulties uses optimal amplification and makes clear their difficulties to the person organising the ceremony. Thus, ideally, it should be held in a facility with good acoustics, together with a loop system or alternative, so that the individual can participate to as great an extent as possible. If they are a key figure in the ceremony, such as a wedding, they will need to discuss with the organiser how the procedure of the ceremony can be made more accessible to them.

Recreation and leisure

This comprises a range of activities, which are listed in Table 9.1, that will present varying degrees of difficulties for those with hearing problems.

Play

This covers 'games and spontaneous recreation', such as chess, card games and other board games in adults. These will usually take place with friends or family of the person with hearing difficulties, who can usually ensure that the other players will be aware of their difficulties and that it will be possible to arrange for these to take place in a room with good acoustics.

Table 9.1 Areas of recreation and leisure based on the ICF.

ICF code	Area
d9200	Play
d9201	Sports
d9202	Arts and culture
d9203	Crafts
d9204	Hobbies
d9205	Socialising

Some problems may arise in the context of a bidding game, such as bridge, in which case the individual must make sure that their partner is familiar with their specific difficulties to be certain that the nuances of the bids are not missed. More of a problem may arise in the context of competitive card games, where the individual may find themselves in a large room with poor acoustics. If they have real difficulties coping there, and there are no alternative venues, it may be necessary to find a quiet alcove and arrange for their games to be played there. Alternatively, it may be necessary to restrict their games to smaller groups. The same may be true for gamblers, who may find it difficult to cope with large casinos and may need to find more intimate venues to indulge their interests.

Sports

Within this context, there is a considerable difference between various sports. Some, like most of athletics, are individual-based; others are team-based, sometimes involving physical contact. In the context of the open-ended reporting of difficulties, problems in sport are rarely found. Meehan *et al.* (2002) found some difficulties reported for hearing impaired teenagers not being able to use their hearing aids in such activities, particularly in swimming, where they were unable to hear their instructor. However, such reports came from the parents rather from the youngsters themselves, who tend to deny any real problems.

In contact team sports, such as rugby, football or Gaelic and American football, there can be real difficulties for any enthusiast with hearing problems as they are unable to hear calls or the referee without a hearing aid and it is potentially dangerous to wear such an aid, even with an in-the-canal fitting. The only way that this has been effectively addressed has been by the formation of Deaf teams, although that presupposes a critical mass of such hearing impaired enthusiasts in a particular area. However, despite this, Dye and Kyle (2001) found 56% of Deaf respondents agreeing with the statement 'Deaf people are less likely to take part in sports and games than hearing people.'

Hearing aids can be used in other open-air team sports which are not usually so violent, such as cricket, baseball and hockey, although it is a sensible precaution to use small in-the-ear aids to minimise any risks of trauma. For other team sports such as bowls, boules and archery, normal hearing aids and hearing tactics can be used. However, it is important to develop a specific alerting system with fellow participants to ensure that the individual can be made aware of any potential dangers.

Indoor team sports such as basketball may be more problematic, as indeed can such sports as squash and badminton. In those entailing only a few other participants, it is usually possible to use hearing aids or to develop a technique to communicate with the other players. However, in a large enclosed stadium, there can be more problems related to the poor signal/noise ratio, which cannot be adequately overcome by the use of hearing aids, so that where possible some visual signalling technique may be necessary.

In individual sports such as athletics, there are generally no problems if hearing aids are used. However, as Meehan *et al.*'s study (2002) shows, there may be difficulties with swimming, where it will be impossible to use hearing aids. Some form of visual signalling may be necessary, and it is essential that the individual is aware of the signal starting any race. The same will be true of individual contact sports like wrestling or boxing, where it is essential that the referee is aware of the individual's problems and so can indicate to them the end of rounds or any other intervention they may wish to make. Horse riding and other activities requiring the use of helmets may necessitate the use of small in-the-ear hearing aids. However, even with such an approach, the rider may be dependent on the horse's awareness of potential dangers (see Chapter 10).

Arts and culture

This area covers participation in or appreciation of fine arts or cultural events including the cinema, theatre, opera, concerts, museums and art galleries. In general, visits to art galleries and museums present no real problems for people with hearing difficulties. Theatre, opera, concerts and cinema may be a different matter.

In most studies using the open-ended reporting of problems, concerts and opera are not specified, and generally the cinema and theatre have been grouped together with a prevalence of reported difficulties of the order of 10% (Barcham and Stephens, 1980). These reported difficulties are more common in workers than pensioners (Golabek *et al.*, 1989) and among people of higher social classes (Stephens, 1987b). Tyler *et al.* (1983) found that problems in the theatre (9%) were more commonly reported than those in the cinema (2%) were and that the latter were more common among hearing aid users (4%) than among hearing aid candidates, possibly owing to the high sound levels experienced. Those complaining of difficulties hearing music ranged from 4–7% in hearing aid candidates, although Tyler *et al.* (1983) found that more hearing aid users (12%) complained of this problem.

Stephens *et al.* (2001), using the Life Effects questionnaire found that 10% of their respondents reported participation restrictions related to recreation and leisure, compared with 1% reporting activity limitations. The former described withdrawal from or reduction of such activities, whereas the latter described difficulties with such activities. In a qualitative study of older people, some 40% of men and 25% of women agreed with the statement 'I avoid going to the theatre and the cinema', although the figures for the male respondents with hearing difficulties did not differ significantly from those with no hearing problems (Karlsson-Espmark *et al.*, 2003).

Stephens and Meredith (1991b) found that 8% of hearing aid users reported benefits in the theatre, lectures or bingo and 3% that they were 'able to sit at the back in concerts'. Cochlear implant users rarely mentioned the theatre or cinema, but 13–18% reported benefits with listening to music (Tyler and Kelsay, 1990; Tyler, 1994; Stephens *et al.*, 2008). However, all three studies report that 7–8% of the respondents reported shortcomings with their implants in the context of music. Zhao *et al.* (2008) found that improved enjoyment of music post-implantation was a predictor of improved quality of life for many of their patients, although, interestingly, Bai and Stephens (2005), looking at group measures, found that the relationship was stronger in the first year after implantation than later. It is possible that, initially, they were happy to hear music at all, but later found the sound quality unsatisfactory.

For theatre and opera, in which amplification is not usually used by the performers, personal amplification together with the use of a loop or infrared system can be of great help. In addition, as many operas are now performed in their original languages, supratitles, giving the translation in one or more other languages and displayed above the stage, are helpful for people with hearing difficulties. In the absence of these, use of the written text or a synopsis, sometimes provided in the programmes, can improve

Figure 9.1 Sign indicating the availability of a loop system.

the individual's understanding of the proceedings. Less commonly, the theatre may provide simultaneous signing, particularly for plays of interest to Deaf people.

However, there will remain problems for some people whose speech recognition ability or musical discrimination ability is impaired. There can also be problems understanding the words of songs in the presence of background music. Without a copy of the score or the words of the song, this can reduce the enjoyment of any such performances. Similarly, the words of stand-up comedians whose catchphrase may be uttered softly or very rapidly may cause problems.

Much the same applies to concerts and live performances in which the external amplification system or the acoustics of the theatre or concert hall are poor, although, in these circumstances, loop or infrared systems can reduce the difficulties. If the listener is familiar with many of the songs, that can be less of a problem. Thus, listening to a CD of the performer on the individual's own hi-fi before going to the show may be helpful. The same can be true of orchestral performances and oratorios.

The cinema usually presents less of a problem, particularly when subtitling is available. In addition, many cinemas have loop systems, although these are sometimes restricted to limited areas, where the person may not want to sit. The presence of loop systems is usually indicated by the use of an established sign (Figure 9.1). In addition, most modern cinemas have good-quality sound systems that provide a loud, clear output, although the loudness itself may present a problem for some individuals with hyperacusis or with inadequately set output limitations on their hearing aids.

For film buffs for whom such cinemas still represent a problem, the development of good-quality DVD systems with a range of subtitles, even in the language of the film, can be a boon. However, it may detract from the enjoyment of going out with a partner, family or friends to the cinema.

Crafts and hobbies

These can include such activities as pottery, carpentry or knitting in the former case and metal detection, stamp collecting, hunting or flower arranging in the latter. Most of these pastimes present little in the way of hearing difficulties except, perhaps, when the individuals meet and interact with other people with similar interests. For metal detector enthusiasts special headphones with additional amplification may be necessary.

However, those involving exposure to potentially damaging noise can be more problematic. Thus, those involved in carpentry or metalwork will need hearing conservation advice with regards to the use of loud tools in order not to exacerbate their hearing problems. A range of other hobbies may result in damaging noise levels (Davis *et al.*, 1985) and some of these are shown in Table 9.2.

Table 9.2 Leisure activities entailing potentially damaging noise levels.

General leisure activity	Specific activities
Music	Discotheques
	Live amplified pop/rock music
	Earphone listening from personal cassette players, iPods etc.
	Classical music
Fireworks	
Sports guns	
Vehicles	Motor cycles
	Snowmobiles
Model aircraft	

For amateur musicians who develop a hearing impairment, there may be a problem, particularly if it is likely that the impairment can be due to excessive exposure to the music itself. While this is more common amongst those using amplified music, there is increasing evidence of classical musicians being affected (Sataloff, 1991; Meyer-Bisch, 2007). Counselling as to possible ways of reducing any potentially damaging noise exposure is essential, as is the use of personal noise protection. Indeed, there is now a range of musicians' earplugs, which provide flat attenuation, so protecting the perceived sound quality. In addition, in some cases, sound barriers may be placed in the orchestra, separating different groups of musicians. However, if the individual experiences considerable sound distortion, relatively little can be done to overcome this.

Hunting can be a particular problem. While the individual will want to use as good hearing as possible in order to hear their prey or signals from other hunters, they will also need protection from the noise of any firearm which they use. While there is hearing protection which can provide limitation of the excessive impulse noise involved while permitting conversation, such devices are more aimed in the context of people on a firing range who are not stalking their prey and who have relatively good hearing. The compromise between the need for such sensitive hearing and appropriate hearing protection is very difficult to achieve and such individuals should be steered as far as possible in the direction of other, less damaging pastimes. Hearing protectors which allow speech to be heard while providing protection against high-level impulsive noise may be of some help (Toppila and Starck, 2004). In addition, a change to hunting with crossbows or some form of trapping may be acceptable, although this is unlikely.

For those who enjoy flying or diving, care needs to be taken to reduce the likelihood of dysbarisms, which could aggravate any hearing impairment. This is particularly important if the individual has an upper respiratory tract infection; in which case, the person should avoid such activities.

Socialising

This is defined in ICF as 'engaging in informal or casual gatherings with others'. As such, it will usually entail meeting in small groups, although the environment in which such meetings take place can be very variable. Some may take place in quiet, low-reverberation environments, and others may not. The size of the group can vary and have an impact on the person with hearing difficulties.

This is reflected by the fact that Tyler *et al.* (1983) found 10% of respondents reporting problems with large meetings, but only 5% for small group meetings. Overall, some 20–30% of people report problems in groups, with similar results for cochlear implant candidates (Zhao *et al.*, 1997). The one patient category reporting such difficulties much more commonly are those with King-Kopetzky syndrome, among whom 56% report such problems (Zhao and Stephens, 1996a). Golabek *et al.* (1989), however, did find some 49% of their respondents reporting difficulties at social gatherings. This was significantly higher among those of working age than pensioners, and Stephens (1987b) found that such problems were more likely to be reported by those of higher social classes.

While a number of outcome studies show that cochlear implants are reported as helping in social activities by 17–26% of patients (e.g. Stephens *et al.*, 2008), they all show patients to consider the implants to be a shortcoming in group situations. This finding is also reflected in responses from hearing aid users (16%; Stephens and Meredith, 1991b). However, Bai and Stephens (2005) found little overall relationship between improvements in social life and those in rated quality of life following cochlear implantation.

Jones *et al.* (1987) asked their subjects with hearing impairments why they refused invitations to visit friends and found that the commonest reason was conversational difficulties, followed by 'being tired of conversation' and because they felt that the friends were not sympathetic to their hearing problems.

Hearing aids, together with hearing tactics, are likely to facilitate communication and socialisation in small groups in acoustically friendly environments, resulting in few residual problems. More noisy and reverberant situations are likely to be more problematic, particularly when most of the background noise is from different conversations of other people. In these circumstances, it may be necessary for the patient to encourage the others to move to a less noisy place, where they can have a conversation with a smaller group of their particular friends.

Religion and spirituality

This section comprises organised religion and spirituality. It is predominantly the former which will be affected by any hearing impairment. The latter consists of the implementation of beliefs, prayer and meditation, which are largely personal activities and independent of any hearing problems.

Religion is rarely mentioned in response to any open-ended questionnaires, although in Poland, Golabek *et al.* (1989) found that some 30% of responses mentioned it as being a problem, with 48% of pensioners and 16% of working people listing it. In Wales, with the Life Effects questionnaire (Stephens *et al.*, 2001), 4% of respondents listed *participation restrictions* (unable to take part in religious services) in the context of organised religion and 2% *activity limitations* (difficulty hearing in church/chapel).

The only mention of religion in terms of benefits from hearing aids or cochlear implants was found by Stephens and Meredith (1991b), with 13% of their respondents reporting their hearing aids to be helpful in church or chapel services. None of the respondents in cochlear implant studies in Sweden, the United States or Wales mentioned benefits in terms of religious practice.

In a study of severe to profound acquired hearing impairment in Belfast, Stewart-Kerr (1992) asked her subjects, 'What effect has your deafness had on your religious feelings and beliefs?' Thirty-one per cent reported that such beliefs were strengthened as opposed to 13% weakened. Forty-one per cent said that they felt this made their life better as opposed to 9% whose life was worse. Furthermore, this question loaded on a factor reflecting positive experiences associated with hearing impairment (Kerr and Cowie, 1997). However, in subsequent, open-ended, studies in Wales, religion was never mentioned as a positive experience (Stephens and Kerr, 2003).

Morgan-Jones (2001) reports that a high proportion of her study population with hearing impairment attended organised religious services compared with the general population and suggests that this was to do with the levels of social support offered. In addition, the concepts of fellowship versus solitude, the tradition, a feeling of belonging and the presence of loop systems were important.

Within many places of worship, there has been an awareness of hearing problems among the (often much older) worshippers for some time and many have installed loop systems in addition to microphones and loudspeakers. The latter may present problems in a number of buildings because of their reverberant characteristics, but the former can be particularly helpful for hearing aid users. FM radio or infrared systems can also be helpful, but are rarely used. Besides these, some churches have designated services for Deaf people with interpretation into sign language.

Some individual members of the Catholic Church may have difficulties in confessionals. The use of appropriate hearing aids can generally be helpful in this context, except for those with profound hearing impairments.

For private prayer, meditation and one-to-one interaction with the priest, there should be no real difficulties, provided that the patient has appropriate instrumentation and the priest is aware of the individual's hearing problems.

Human rights, political life and citizenship

This entails, in part, ensuring that the individual with hearing difficulties has the same rights and equality of opportunities as those with normal hearing. In addition, they should be able to participate in an active way in politics. In some respects, the first is dependent on the second, although hearing health care professionals should also be concerned about such rights to equal opportunities and their implementation.

In general, the question of equal opportunities for people with hearing disabilities should be enshrined in national law and covered in the United Nations Standard rules for the Equalisation of Opportunities for Persons with Disabilities (1993). However, local authorities and other owners of public places may not always be obliged under law to implement such legislation, or may not know how to implement it. In other cases, they may focus entirely on people with physical disabilities, such as wheelchair users and not consider those with sensory problems. In all circumstances, it is incumbent on both people with hearing impairments, either as individuals or via voluntary organisations, as well as on the professionals helping them to lobby the legislators to ensure that there is a legal framework and, more locally, to see that this is subsequently implemented.

In terms of participation in political life, people with hearing difficulties may have considerable problems hearing in council chambers, parliaments and even at local branch meetings of their particular political organisation. Particularly in local government in many countries, this can be a significant problem given that many councillors are older people.

Thus, in order for such people to play a full part in the activities of the organisation, they may need considerable support. While personal hearing aids can reduce the problem, as many of the rooms in which their meetings are held have poor acoustics, some augmentation of the signal/noise ratio is necessary. Usually, this can be achieved by the installation of a loop system and in other cases an FM or infrared system may be used. In addition, in order to overcome the poor clarity of the speech of some participants as well as the distortions inherent in their hearing impairment, reinforcement by as much printed matter as possible can be invaluable. Other hearing tactics can be used including positioning themselves so that they can clearly see the faces of important participants and, where necessary, by seeking clarification and help from officers of the council.

For those with the most severe problems, as in the case of Jack Ashley, a former MP in the Houses of Parliament, the text input from an electronic system such as Pallantype, with an operator listening closely to the proceedings, can be essential. Such an approach, in principle, is no different from having simultaneous interpreters in a multilingual parliament, such as that of the European Union. There is nothing to prevent a similar approach with a sign language interpreter for a Deaf councillor or legislator, should they be elected to such an office. This would reflect equal opportunities in practice.

Conclusion

Problems with leisure activities are less frequently reported than those concerned with work, education and family life. However, for many people, difficulties in this domain have a significant impact on their quality of life. There is a commonality of problems across different aspects of social and religious domains, dependent on the environmental circumstances and the number of people involved. Among leisure activities, sporting environments can result in particular problems, especially in the context of contact sports. Special arrangements may need to be made for people with severe hearing difficulties, although in certain cases this may not be possible. Particular care is also necessary for hobbies, such as hunting, that entail significant noise exposure in order to avoid any aggravation of the underlying hearing impairment. Changing to more solitary or acoustically friendly activities may be acceptable to some people, but not to others. Such acceptance must be encouraged when all other attempts to reduce the problems fail.

10 The process of enablement 1: Evaluation and decision-making

Introduction

The aim of this chapter is to provide an overview of the process of audiological enablement with cross-references to aspects of the process which are dealt with in detail in other chapters. It has five key sections, those of *evaluation, integration and decision making, short-term remediation, ongoing remediation* and *outcome assessment*, with subsequent decisions based on the results of those. This is summarised in Figure 10.1. A more detailed outline of the pathways within the enablement process is shown in Figure 10.2.

The remediation process is deliberately split into two components, with the short-term aspects being applicable to all individuals presenting to the process, and the ongoing remediation being applicable at length to those individuals with more complicated problems. This does not, however, preclude those with relatively straightforward problems from participating in at least part of the process, but their needs are likely to be met by a relatively short session.

Within the outcome assessment component, decisions have to be made by the patient and professional together as to what, if any, further action needs to be taken in light of the various measures. This may entail a return to the remediation process to meet any needs not adequately addressed, arrangements for a routine review either after a certain period or when the individual perceives that they have further problems, or the patient may decide that they want no further contact. The work that we have done with Louise Hickson (see the Appendix) has highlighted the fact that managing certain aspects of the patient's problems may highlight or even provoke further problems of which neither the patient nor the professional was aware before. The outcome assessment process needs to take such developments into consideration.

The evaluation process

The aim of this is to ensure that any remedial intervention is relevant, appropriate and acceptable to the individual seeking rehabilitative help. The process of evaluation may be accomplished in many different ways which are relevant to the aspect being evaluated and the facilities available for the evaluation.

Approaches to evaluation

The possible approaches which may be used come within the three broad categories of *observation*, *questioning* and *testing*. These approaches are shown in Table 10.1.

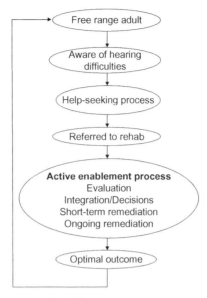

Figure 10.1 Summary of the process of enablement.

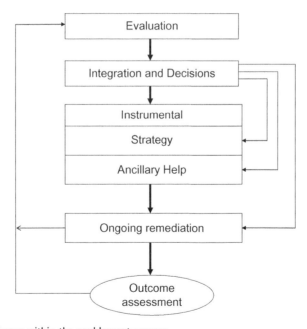

Figure 10.2 Pathways within the enablement process.

The particular approach to evaluation to be used will depend on the element of the evaluation process which is being evaluated, the nature of their problems and, to a lesser extent, the circumstances in which the evaluation is taking place. In addition, the nature of the particular evaluation will vary along the following dimensions:

Table 10.1 Approaches to evaluation.

Evaluation mode	Approaches
Observation	Direct
	Video-recorded
	Reports by family, friends and professionals
Questioning	Direct – Person to person
	– Significant others
	Questionnaires – Open-ended
	– Structured
	Questionnaires to significant others
	Computerised questioning
Testing	Subjective
	Objective

▨ Formal–Informal
▨ Systematic–Non-systematic
▨ Qualitative–Quantitative
▨ Binary–Multivariable
▨ Standardised–Non-standardised.

In every case, the approach used must be relevant to the enablement of the individual concerned.

Thus, a direct, informal, observation that the patient has absent or severely deformed auricles (pinnae) will have implications for their management. A more systematic formal observation prior to otoscopy may reveal minor auricular abnormalities, which can be of relevance to the particular hearing aid fitting to be undertaken.

Knowledge of sign language may be approached using a systematic binary question, 'Do you use any form of sign language?' If the answer is 'No', that will be the end of this aspect of the evaluation process. However, if the answer is 'Yes', further direct questioning may be undertaken to determine the type(s) of sign language known, and this may be followed by non-standardised testing of the individual's fluency in that sign language and, perhaps, standardised testing of their receptive abilities for that sign language system, using video-recorded test material.

The hearing itself will be assessed using a combination of approaches ranging from informal, systematic, qualitative, binary non-standardised clinical testing followed by different forms of audiometry. The latter will be formal, systematic, quantitative, multivariable and standardised. However, the clinical approach may be all that is possible under certain circumstances, for example if the patient is seriously ill or intellectually disabled; but, carefully performed, this may still provide useful information to guide the necessary approach to amplification. The overall components of the evaluation process are shown in Figure 10.3.

While some elements of this process may appear irrelevant to certain patients, for example *manual communication* in an older person with a moderate hearing impairment, it is important to consider all aspects, even if only to rapidly dismiss them in the context of the individual concerned. In that way, elements which may have a bearing on the successful enablement of the individual will not be missed.

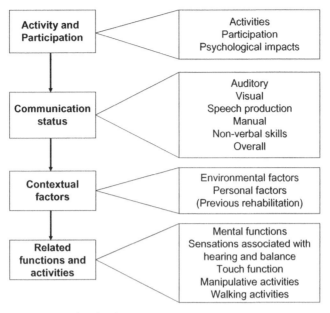

Figure 10.3 The components of evaluation.

Activity and participation

This section essentially addresses an assessment of the problems that the individual experiences as a result of their hearing impairment. It is obviously the key area in terms of defining the enablement that is necessary.

Traditionally, this is addressed by simply asking the patient in a clinical interview what their problems may be. Unfortunately, many are overawed and anxious during such a session and find it difficult to articulate such problems. In addition, they may think of their immediate difficulties and overlook key problems.

In this context we have found it helpful to send the patient a Problem Questionnaire (Barcham and Stephens, 1980; Stephens, 1980; Tyler *et al.*, 1983) with their appointment letter asking them to write down their problems. It was worded as follows: 'Please make a list of the difficulties which you have as a result of your hearing loss. List them in order of importance, starting with the biggest difficulties. Write down as many as you can think of.' This gives the patient a chance to reflect on their problems and to discuss them with significant others prior to their appointment. It also helps them to focus on their problems rather than on other preconceptions of what the clinician might want to know, when they arrive for their appointment.

Several analyses (e.g. Stephens, 1987b; Stephens *et al.*, 2001) indicate, however, that responses to this question tend to focus on *activities* rather than on *participations* and *psychological impacts*, which are more key drivers to help-seeking (Stephens *et al.*, 1991a). This led us to change over to the Life Effects questionnaire, worded, 'Please make a list of the effects your hearing problems have on your life. Write down as many as you can think of.'

Using this measure, as shown in Figure 10.4, significantly fewer responses listing impairments ($p < 0.01$) and significantly more listing participation restrictions, environmental and personal contextual factors (all $p < 0.001$) were found. There was no

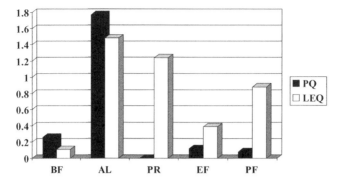

Figure 10.4 Mean number of responses per patient in each ICF (WHO, 2001) category on the x axis. (Black bars indicate responses to the Problem Questionnaire, white to the Life Effects questionnaire.)

significant difference in the number of activity limitations listed using the two measures (Stephens *et al.*, 2001).

When the clinician sees the patient, they can request clarification of particular aspects of the responses, such as 'hearing speech' by enquiring as to whether this was under any particular circumstances or with any particular person. What they should *not do* is to force the patient to tell the clinician what they think they want to hear by specifying particular circumstances, as this will change the concept from one expressed by the patient to one fitting the audiologist's preconceived ideas. In other words, the response evoked becomes a semeion rather than a symptom.

As well as being used to guide the enablement process, the ultimate patient-generated response can then be fed into the first stage of appropriate outcome measures such as the Client-Oriented Scale of Improvement (COSI; Dillon *et al.*, 1997) or the Glasgow Hearing Aid Benefit Profile (GHABP; Gatehouse, 1999).

In addition, by asking the patient to rate the importance of each problem using a visual analogue scale, it is possible for the patient to generate their own baseline for relevant outcome measures, which can be applied repeatedly in long-term interventions (e.g. Bai and Stephens, 2005). While earlier studies (e.g. Barcham and Stephens, 1980) had asked patients to list their problems in order of importance, starting with the biggest difficulty, as a way of assessing their relative severity, in practice this was found to be an unreliable measure and this approach was discontinued.

A wide range of structured questionnaires asking about specific hearing difficulties have been described over the years, dating back to the Hearing Handicap Scale (High *et al.*, 1964). Many have been reviewed by Bentler and Kramer (2000) and by Noble (1998). They may be useful in highlighting specific areas of difficulty, although the majority of questionnaires predominantly focus on speech communication. Some also include impairments, such as localisation, detection of sounds and identification/discrimination (Kramer *et al.*, 1996), and disabilities, including aversiveness of loud sounds (Cox and Alexander, 1995). Gatehouse and Noble (2004) suggest an extension towards other aspects than speech relevant in hearing, such as 'effort' and 'segregation of sounds'.

Nevertheless, these structured types of questionnaires tend to approach the patient's problems from the standpoint of the professional rather than of the patient. In many there is terminological confusion as they use terms such as 'Handicap and Disability' in ways which bear little relationship to an ICF-based approach. In addition, there is little emphasis on the psychological effects of the hearing impairment, although some measures, such as the Hearing Measurement Scale (Noble and Atherley, 1970a), do have useful sections on the 'emotional response' to hearing impairment. Generic health-related quality of life measures (e.g. SF-36, EuroQol) seem to be insensitive to the specific communicative and emotional difficulties experienced by individuals with hearing impairment.

Communication status

This is a key area of the evaluation, focusing essentially on the raw materials with which the audiologist will have to build in the process of enabling patients to achieve what is important for them. It focuses on different and relevant aspects of their existing sensory and communication functions. In each case, the evaluation will concentrate on the aspects of these which will have a direct bearing on the enablement process.

Auditory
The elements of this are shown in Table 10.2, together with their relevance to enablement.

There is a range of measures which fall in each of these categories. Thus, as measures of sensitivity, while pure tone audiometry is almost universally used in this context, it generally only measures at octave or half-octave intervals, and may not indicate features of the audiogram which may be important to sophisticated hearing aid fitting. Arguably, a sweep-frequency approach, such as the Békésy audiometry or Audioscan (Meyer-Bisch, 1996), would be more relevant in this context. They can be particularly relevant for defining 'peakiness' of audiograms, which, if ignored, may lead to the patient rejecting their amplification because of tolerance problems.

In addition, as mentioned earlier, certain individuals (e.g. those with intellectual disabilities) may be unable or unwilling to cooperate with formal audiometry, and so either carefully performed clinical tests and/or auditory evoked response measures or otoacoustic emissions may be used in this situation.

Table 10.2 Relevant elements of audition.

Element	Example	Relevance
Auditory acuity	Pure tone threshold	Broad measure of impairment and indicator of type of approach necessary
Dynamic range	Uncomfortable loudness level (ULL)	Indicates gain and maximum output for hearing aid fitting
Speech recognition	PB word list	Governs selection of instrumentation type and approach
Binaural interaction	Masking level difference	Predictor of benefit of bilateral fitting
Other signal processing abilities	To be defined	Of more relevance as signal processing techniques become better tailored to the individual
Dynamic range for electroauditory stimulation	Threshold and ULL	Appropriate fitting of cochlear implants

In addition, there is the question of bone-conduction thresholds, which have little bearing on the majority of hearing aid fittings, provided that uncomfortable loudness levels (ULLs) are measured. However, in those patients with chronic suppurative otitis media or congenital atresia of the external acoustic meatus, they may have a vital role in defining the appropriate fitting of bone-conduction or bone-anchored hearing aids.

Traditionally, the dynamic range is measured using the ULL in conjunction with the pure tone threshold. The ULL is generally measured with pure tone stimuli using a technique similar to that for determining the pure tone audiometry (PTA). However, sweep-frequency testing may be used with Békésy audiometry or the ULL may be determined using broad-band noise or even speech stimuli. Its particular importance is to ensure that any hearing aid output does not exceed the patient's ULL and so lead to the rejection of the hearing aid fitting.

For gain determination, what is important is the patient's most comfortable listening level (MCL) or the range of comfortable levels. Unfortunately, measures of these show great intra- as well as intersubject variability (e.g. Stephens *et al.*, 1977) and a reasonable approach is to take the MCL as about two-thirds of the range (in dB) between the threshold and the ULL (Keller, 1971; Lundborg *et al.*, 1973).

Speech recognition has its advocates as a more 'natural' test of hearing. However, its relevance to enablement decisions is somewhat limited. Two key areas in which it impacts on such management decisions are concerned with unilateral hearing aid fittings and the decision as to whether a cochlear implant may be more relevant for the patient than a powerful hearing aid.

Even when hearing aids are provided free of charge, almost one half of potential hearing aid candidates prefer to have one hearing aid rather than two (Stephens *et al.*, 1991b). Furthermore, on a long-term follow-up, about a third of those originally opting for two aids reverted to a unilateral fitting (Gianopoulos and Stephens, 2002).

When given the choice as to which ear to be fitted, most individuals prefer to use a hearing aid on their worse hearing ear. This is reasonable when the speech recognition score in that ear is good. However, when the speech recognition score is markedly better in the better ear, the patient should be encouraged to use an aid on that ear rather than the poorer hearing ear.

The other management decision in which a measure of speech recognition is important is the decision as to whether to fit a patient with powerful hearing aids or with a cochlear implant. When single-channel cochlear implants were first developed, the presence of any significant speech recognition was regarded as a contraindication to implantation. However, as signal processing in multichannel implants has improved, the criterion has become more lax with the demonstration that those patients with some unaided speech recognition of up to 30–40% are likely to perform better with an implant than with hearing aids. This is obviously only one factor, together with general health, personal and financial conditions, which may influence such a decision.

In all cases, such testing can be performed using either phonetically balanced word lists or sentence lists. In the context of cochlear implant candidates, it is important to consider the differences between the results obtained with the two techniques, given the higher redundancy of the test material in the sentence lists.

Bilateral hearing aid fitting will also be influenced by the individual's bilateral signal-processing abilities. While measures of masking level difference have been shown to provide a useful indication of such abilities, no tests have reached the level of being incorporated into regular clinical practice. Markides (1977b), in his study on bilateral hearing aids, found that an audiometric measure of diplacusis binauralis provided a good predictor of bilateral hearing aid benefit. While such audiometric measures, in which a frequency match of the pitch in the two ears is performed, are rarely used clinically, the use of a 512 Hz tuning fork presented alternately to the two ears, with the patient asked whether the pitch is the same or different, may provide a useful pointer.

At the time of writing, while the current generation of digital hearing aids has far more potential capacity for signal processing than is actually used, there is little evidence to indicate useful psychoacoustical tests that could be used to predict a particular optimal signal-processing strategy for the individual patient. Undoubtedly, this will come in the not-too-distant future when certain measures will be found relevant to specific strategies.

Finally, the dynamic range for electroacoustical stimulation is important in the programming of cochlear implants. While it is normally performed following implantation, in patients suspected of having a very limited dynamic range, such testing may be performed using a transtympanic electrode placed on to the bony promontory, prior to any surgical intervention. The normal measures used will be threshold and ULLs for stimuli of different frequencies throughout the speech range.

Visual

This may be regarded as having two main components: first, visual acuity and discrimination ability and, second, speechreading (lipreading) ability. In addition, the concurrent use of spectacles, which may have an influence, can be considered here.

Visual acuity, normally measured using Snellen charts, can have an influence in two ways, of which the most important will be distance vision and its effect on speechreading. In addition, close vision can be important when it comes to making adjustments to hearing aids, although with the advent of programmed signal-processing hearing aids this has become less relevant.

A number of studies have indicated that the degree of visual acuity is one of the most important determinants of speechreading performance (e.g. Hardick *et al.*, 1970). This is particularly important in the case of those with a hearing impairment affecting mainly the high frequencies, which are particularly important for discriminating fricatives. In turn, such fricatives are reasonably easy to discriminate visually, and such visual cues reduce the impact of the hearing impairment.

In clinical practice it is relatively easy to screen for any significant visual impairment combining some questioning about recent tests of vision and renewal of spectacles, coupled with a simple check using a Snellen chart or equivalent in the clinic room. If the patient's vision is poor and not adequately corrected, they should be encouraged to consult an optometrist or ophthalmologist. If the person has spectacles but rarely uses them, emphasis on the importance of regular use will be essential in terms of facilitating their receptive communication.

Some patients with hearing difficulties will also suffer from more severe visual disorders such as retinitis pigmentosa, glaucoma or macular degeneration and may be designated as having an irreversible visual impairment. This will have important implications for the management of the person concerned in terms of the implementation of the enablement process, including the discussion of expectations and emphasising the use and benefits of bilateral amplification.

The physical interaction between spectacles and hearing aids was more important at the time when both hearing aids and spectacle arms were more bulky. Indeed, at one time some patients would use such spectacles with the hearing aid mechanism

Table 10.3 Screening test of speechreading.

Self-rating (%)	
Digits	**Questions**
561	What did you have for breakfast?
312	Have you had any coffee today?
479	When do you have your lunch?
854	Do you take sugar in your tea?
906	Where do you do your shopping?

(*Source:* after Stephens, 1987.)

built into the arm of the device, together with clear lenses, as a way of disguising the fact that what they had was a hearing aid. Attitudes towards the stigma of spectacles were less negative than towards that associated with hearing aids. Now, however, hearing aids built into or fixed to spectacle frames are rarely used, although experiments with a multi-microphone array (Verschuure *et al.*, 2007) may lead to some renewal of interest in such devices.

With more modern spectacle arms together with smaller postaural hearing aids, there is less difficulty associated with fitting both to the same ear or ears. In certain cases, however, it will be necessary to consider in-the-ear hearing aids, particularly when the pinna is small and closely bound to the side of the head.

Speechreading ability can be assessed in a range of different ways. There is, however, often a great discrepancy between self-rated ability and that measured in a variety of tests. It can be useful, therapeutically, to ask the individual to rate their ability using a visual analogue or other scale and then confront them with the discrepancy between such a rating and the test results. Most commonly, individuals will state that they have no or very poor speechreading ability, whereas the tests will indicate moderately good performance.

A simple screening test of speechreading is shown in Table 10.3. While it obviously has an evaluative component, it furthermore serves to convince the patient that they are in fact able to perceive speech signals visually.

Initially, the patient is asked to rate their speechreading ability either on a scale from 0 to 100 or using a visual analogue scale. They are next given groups of three digits to repeat and most are able to score 12 or more out of 15 digits correctly. That gives them confidence in their ability to speechread when they are given the questions, shown on the right part of the table. The context of these is introduced as 'questions about food, meals and shopping', and the patient is asked to guess even if they are unsure. This screening test is based on the earlier work of Skamris (1974), and may be followed by some sentences without context either by speechreading alone or, in people with severe or profound hearing impairment, audiovisually.

As well as giving the clinician an idea of the patient's speechreading ability and providing a therapeutic boost to the patient, this test may provide information as to what more detailed, systematic tests may be indicated in those patients who are particularly dependent on speechreading.

Formal tests of speechreading range from tests of phoneme recognition up to continuous discourse. Some examples of these are shown in Table 10.4.

The choice of test depends on the communication needs of the patient and the type of intervention(s) being considered. Such testing will be particularly important in

Table 10.4 Types of speechreading tests.

Test group	Example
Consonant confusion tests	/aba/, /apa/, /ata/
Vowel confusion tests	/bid/, /bad/, /bud/
Word recognition tests	Boothroyd (Boothroyd, 1968); NU6 (Tillman and Carhart, 1966)
Sentence recognition tests	BKB sentences (Bench and Bamford, 1979); CID sentence tests (Hirsh *et al.*, 1952)
Connected Discourse Tracking	(de Filippo and Scott, 1976)

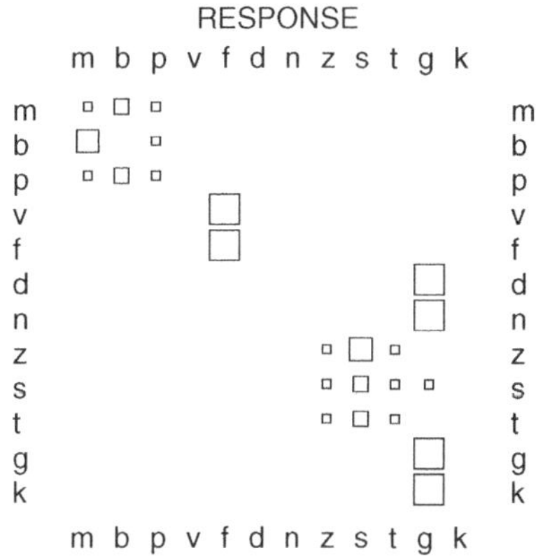

Figure 10.5 VCV confusion matrix in a patient following brainstem trauma.

people with severe communication difficulties. Thus, it may be necessary to delineate the problems experienced by an individual with specific difficulties in terms of what consonants and vowels they are able to recognise and which pairs or clusters they confuse with each other using vowel–consonant–vowel (VCV) confusion tests. An example of such a plot from a patient with brainstem trauma is shown in Figure 10.5 in which the responses are broadly correct in terms of place of articulation, but confused with regards to voicing and nasality.

Similar plots can be made for vowel tests, although in practice they are used less frequently. Likewise, word recognition tests are infrequently used as they provide little information which cannot be obtained from sentence lists and VCV tests.

Balanced sentence lists are the most frequently used in assessing speechreading ability before, during and after the enablement process. Those used in an American context date from the Utley test (1946) and are discussed by Hipskind (2007), who also lists some of the more important tests. Within the United Kingdom, focus has largely been on the BKB test (Bench and Bamford, 1979) with a standardised recording and corrections for list and practice effects presented by Foster *et al.* (1993). Overall, such measures performed carefully with well-structured tests provide a valuable overall assessment of the speechreading, auditory and audiovisual abilities of the patient. There may, however, be some problems with multiple repeat measures, as in some patients with cochlear implants, in which case Connected Discourse Tracking comes into its own. A further problem, common to all low-redundancy tests of speech,

Table 10.5 Elements of speech production skills relevant to audiological enablement.

Impact	Aspect of speech
May be affected by both pre-lingual and post-lingual hearing impairment	Phonology Pragmatics
Normally affected only by pre-lingual hearing impairment	Morphology Syntax
Effects on the enablement process but essentially independent of hearing impairment	First language Dialect Lexicon

is in the context of testing a patient for whom the test is not their maternal language, a matter highlighted by Plant *et al.* (1980) in the context of the Utley test.

The Connected Discourse Tracking technique was developed by DeFilippo and Scott (1978) and, as currently used, entails the tester reading a text within the vocabulary range and interests of the patient. This is presented a phrase at a time; if the patient is unable to correctly repeat it, the reader repeats it with increasing cues. This is normally performed over 3–5 minutes and the patient is scored in terms of the number of words per minute correctly identified. This may be presented visually, auditorily or audiovisually, from the same text and repeated on as many occasions as may be necessary during and after the enablement process. Thus, the individual's progress may be plotted using texts which are broadly equivalent but without the need to repeat the same test.

Speech and language production skills

This section is concerned with those aspects of speech and language production that are directly related to hearing impairment and its management rather than those, such as *specific language impairment* or *stammering*, which are essentially independent of any hearing impairment. The elements of speech which are particularly relevant in this context are shown in Table 10.5. We consider first those that may affect anyone with a hearing impairment, followed by those essentially affected only in people with pre-lingual hearing impairments and finally those background effects important to the enablement process. It is important to assess any speech production deficits, which can normally be done informally during a clinical interview. In addition, the background effects (first language etc.) can be tapped by a few relevant questions, coupled with local knowledge on the part of the clinician.

Phonology

The phonological aspects of speech are those concerned with the sound pattern of the language, and these may show relatively minor and very variable changes in people with late-onset hearing impairment. In particular, in people with bilateral high-frequency hearing impairment, there can be difficulties in the pronunciation of voiceless consonants such as /s/sh/f/th/ when the speaker has no acoustical feedback with regard to the sounds that they are producing. In addition, they may have further problems when they are learning a new language, which may include phonemes not found in their maternal language.

Pre-lingually hearing impaired individuals will generally have much more severe problems in producing most of the spoken language. This will depend much on the severity of their hearing impairment, the educational approach they have received and the instrumentation (e.g. hearing aids and cochlear implants) they use. Their exposure to good-quality speech from their parents and family at a young age can also be particularly important here.

Pragmatics

Pragmatics comprises the social use of language. Thus, the use of the same word or expression can carry very different meanings according to what the speaker wishes to convey. This will depend both on the context and on the intonation used. For example, 'He is going out' can be a simple statement, a question or a command, according to the intonation used.

A severe hearing impairment affecting particularly the low to mid-frequencies can interfere with the individual's ability to monitor their production of such intonation and may lead to the listener receiving misleading information. In addition, most pre-lingually hearing impaired people are unlikely to have learnt such intonation and their significance in the first instance, and hence find it difficult or impossible to produce the relevant nuances in their speech.

Morphology

This concerns the lexical and grammatical structure of words. Most people with hearing impairment have no difficulty with lexical morphology. However, grammatical endings may present a problem for those with pre-lingual hearing impairment. An example of the sort of speech production problems which a pre-lingually hearing impaired person may experience in this respect is differentiation between the production of 'a wick*ed* man' and 'a leak*ed* document'.

Syntax

Syntax is the grammatical structure of the language. Again, apart from patients whose hearing impairment is associated with a stroke or other severe brain damage, this will be essentially normal in those with a late-onset hearing impairment. In many sign languages (e.g. BSL, ASL), the syntax is different from the local spoken language. This may lead to confusions on the part of pre-lingually hearing impaired people, who are primarily sign language users. The development of syntax in pre-lingually hearing impaired children who are cochlear implant users broadly follows that of hearing children, although they may have problems with more complex sentence structures (Stephens, 2006).

First language

In any rehabilitative intervention, it is essential that the therapist is aware of the first language of the patient and arranges, as far as possible, for any enablement to be offered in that language. In the case of immigrant populations this may not be possible; in such situations, it is essential that an experienced interpreter, ideally from outside the family, be present throughout the process.

Many people who have immigrated to a new country may be able to cope with the language of their new environment as long as their hearing is good. However, there will be less redundancy present for them in the new language, so that when they subsequently develop a hearing impairment they can experience far greater problems, both productive and receptive, in that language.

Dialect

Dialectal differences are generally less important, but can still be very relevant for the acceptance and lack of stigmatisation of the individual within their society. It is therefore important for the therapist to bear this in mind when providing any communication training for the individual concerned.

Lexicon

This comprises the range of the vocabulary and specific aspects of the vocabulary used by and important for the particular patient. Thus, for a meteorologist the use and recognition of climatic terms will be particularly important, whereas a computer programmer will have a very different lexicon. It is essential that this be taken into account in the planning of any communication training.

Manual communication

The knowledge and use of various types of sign language systems is very important to many patients with severe to profound hearing impairment, particularly those with pre-lingual impairment. The attitudes towards sign language vary considerably between different individuals, even among those born with severe hearing impairments. It is, however, important to obtain some idea of the individual's attitude towards such systems as well as their knowledge and skills in any particular system. The assessment of the individual's ability in any particular sign language system will normally be assessed informally, ideally by a member of the department who has good signing skills themselves. Formal testing, as reviewed by Hatfield (1982) and by Singleton and Supalla (2003), may be used in a small minority of cases, when considered relevant. While most such tests are designed for use with children and college students, they can generally be applied to adults as well.

The different types of sign language are summarised in Table 10.6. Within this table, we present those which constitute a supplement to speechreading and audiovisual communication and are the most relevant to people with acquired hearing impairments, autonomous sign language systems with their own syntax and, finally, modi-

Table 10.6 Types of sign language.

System type	Examples
Supplements to speechreading and audiovisual communication	Danish mouth–hand system
	Cued speech
Supplements to both speechreading and generic sign language systems	Finger spelling
Autonomous sign language systems	British Sign language (BSL)
	French Sign language (LSF)
	American Sign language (ASL)
Sign language systems based on the syntax of the local spoken language	Signed English (USA)
	Sign Supported English (UK)
	Paget Gorman
Informal gesture systems (Home signs)	Developed within the family or community

fied or independently generated sign languages that use the syntax of the local spoken language.

Supplements to speechreading

The mouth–hand system was developed in Denmark to help individuals with a severe acquired hearing impairment to help them recognise aspects of speech which they cannot see on the speaker's lips, particularly differentiating voiced, voiceless and nasal consonants (Forchammer, 1903). For the speech to be understood, the listener/ viewer needs to be speechreading at the same time.

Cued speech, a rather more complex system, was developed in the United States (Cornett, 1967) primarily for use in the education of hearing impaired children, although it has been used with adults with late-onset hearing impairment as well. With improvements in amplification systems and cochlear implantation, the use of both cued speech and the mouth–hand system has declined in recent years.

Finger spelling

Finger spelling methods differ between countries, but the general principle behind them is to supplement traditional sign language systems by providing signs for real names and other words for which the sign may be unknown to the signer or to the receiver. British finger spelling uses both hands, whereas the American and French systems are essentially based on one hand.

In addition, finger spelling can be used with patients and their significant others to supplement speechreading in contexts where the patient has difficulties. An example of this is the differentiation between 'pan', 'ban' and 'man', which may be facilitated by teaching both the significant other and the patient the signs for /p/, /b/ and /m/ respectively, to be used when there is any confusion. Most people find this more acceptable than using a formal system like the mouth–hand system.

Autonomous sign language systems

These have been developed in Deaf communities over the centuries and have become modified and standardised, particularly through the influence of schools for the Deaf over the past two hundred years (Armstrong and Wilcox, 2003). Those found in different countries (e.g. the United Kingdom, France) differ markedly from each other, but there exist similarities between some, largely derived from the influences of one country on Deaf education in another. Thus, there are considerable similarities between French (*Langue des signes française*, or LSF) and American Sign Language (ASL).

While the great majority of users of such systems have pre-lingual hearing impairment, there has been increasing interest among both hearing people and some people with acquired hearing impairment in learning such systems, although knowledge of and fluency in the local sign language is not always synonymous with acceptance by the Deaf community. There have been cases, such as in Martha's Vineyard in the United States (Groce, 1985) and Bengkala in Bali (Branson *et al.*, 1996), where, resulting from a significant proportion of the community having a congenital hearing impairment, the majority of the hearing people also sign.

Sign language systems based on the syntax of the local spoken language

A number of efforts have been made by educationalists to make the syntax of sign language identical to that of the local spoken language. The aim of this was to help the children in their understanding and acquisition of the spoken language. This resulted in the development of signed English and Sign Supported English by modification of ASL and BSL respectively. In addition, a few completely new systems such as the Paget Gorman system (Craig, 1973) were developed. However, in recent years, the approach has been more to stick to the traditional sign language systems and encourage the development of true bilingualism (signing and spoken language).

Informal gesture systems (home signs)

These have been developed within families and communities, particularly where there have been a number of Deaf people. They, almost certainly, date back to early historical times and some of these, such as that used in Martha's Vineyard, have contributed to the development of formal autonomous sign languages (e.g. Armstrong and Wilcox, 2003). In isolated communities and families excluded from Deaf education, these continue to appear and it is important for the clinician to be aware of such systems within individual families.

Non-verbal communication

This is generally taken to refer to the aspect of communication between two or more people that occurs independently of the use of words, either spoken or signed. It can, however, be used to facilitate speech and sign language communication. In particular, it is used to express emotions and interpersonal attitudes. In addition, Argyle (1988) argues, it is used for self-presentation of one's personality and for rituals, such as greetings.

Non-verbal messages may be presented through body language or posture, facial expression, gesture, eye contact and choice of clothing, hairstyles etc. The meaning of such forms of communication differ somewhat from culture to culture and most people with acquired hearing impairment will be familiar with the various implications of its different elements. However, Rustin and Kuhr (1989) ague that certain paralinguistic elements of communication, such as the use of silence (Jaworski, 1993), emotional tone and timing of speech may degrade following the loss of auditory feedback in individuals with acquired hearing impairment. This may present a problem for some individuals with pre-lingual hearing impairment, although it is usually an integral part of their communication styles.

More particularly, it may present a problem for immigrants who develop hearing impairment, and who may be familiar with a body language with meanings and implications which may be very different from those of their adopted home. In such a case, the provision of information on the main elements of non-verbal communication within their new society can reduce their communication disability.

A patient's non-verbal communication skills and their appropriateness within the particular society can be generally assessed informally during the clinical interview. This will be complemented by further information acquired through the course of the enablement process.

Overall

In the previous sections, individual elements of the communication process have been discussed. It is essential, however, that these are not considered in isolation but be regarded as parts of the individual's overall ability to communicate. This may be equal to the sum of the components, it may be poorer than such a sum and it may be better. Thus, certain individuals with relatively poor auditory discrimination abilities and only moderate visual discrimination ones, may have extremely good speech recognition when the speech is presented in audiovisual mode. Others, with good speechreading ability, when an auditory input is added, may experience a degradation of their performance. Interaction between auditory and visual inputs is seen in the McGurk effect (McGurk and MacDonald, 1976). It is therefore essential to assess the patient using their optimal mode of communication.

A similar situation arises with the integration of sign language with spoken language and non-verbal communication. Hatfield (1982) discusses approaches to the assessment of such sign language: spoken language bilingualism using rating scales, fluency tests, flexibility test and dominance tests. However, in practice, most assessment of overall communication ability will initially be performed based on the clinical interview session, although any realistic assessment in this context should be performed by a signing professional. A visual analogue scale or a rating scale can be used for such an assessment.

Returning to audiovisual integration used by patients with late-onset hearing impairment, the techniques used will be broadly similar to those used for assessing speechreading abilities, in particular sentence tests and connected discourse tracking. These can provide separate measures of auditory, visual and audiovisual performance which are directly comparable and can be supplemented by the clinician's assessment using a rating or visual analogue scale.

Before concluding this section, it is important to remember the additional effort required by those with hearing impairments in the communication domain (see also Chapter 5). Such individuals have to listen intently rather than passively hearing any speech. The degree of such effort can be assessed clinically, but in certain individuals additional techniques such as pupillometry or choice reaction times may be used to assess them more formally.

Contextual factors

This section is concerned with the assessment of relevant background factors that can have a major influence on the patient's attitude to and acceptance of the enablement process and different components of it. Hence, it is essential to be aware of such influences in order to be able to help the patient in an acceptable and effective manner.

This section is split into three components: *environmental factors*, particularly those people close to the patient and their attitudes, *personal factors*, within the patient and, finally, a consideration of any *previous enablement* that they might have received, its effectiveness and their reaction towards it.

Environmental factors

Within this section, while the support, relationships and attitudes of those around the patient can have a major influence on the enablement process, other elements contained within ICF (WHO, 2001) must also be taken into consideration. These include 'Products and technology', 'Natural environment and human-made changes to the environment' and 'Services, systems and policies'. Thus, for example, someone living in a small urban apartment may have very different needs from one living in a farmhouse in the middle of the country. Furthermore, the nature of the transportation and health care provisions and whether they are free of charge can affect the person's willingness to undergo a programme of enablement covering a number of sessions.

Products and technology

The key areas here are those 'for personal use in daily living' (e115), for 'mobility and transportation' (e120) and 'for communication' (e125) (WHO, 2001). The first of these will include environmental aids, which will be addressed later in the section on previous enablement. Here, it is important to think of various units within the patient's home such as smoke alarms, doorbells and burglar alarms. The inability of the individual to hear these can result in major feelings of insecurity. Similarly, in transportation, the inability to hear indicators in the motor car can have similar effects.

Communication devices, however, constitute the most relevant area, comprising particularly the television and radio, telephones and music systems, and it is important to know what types of devices the person has and which create difficulties for them. Again, hearing aids and environmental aids within this context will be considered later.

Natural environment and human-made changes to the environment

Within this context, the most relevant areas are 'Light' (e240) and 'Sound' (e250) (WHO, 2001). The kind of lighting which the person has in their normal environment and its orientation can have a major impact on their speechreading ability and hence on their overall communication. Poorly lit rooms with any light focused on the listener rather than on the speaker will result in major difficulties.

In this context, sound is even more important, particularly given the difficulties experienced by most people with hearing impairment in noisy or reverberant places. People living by a busy street and having only single glazing on their windows will have far more problems than those with double or treble glazing or living in the country. In addition, rooms with hard bare walls and floors will create considerable problems with reverberance, making it difficult for individuals with hearing impairment to hear what is said on the radio or by live speakers.

Support and relationships (and attitudes)

These two sections are considered together as it is very much the attitudes of those around the patient as well as their mere existence which will affect the difficulties experienced.

While ICF (WHO, 2001) concentrates on different groups of people, including 'Immediate family' (e310), 'Extended family' (e315), 'Friends' (e320), 'Acquaintances, colleagues, neighbours etc.' (e325), the key element in all these groups is whether the individual plays an important role in the life of the patient and can hence be defined as a *significant other* (or SO). Such individuals may include carers, who came under the categories 'Health professionals' (e355) or 'Other professionals' (e360). Whether the patient has regular contact with any significant others and which have the most influence on them is the first question. The second will be the attitudes of any such significant others towards the patient in general and towards their hearing impairment in particular, which can have most important effects on the patient and their attitude towards different aspects of the enablement process. Contact with health professionals and, especially, their general practitioner (primary physician) and the attitudes of these people will also very much colour the patient's approach. The influence of wives of men with noise induced hearing loss (NIHL) and their attitudes toward their partners can be reflected in very different approaches to enablement (Hallberg and Barrenäs, 1993; this book Chapter 7).

Another area of relevance here is that of significant others and various acquaintances who might have received interventions (e.g. hearing aids) themselves. In some, this might have been successful and will consequently encourage the patient to seek such intervention themselves. In others, such a fitting, inappropriately made, may result in very negative attitudes towards the enablement process and lead to the patient being very reluctant to accept such intervention.

Related to this is the question of role models within the family or among significant others. This has been discussed elsewhere (Chapters 3 and 7) and, in more detail, by Kramer *et al.* (2006b) and by Coulson (2006). These authors found that having such a role model who has benefited from intervention might encourage patients to seek intervention themselves. In addition, having a role model who has resisted any intervention, which has consequently led to major problems, both for themselves and for those around them, may encourage the patient to seek help in a more open-minded way at an earlier stage.

A further category which may be of relevance is that of 'Domesticated animals' (e350; WHO, 2001). While the concept of specially trained 'hearing dogs' may be considered elsewhere in the enablement process, many dogs without such training will indicate to the patient that there is someone at the door or that the telephone is ringing. In addition, one of the authors has a patient with a 'hearing horse' (Figure 10.6). When she rides this horse in her local forests and motor cycles or quad bikes are approaching, the horse will automatically move off the main track to a position of safety, where it stays until the machines have passed. The horse itself had become aware that its rider was unable to hear the bikes.

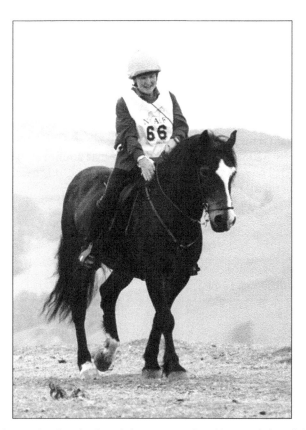

Figure 10.6 A patient on her 'hearing horse'. (*Source:* reproduced by permission of the patient.)

Services, systems and policies (and societal attitudes)

'Societal attitudes' (e460) are included here as they reflect the views of the broader society in which the patient lives (WHO, 2001). The important area in this context is the question of stigma of hearing impairment and, further, of hearing aids, which will influence the approach of the patient towards aspects of the enablement process.

The more general areas which impact on the patient are particularly those of 'Communication services, systems and policies' (e535), 'Social security services, systems and policies' (e570), 'General support services, systems and policies' (e575) and 'Health services, systems and policies' (e580). In addition, 'Transportation services, systems and policies' (e540), 'Education and training services, systems and policies' (e585) and 'Labour and employment services, systems and policies' (e590) will be of relevance to the extent that they include provisions for people with hearing impairment, both childhood and of later onset.

'Communication services' will define which modes of communication are available to people with hearing impairment within the particular society. This can include fax machines, e-mails, Teletext and mobile phones, including inbuilt digital cameras, which people with hearing difficulties but who are fluent in sign language can use to communicate with each other.

The nature of the 'Social security services' within a particular society will determine the support given to people with hearing difficulties and, in particular, to the provision of 'General support services'. This is important for people with severe problems as it may include the provision of carers, where relevant.

The final area of 'Health services' is the domain which, in most countries, provides the enablement service for people with hearing difficulties. This may be provided free of charge from the general taxation, from insurance-based provisions or the patient may have to pay part or all of the costs of the enablement. This will inevitably influence the patient's acceptance of elements of the enablement programme, or even of the entire programme. In addition, the geographical accessibility of appropriate services for the patient may also have a major impact on its acceptability.

Personal contextual factors

These are not clearly defined in ICF, which merely lists a number of relevant components (WHO, 2001). The factors listed can be seen in Box 10.1, based on ICF and on Stephens and Danermark (2005).

Box 10.1 Personal contextual factors.

Gender, race, age	Other health conditions
Lifestyle	Fitness
Habits	Upbringing
Coping styles	Social background
Education	Past and current experience
Profession	*Positive experiences*
Overall behaviour pattern and character style	
Individual psychological assets and other characteristics	

While all the factors listed above may have an influence on the individual and their approach to the enablement process, those indicated in italic type in Box 10.1 would seem to be the key areas. 'Past and current experience' will be covered in the next section.

The individual's lifestyle, whether gregarious or solitary, will have a marked impact on whether they think enablement necessary and which aspects of the enablement process may be important for them. This is also reflected in their habits and specific interests.

Different people have different coping strategies, which, throughout their lives, they might have found helpful in other circumstances. They will tend to use such strategies when they experience hearing difficulties, and while some, such as avoidance of challenging situations, may be helpful in saving face, others, if used in an unselective manner, can result in major difficulties for the individual (Jaworski and Stephens, 1998).

The patient's 'Overall behaviour pattern and character style' and their 'Individual psychological assets and other characteristics' concern predominantly their emotional state as reflected in their behaviour and their underlying personality. Both areas can have a major influence on their attitudes towards help-seeking and various aspects of the enablement process such as hearing aids and the adoption of different hearing tactics.

Finally, an area which has not previously been considered in this context is that of *positive experiences* associated with hearing impairment. This has been discussed in Chapter 1, and a relationship has been found between self-reported positive experiences and the patient's attitude towards their hearing impairment (Stephens and Kerr, 2003). Similar findings have been reported in the context of Menière's disorder (Stephens *et al.*, 2009b). These results imply that if the patient feels that their condition is not really severe and they become aware of having developed new skills, they feel that their hearing problems are more acceptable.

Previous enablement

Any interventions in the context of enablement which the patient has previously received can have a major impact on their attitudes towards different parts of the enablement process. Thus, a positive and effective previous intervention will ensure that the individual is receptive to any additional aspects of the process. On the other hand, if the patient has had a poor previous experience, such as being fitted with an inappropriate or poorly fitting hearing aid, they may well have negative feelings about any future prosthetic intervention. They will need a markedly different approach from the audiologist from a patient who has had a good fitting before which merely needs to be updated.

In any case, it is important for the professional to enquire as to any previous experiences the patient has had with hearing aids, environmental aids, speechreading training etc. This knowledge is essential if the professional is to be able to tailor the enablement process to meet the individual's specific needs. Furthermore, the professional must be aware of what effects any earlier interventions might have had on the patient's reported hearing difficulties.

Related functions and activities

While the *contextual factors* will have an influence on the overall approach to be adopted in the enablement process with the particular patient, the present section is concerned with factors which will rather have an influence on detailed aspects of the process, particularly with regard to instrumentation and communication training. In a number of patients, particularly among older patients, several of these functions and activities may be impaired within the same individual. Thus, an older person may have mild impairment of their cognitive function, reduced touch function and limited manipulative activities. Each in itself may have only a minimal impact on their ability to learn to control and effectively use their hearing aid, but the three occurring together can have a major impact on the enablement process.

Mental functions

This section is concerned particularly with the intellectual and cognitive functions of the patients. They may have intellectual disabilities, either congenital or acquired, or may have specific problems with learning and remembering instructions and training programmes. These should be assessed informally and from the patient's files, and will need to be taken into account when planning any enablement programme.

Significant others, either family or other carers, should be much involved in such a programme, which should be presented in as clear and simple a way as possible. In the case of patients with severe intellectual disabilities, much of the individual's hearing difficulties will generally be articulated by their carers rather than by the patients themselves. In this case, it is especially important to ensure that the patient is prepared to accept any intervention, particularly in the form of hearing aid(s). With many individuals, training in the form of communication tactics and the use of environmental aids may be all that can be achieved.

Sensations associated with hearing and vestibular function

These sensations comprise a number of symptoms and signs that can interfere with hearing aid fitting. They include tinnitus, hyperacusis, pressure sensations, otalgia, Tullio phenomenon and otorrhoea. The last, while not strictly within this category, impacts on the enablement process in a similar way. Its history can usually be obtained by an appropriate clinical interview.

Tinnitus, or noise in the ear(s) or head, is usually associated with hearing impairment and is very disturbing for a proportion of patients with the symptom. Its relevance to the enablement process is that it can often be relieved by an appropriate hearing fitting and, when a unilateral fitting is being considered, the ear with unilateral tinnitus should be considered in the first instance. However, this should be tempered with caution, as a small proportion of patients with tinnitus find that it is exacerbated by even a well-fitted hearing aid. In particular, care needs to be taken to ensure that the earmould fitting is as open as possible as occlusion of the external meatus will frequently increase the perceived loudness of the tinnitus.

Hyperacusis is often associated with tinnitus, but may occur independently. It is discussed in Chapter 3, and it is a factor which must be considered in hearing aid fitting to ensure patient comfort and acceptance.

The sensation of pressure or fullness in the ear has been discussed earlier (chapter 4). It may be caused by disorders either of the middle ear or of the cochlea. It is important to be aware of this when assessing the patient in order to be sure that any earmould fitting is as open as possible so as not to exacerbate the sensation.

Pain or irritation in the ears can also be aggravated by an inappropriate earmould fitting. Such fittings may be poorly made, occlusive or may result in a true allergic reaction, which can lead to rejection of any such earmould. Sometimes the pain may be associated with an infection of the ear (otitis externa or chronic suppurative otitis media) with a concomitant discharge. Such infections can again be exacerbated by tightly fitting earmoulds and can lead to a blockage of the earmould tubing or of the output transducer of an in-the-ear hearing aid. In severe cases, such infections or chronic allergic reactions can preclude any air-conduction hearing aid fitting and necessitate the fitting either of a bone-anchored hearing aid or even of a middle ear implantable aid.

Tullio phenomenon is the provocation of vertigo accompanied by nystagmus when the ear is exposed to loud sounds. In certain patients after fenestration surgery on a proportion of those with Menière's disorder, this can occur at relatively modest hearing levels. It is important, if this is suspected, to ask the patient if they become dizzy while walking in the street when a heavy lorry drives past. Other people may report the phenomenon spontaneously as being provoked by specific sounds. The condition can be tested for using a variant of the uncomfortable loudness level test while monitoring any nystagmus using an appropriate technique.

Touch function

Touch function can be affected by a number of diseases, such as diabetes mellitus or multiple sclerosis, and tends to be less sensitive with increasing age. This can have a significant effect on the person's ability to feel the controls of a hearing aid and hence use it appropriately.

It may be assessed clinically or by using a number of structured tests, such as recognising the shape of an object when unable to see it (Stephens, 1997).

Manipulative activities

These concern particularly the person's ability to make fine-controlling movements with their fingers, important for altering the volume control, on/off switch and battery compartment of the hearing aid. This can be impaired by tremor, strokes, a range of neuromotor degenerative conditions as well as, to some extent, age. As mentioned earlier, such impaired manipulative ability may occur in parallel with impaired sensory function and consequently have a more marked impact on the patient's abilities to fit and use a hearing aid.

Again, this may be assessed informally, such as by timing a person when they change a hearing aid battery. In addition, there are a number of more formal tests involving the patient's ability to remove a nut from one bolt and put it on another (Stephens, 1997; Singh et al., 2008).

Walking activities

This section is concerned essentially with the patient's mobility, whether they are bed-bound, house-bound or actively mobile. These will have an impact on the individual's acoustical environment and consequently on their listening and communication needs.

For those who are completely bed-bound, often with a terminal illness, hearing and communication with their loved ones and carers may be the only respite from their condition and it is essential that they are able to hear optimally. However, this will entail the use of appropriate amplification, often in the form of environmental aids as well as acoustical modifications to the room in which they are confined. Such an approach may be more effective and acceptable than introducing a hearing aid system.

Other individuals will have greater mobility but be unable to move out of their house or flat. Such individuals will have a wider range of acoustical environments but far fewer than fully mobile (or wheelchair-mobile) people. The range and nature of their environments will need to be taken into account when planning an enablement programme, using an appropriate balance of hearing aids, environmental aids and environmental modifications, as well as communication tactics for their significant others.

Integration and decision-making

This is the stage of the enablement process in which the information obtained in the evaluation process is pulled together to make some initial decisions regarding the most appropriate interventions for the individual concerned. In the course of this, we consider a pragmatic classification of the patient and his or her attitudes towards the process, discuss how many require in-depth support and address the first stage of goal-setting.

Integration

At this stage, the different elements of information acquired about the patient, their needs and attitudes and those of the people around them are drawn together in order to determine the plan of intervention most likely to help them. The patient or significant others may have been found to have inappropriate ideas as to the benefits and limitations of aspects of the enablement process and an initial attempt may be made at this stage to give them more appropriate information with, ultimately, greater likelihood of a successful outcome.

Thus, the patient may feel that provided they have a hearing aid or aids, they will hear perfectly in all circumstances, much as with a pair of spectacles for myopia. The reality is that, even with the most advanced digital signal-processing systems, they will still have considerable problems hearing in background noise or in a highly reverberant environment. A short discussion of the likely benefits and shortcomings of possible interventions at this stage can result in more realistic expectations and avoid the potential disillusionment which the patient may experience when the intervention does not live up to their expectations. Such disillusionment can lead to the patient rejecting the whole enablement process and hence missing out on a range of potential benefits.

On the other hand, the patient may have heard from friends or associates that hearing aids are likely to be of little or no benefit. They will consequently have limited motivation to persist with the enablement process and may well drop out before benefit has been achieved. Again, a brief discussion of the realistic benefits and limitations of any interventions is valuable here to give them a more balanced view of possible outcomes and hence to persist sufficiently for such outcomes to be achieved.

Patient categorisation

The purpose of this stage is to define the most appropriate and relevant approach to the intervention for the particular patient concerned. It may be regarded as a type of triage and we argue that using the same interventional programme for every single patient constitutes an inappropriate use of the resources available. Some patients require relatively limited intervention, achieved in two or three sessions, whereas others will require far more sustained support. There are yet other individuals for

Table 10.7 Patient category types.

Category	Description
1	Positively motivated and straightforward
2	Positively motivated with complicating factors
3	Want help, but is resistant to certain elements of the enablement process
4	Deny any disability

whom any intervention is inappropriate, although support may be given to their significant others.

Goldstein and Stephens (1981) define four categories of patients, shown in Table 10.7, and this categorisation seems to have withstood the test of time.

Type 1 patients constitute some 40–50% of those seen in clinics. They are positively motivated, with no real complicating factors and have the type of hearing impairment for which an appropriate hearing aid fitting would not be difficult. They will progress rapidly to such a fitting, which will involve a brief discussion of relevant environmental aids. A follow-up session a month or so later will ensure that they are managing well with their aid(s), and possibly include some fine tuning of the aid, a short discussion of any problems which they might have experienced with appropriate counselling, followed by a further discussion of any other relevant environmental aids (e.g. TV devices). They will then be discharged from the clinic in the knowledge that they will return if they have any specific problems. Most patients who have had a previous hearing aid but are returning for an upgrade or because of a change in their hearing impairment will come within this category.

Type 2 patients, who also constitute some 40–50% of those seen, are again positively motivated and acceptant of any relevant intervention. They may, however, have one or more complicating factors, which will result in the enablement interventions being more prolonged. Such complicating factors may relate to their type of hearing impairment, to related ear conditions, to their handling skills, mild confusion or to relatively low overall motivation with little support from significant others.

Types of hearing impairment leading to the patient needing more prolonged attention are the more severe, where there will be a question of the most appropriate types of intervention, and the very mild (e.g. King-Kopetzky syndrome). For these, hearing aids will not necessarily be appropriate but the patients will need psychological support. Those with a low-frequency sensorineural impairment, for whom an appropriate hearing aid fitting may be difficult to achieve, will also need more attention. Patients with otorrhoea or disturbing tinnitus will require considerable care with their fitting, and a number of the former group may end up with bone-anchored hearing aids. Commonly, given that most patients seen in enablement clinics are older people, the patient may have a combination of tremor, poor sensation in their fingers and mild confusion, leading to the need for a greater degree of training before they are able to use any hearing aid adequately.

Type 3 patients, who constitute up to 10% of those seen, most commonly are resistant to any hearing aid fitting. However, others may have a very inappropriate expectation of hearing aids, feeling that such a fitting will solve all their psychosocial problems, even if those have little relationship in reality to their hearing impairment. Such patients will require a sensitive approach from the professional, and the use of group sessions including patients with less complicated problems can be helpful. In the case of those resistant to hearing aids, a combination of peer group pressure coupled with an offer of a trial of hearing aids in a relaxed manner can be helpful. In the other group of patients, individual counselling developed from their reactions within a group situation may be the most effective approach. In such patients, the 'Instrumentation' stage of the enablement process will be bypassed, moving straight to 'Strategy' or even to 'Communication training'.

Type 4 patients (up to 4%) are resistant to intervention, usually having attended the clinic as a result of pressure from significant others. When they deny any problems or are frank that they do not want any kind of intervention, they should be discharged from the clinic and reassured that should they find their condition to be problematic in the future or change their minds regarding intervention they would be welcome to return to the clinic. At the same time, it is often helpful to see the significant other, separate from the patient, and to provide them with information on environmental aids and communication tactics, which can be introduced in a non-threatening manner to reduce domestic stresses.

The benefits of such a categorisation, which should not be applied in too rigid a manner, can enable the clinic's resources to be planned and used most effectively. It is important, however, to be aware of the patient population seen in any particular clinic and the demographics of that population. Elsewhere (Stephens and Meredith, 1991a), it has been found that the proportion of patients in the different categories will differ as a function of the age group seen, with more complicated problems generally found amongst older patients. In addition, the situation will differ according to whether the clinic concerned is a second-tier basic referral clinic or a third-tier clinic that receives only those patients with more complicated problems.

Initial goal-setting

At this stage, the time has come for the first approach to goal-setting, which will take as a starting point the disabilities reported by the patient. They will be asked to prioritise these in terms of the effects on their life and then to discuss with the professional how and whether such goals may be approached. Most will be potentially achievable to a greater or lesser degree, whereas some, such as the desire to localise sounds by a patient with a total unilateral hearing impairment, may be largely impossible.

The most important goals at this stage can be fed into the COSI assessment (Dillon *et al.*, 1997) to provide a basis for the assessment of the effectiveness of the enablement programme for the individual concerned. While the goals will be essentially driven by the patient, a significant other may be involved at this stage to help in their definition and prioritisation. However, such significant other participation must depend on the wishes of the patient. In some cases where the significant other is a very dominant person, they may be held at a distance. In cases with a very supportive significant other, such an individual can provide much insight into the patient's specific needs and relevant goals.

Once the integration, categorisation and goal-setting have been accomplished, a decision has to be made about to which part of the enablement process they should proceed. The majority will go to 'Instrumentation', although others will proceed to 'Strategy', 'Ancillary help' or even to elements of 'Ongoing remediation', bypassing the intermediate stages.

Conclusion

The first stage of any enablement process is the evaluation of the problems experienced by the patient and of relevant factors which may influence the process. The exact methods used in any such evaluation will depend on the patient and the socio-medical system in which they live. However, they should always entail an assessment of the patient's problems, their communication status, their psychosocial background and related conditions, which can influence details of the enablement process.

Assessment of the patient's problems must be performed using an open-ended approach, rather than imposing the constraints of structured questionnaires which may or may not be relevant to their needs. The responses can be elaborated on in an interview and fed into a patient-relevant outcome measure such as COSI (Dillon et al., 1997). Any evaluation of audition must be related to tests which will influence decision-making in the enablement process. The approach to evaluation of vision, speech production, sign language use and non-verbal communication will depend on the patient's needs and status, but all must be considered. The psychosocial status of the patient and of the results of any previous interventions will determine their attitude towards different parts of the enablement process. Assessment must include appraisal of the role and attitudes of significant others. Finally, related functions and activities cover domains such as tinnitus and ear discharge, which can influence the details of any instrumentation. The handling skills of the individual are important in this context. The mental and mobility status of the patient will have a broader effect on different parts of the enablement process.

Such evaluations must then be drawn together and decisions made as to the approach to be used with the particular patient. This will follow an agreement between the professional and the patient on the relevant goals that should be achieved.

11 The process of enablement 2: Short-term remediation

Introduction

The short-term enablement intervention has three components, which are outlined in Figure 11.1. This stage comprises elements which can normally be covered in one or two sessions, with the possibility of returning to one or more of the components at a later stage if that is indicated. As shown in Figure 11.1, it comprises *instrumentation*, generally hearing aid fitting and consideration of environmental aids, *strategy*, which entails a broader approach than hearing tactics alone, and referral for *ancillary help*. This last covers areas related to the enablement process that come outside the scope and expertise of the audiologists caring for the patient.

Instrumentation

Most publications on audiological enablement (rehabilitation) focus on aspects of hearing aid fitting and, in particular, on the electroacoustical aspects of such fitting. While we agree that this constitutes a very important aspect of the process, we shall seek here to put the instrumentation in a broader psychosocial context and refer the reader who requires more detail on that respect to a number of more detailed publications (Dillon, 2001; Kates, 2008).

As shown in Figure 11.1, we subdivide *instrumentation* into two main sections, the first concerned with instruments adjusted for and particular to the patient concerned, and the second covering more general instrumentation in the form of environmental aids. The selection of any and all of these will depend on the problems reported by the patient, modifying factors identified in the evaluation process and the degree and configuration of the hearing impairment. In all cases, any fitting will be accompanied by the relevant instructions as to the use of the instrument(s), presented in a way that is clear and comprehensible to the patient.

Personal instrumentation

The range of personal instrumentation is shown in Table 11.1.

Within this context, by far the most common instruments fitted are hearing aids, some half a million of which are fitted annually in the United Kingdom (population *ca.* 60 million). After hearing aids, the next instruments to be considered are cochlear implants, although fewer than 500 of these instruments are fitted annually in the same

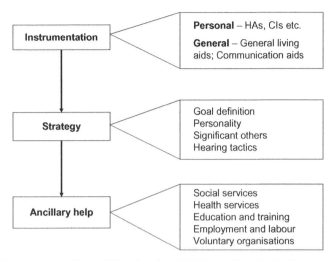

Figure 11.1 Short-term remediation. (HA = hearing aid; CI = cochlear implant)

Table 11.1 Types of personal instrumentation.

Group	Examples
Hearing aids	Orthodox
	CROS
	Frequency transposition
Implantable aids	Bone-anchored hearing aids (BAHA)
	Middle ear implants
	Cochlear implants
	Brainstem and mid-brain implants
Tactile aids	Vibrotactile
	Electrotactile

population. Less commonly, auditory brainstem implants may be considered for a select group of patients with specific needs, but only some 10–20 of these are fitted annually. The number of bone-anchored hearing aids (BAHAs) fitted annually is somewhat smaller than the number of cochlear implants, but of the same order of magnitude. Finally, tactile aids and middle ear implants may be considered, although the former are used much less frequently than previously, and very few middle ear implants have been inserted in the United Kingdom, although they are used more frequently in certain countries of Continental Europe and Japan.

The overall concept behind the fitting of all such devices within the framework of audiological enablement follows the same general principles. These have been discussed in some detail elsewhere in the context of hearing aids (Stephens, 1984), and relevant elements of this will be picked up in the following sections.

Hearing aids

Within the area of hearing aids, the first decisions to be made are whether such a device or devices are likely to be beneficial to the individual and whether they are likely to be acceptable. If they are unlikely to be beneficial because of the severity of the person's hearing impairment or the mild degree of impairment, other approaches must be considered, such as cochlear implants in the former case and communication training in the latter. Similarly, if a hearing aid fitting is considered likely to be beneficial to a certain individual but is unacceptable to them at this stage, the patient should proceed to communication training, with the option of returning to this hearing aid fitting at a later date, should they change their minds.

Once the decision has been made between the patient and professional to proceed with a hearing aid fitting, the process of selection begins, both with regard to the electroacoustic characteristics of the device(s) and with regard to the type of fitting (e.g. behind-the-ear (BTE) vs in-the-ear (ITE) vs body-worn; one aid vs two; plain vs coloured aids etc.).

Audiometric candidature

The optimal electroacoustic characteristics of the fitting will be defined by a range of audiometric variables, in particular the threshold and uncomfortable loudness levels. In addition, the introduction of the threshold-equalising noise (TEN) test to define dead regions of the cochlea (Moore *et al.*, 2000, 2004) can provide indications as to whether high-frequency amplification or frequency transposition may be the most promising approach in an individual patient (Robinson *et al.*, 2007).

Furthermore, it is likely, given the flexibility of digital signal processing hearing aids, that other psychoacoustical tests will be found in the future to be relevant predictors of optimal parameters of hearing aid fitting. In an initial study, Gatehouse *et al.* (2006a) provide evidence that susceptibility to spectral and temporal smearing and to the upward spread of masking can differentiate between the performance with different compression systems.

The position of speech recognition tests in this context is more problematic as, while they can provide guidance for decisions concerning unilateral versus bilateral fitting, or hearing aid versus cochlear implant fitting, they do not provide guidance as to the specific electroacoustic parameters to be used in any individual fitting.

In earlier times, the hearing aid paradigms indicated by these were calculated manually, based on a range of fitting programmes such as NAL (Byrne and Tonisson, 1976) and its derivatives. Now, however, following the advent of digital signal processing hearing aids with real ear insertion gain measures, appropriate fitting programmes (e.g. NAL-NL1 and DSL – see Dillon, 2001) are included in the electronic fitting protocol, which operates almost independently of the audiologist.

This approach can, however, have its own risks, with most fitting programmes being based on the hearing aid settings preferred by experienced users. This stems from the fact, first highlighted by Barfod (1979), of the question of adaptation to the frequency characteristics of the hearing aid. Thus, patients without previous experience of hearing aids prefer a sound equivalent to that which they are used to hearing with, for example, their high-frequency impairment. A hearing aid providing more high-frequency emphasis, and which could theoretically give them better speech recognition, will be reported as sounding 'tinny' and may be rejected. An effective fitting needs to start with an acceptable compromise between the sound preferred by the patient and the ideal for speech recognition. As they become used to this fitting, the degree of high-frequency emphasis can be gradually increased to approach the ideal fitting in a way acceptable to the patient. Such adaptation to hearing aids was subsequently studied by Gatehouse (1992), Lindley (1999) and others, also in the concept of the loudness levels acceptable to the patient.

These findings must be borne in mind by the audiologist performing the fitting, using the fitting program to define the broad area of the hearing aid response, with fine-tuning according to the responses of the patient to the sound quality experienced. These can then be altered on subsequent visits. The need for such adjustment and the amount of adjustment required can vary from subject to subject.

Other determinants of optimal electroacoustic characteristics

Gatehouse *et al.* (2006a) highlight the fact that cognitive factors (visual digit and letter monitoring tasks) as well as a number of 'Auditory ecology' measures, reflecting the complexity and variability of the auditory environment to which the individual is exposed, can influence the benefits of different signal processing systems. Broadly speaking, listening in fluctuating types of noise (those that are generally met in daily life) impose a larger involvement of an individual's cognitive capacities than situations with more steady-state types of background noises (Lunner and Sundewall-Thorén, 2007). Hence, people with relatively poor cognitive function perform better with linear systems and those with high cognitive capacity derive most benefit from wide dynamic range compression systems (Foo *et al.*, 2007). The relationship between auditory ecology and the most beneficial processing system is more complex and is discussed in Chapter 5.

One hearing aid or two?

Discussion as to the relative benefits of a bilateral (binaural) hearing aid fitting date back to the 1950s and certainly achieved prominence when head-worn aids became available. Koenig (1950) wrote of the advantages of bilateral hearing aids particularly in terms of improving the recognition of speech in noise. A number of other advantages, particularly in relation to directionalisation and ease of listening, were highlighted over the following twenty years and are discussed by Markides (1977b).

The most enthusiastic of the early advocates of bilateral hearing aid fittings was Ole Bentzen who, in the early 1960s, insisted that all hearing aids delivered to his department in Århus be provided in boxed pairs, and later reported a range of benefits from such fittings (Jordan *et al.*, 1967). However, in 2003, a review in Scandinavia (SBU, 2003) reported that, despite the evidence of benefits of bilateral fittings in laboratory studies, there was a dearth of evidence indicating their benefit in clinical studies.

Subsequently, Mencher and Davis (2006), reviewing the evidence at the International Binaural Symposium, adduced support for the clinical benefit of bilateral fittings in terms of:

▓ speech recognition in noise
▓ localisation/directionalisation
▓ perception of sound quality
▓ tinnitus suppression
▓ binaural integration
▓ reduction in auditory deprivation
▓ ease of listening.

In addition, there is evidence for patient preference for bilateral fittings with, for example, 60% of those who had taken part in a cross-over study with one or two hearing aids opting to continue using two (Stephens *et al.*, 1991b). A long-term follow-up of these patients indicated that these individuals were more likely to continue using their hearing aids than those who had opted for one, suggesting that such a choice may be a reflection of patient motivation (Gianopoulos and Stephens, 2002).

In current clinical practice, it is generally wise to follow the principle of first considering a bilateral fitting, but accepting that probably in a majority of patients a unilateral fitting will be most appropriate for reasons of patient choice, manipulative skills, related aural conditions (e.g. discharge, pressure) or pronounced hearing asymmetry.

Hearing aid colour

Coloured and bejewelled hearing aids have been available since the early 1980s and, subsequently, coloured aids have become popular among children. Bejewelled aids never achieved much market penetration, partly because of cost and partly because of the reluctance of distributors, hearing aid dispensers and audiologists to publicise their availability.

The advantage of such coloured devices, apart from aesthetic considerations, is that they can contribute to destigmatising the concept of hearing aids, moving away from the view that they are something to be hidden. In the same way, spectacles are available in frames of many different colours and forms, and recent trends using first Walkmen and subsequently iPods in the ears should facilitate the use of such an approach. Nevertheless, coloured aids are rarely offered to, let alone used by, adults, an approach for which audiologists and dispensers have a considerable responsibility.

Major manufacturers such as Phonak, who first introduced coloured and bejewelled hearing aids, and Siemens, who introduced hearing aids of an aesthetically attractive design, are to be applauded in this context, but a more imaginative approach is needed on the part of those involved with fitting and dispensing hearing aids to the public.

Choice of earmoulds

Earmoulds comprise the crucial link between any air-conduction hearing aid and the ear. A poor earmould can negate the benefits of a good hearing aid and a good earmould can enhance the qualities of an aid.

Since the turn of the century, earmoulds have became available in different colours, with glitter or with various emblems incorporated in them such as those of football clubs, national emblems etc. However, again, these are normally offered only to children and their availability should be more publicised among adults.

However, the main consideration about earmould concerns their acoustical qualities and the effects that these can have on hearing aid performance. The advocacy of open (non-occlusive) earmoulds has been made since the early 1970s (Courtois and Berland, 1972), but this was largely limited to patients with mild hearing impairments by problems with acoustic feedback. They had earlier been used with CROS (contralateral routing of signals) hearing aid fittings (Harford and Barry, 1965) and fittings of the aid to the same ear as the earmould were sometimes known as IROS (ipsilateral routing of signals) in North America. More recently, the introduction of various electronic feedback suppression systems, particularly since the development of digital signal processing hearing aids, has led to the applicability of such systems to patients with more severe hearing impairments.

The advantages of open-mould fittings are the lack of occlusion influencing both pressure sensation and any discharge from the ear, comfort and facilitating a one-stop fitting. The last has implications in terms of waiting times and the number of appointments necessary for a particular patient, and is applicable in both state health care provision and the private sector.

If feedback problems preclude such a fitting, a vent can be made in the earmould to allow ventilation of the ear canal and prevent sensations of occlusion. Should even this be impossible, as in some cases of mixed or profound hearing impairment, a vent can be made with a sintered filter inserted, which can permit aeration and relief of pressure in individuals with a tendency to discharge or a sensitivity to pressure sensation (French St George and Barr-Hamilton, 1975).

Another form of earmould that was advocated for improving sound quality and advocated, particularly before the development and introduction of digital signal processing aids and routine measurement of sound pressure at the eardrum, was the horned mould (Killion, 1981; Dillon, 2001). The sound tube of this mould is shaped so that its diameter is greater closer to the tip (and hence to the eardrum) than in the outer part of the ear canal. This approach can also be applied to open ear fittings, where it was pioneered as the Libby Horn (Libby, 1982).

The other important aspect of earmoulds, apart from the extent to which they fit well to the ear, is the material from which they are made. Typically, they are made from hard acrylic, with soft acrylic, silicone or a variety of other materials used for moulds which need to be tight fitting to avoid feedback. Some patients develop reactions to their earmoulds, although this is most commonly due to poor hygiene. True allergic reactions do, however, occur often to the catalysts involved in the production of the acrylic moulds. Apart from silicone, there is a range of hypoallergenic materials from which earmoulds can be made to replace those provoking a skin allergy. In certain hypersensitive cases, it may be necessary to use either silver, titanium or porcelain moulds.

Among the most common problems which many first-time users have in fitting a hearing aid to their ear is a difficulty with the 'top prong' (Helix lock or top lock), the upper part of the mould that fits into the upper recess of the ear to provide stability. This applies to 'standard' or 'skeleton' moulds. However, Meredith *et al.* (1989) show that by merely cutting off the top prong it is possible to minimise such fitting problems. Such a modified skeleton mould was more effective in this respect than a meatal tip or 'canal mould' fitting. The only problem is an increased likelihood of feedback in patients with more severe hearing impairments, but this problem has been lessened by digital feedback suppression techniques.

Type of hearing aid
Since the 1950s, when the first head-worn hearing aids were developed, with the progress in electronic technology, hearing aids have become smaller and more sophisticated. One major driver for this has been the stigma associated with such aids and the 'need' to make them more and more invisible. This has led to the development of behind-the-ear (BTE) aids, spectacle aids, in-the-ear (ITE) aids, in-the-canal (ITC) aids and completely-in-the-canal (CIC) aids.

Essentially, with modern technology any one of these can incorporate the basic processing systems available, although high-gain hearing aids do need some separation of the microphone from the output transducer (telephone) in order to avoid problems with feedback. Thus, for patients with severe to profound mixed hearing impairments, a body-worn hearing aid may still be appropriate.

While through the 1980s and 1990s there was a move towards ITEs, ITCs and CICs, with the development of digital signal processing aids with dual microphone systems to improve speech recognition in noise, the use of BTEs increased again. The choice of aid type will also depend on the health care provision system, any deformities of the ear, whether the hearing impairment is congenital or acquired and on the manipulative skills of the patient. In addition, for patients with severe conductive hearing impairments, bone-conduction transducers may be used, generally in association with a body-worn hearing aid, although devices built into spectacle frames and into headbands have been widely used. These will be discussed further in the section on bone-anchored hearing aids (BAHAs).

Specific hearing aid systems: CROS and frequency transposition

Certain systems have a particular relevance to specific types of hearing impairment. Among these are the CROS (contralateral routing of signals) system, which was developed for people with unilateral hearing impairments (Harford and Barry, 1965) and a variety of frequency transposition systems developed for people with relatively good hearing at the low to mid-frequencies, but no useful hearing in the high frequencies.

The CROS system has a microphone on the side of the non-functioning ear, which feeds into a hearing aid on the good ear. They may be linked either by a hard wire connection, via a loop around the back of the neck or via a spectacle frame, or have a radio link. The principle is to overcome the head shadow effect and improve the patient's hearing for sounds arriving at their non-functional ear. Inevitably, it can have a detrimental effect on directionalisation, but many people with unilateral impairments find it helpful.

A range of variations on the CROS were subsequently developed including POWERCROS, CRISCROS, BICROS and IROS (Hodgson and Skinner, 1977). The first two were designed to overcome feedback problems and have been rarely used. IROS was discussed earlier and is, essentially, just an open earmould fitting. BICROS is a system with standard amplification on one moderately impaired ear with an additional input from the opposite, profoundly impaired, ear.

CROS and BICROS aids have largely stood the test of time for patients with profound unilateral hearing losses (Dillon, 2001). They can be very helpful in moderately noisy situations when the background noise is predominantly on the side of the better ear and the speech is coming from the impaired side. If the reverse is true, use of such aids can further impair speech recognition. Many people find them particularly helpful in meetings.

Frequency transposition aids entail the shifting of sounds from frequencies inaudible to the listener to those they can hear. They have been tried for many years (Bennett and Byers, 1967; Velmans, 1973) and much of the early work concentrated on individuals with profound hearing impairments, often with limited success. However, there was increased realisation, particularly with the demonstration of 'dead regions' in the high frequencies of the cochlea (Moore *et al.*, 2000) that this approach might be more useful for those people with a severe high-frequency hearing impairment and good hearing in the low to mid-frequencies.

A number of hearing aids transposing high-frequency signals to lower frequencies were developed in the 1960s and 1970s. However, following the poor results obtained with these, there was little further development in this field until the first decade of the present century. Robinson *et al.* (2007) discuss some of the factors behind the earlier failures and more recent developments, and present some limited evidence for benefit in consonant discrimination. At the same time, some of the leading hearing aid companies have produced hearing aids incorporating frequency transposition systems and it is likely that an effective system with indications for candidature will be developed in the near future.

Implantable aids

A range of implantable hearing aids have been developed, often in the context of providing a hidden device and that requires a surgeon to fit it. At the time of writing, the most widely used and accepted of these is the bone-anchored hearing aid (BAHA), with one or two middle ear implants, particularly the Vibrant Soundbridge, having received some acceptance. Efforts continue to develop other aids of the latter type, even if, realistically, they are clinically valuable only for patients with intractable otitis externa.

Bone-anchored hearing aids

This percutaneous device was developed in the early 1980s and comprises a titanium screw inserted into the mastoid bone behind the ear, to which is linked a vibratory transducer (Håkansson *et al.*, 1985). An example of a BAHA is shown in Figure 11.2.

Following a skin incision, a titanium screw is inserted into the skull, usually behind the upper part of the auricle. The surgery may take place in one or two stages, and following healing the transducer is attached to the screw via a titanium abutment and various connections. This approach proved to be more effective than the transcutaneous device, the Xomed Audiant, developed by Hough *et al.* (1986), but which is no longer used.

The BAHA is invaluable for those with congenital abnormalities of the outer and middle ears (e.g. Treacher-Collins syndrome) as well as patients with intractable chronic suppurative otitis media, and some with intractable chronic otitis externa. There has been a move to use bilateral BAHAs that, despite the potential problems with cross hearing (stimulation of both cochleas), would appear to provide some

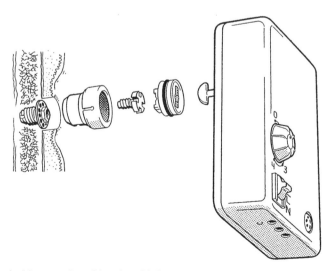

Figure 11.2 Typical bone-anchored hearing aid. (*Source:* derived from Carlsson, 1990.)

additional benefit to the patients (Bosman *et al.*, 2001). However, there do not appear to have been any cost-benefit studies in this respect.

Over the years, many studies have documented the audiometric benefits of the device in both children and adults (e.g. Snik *et al.*, 2008). Furthermore, patients report greater benefits than shortcomings compared with other types of hearing aid fittings, particularly in the context of their practicality as well as acoustical benefits (Stephens *et al.*, 1996).

Middle ear implants (e.g. Vibrant Soundbridge)

A number of different semi-implantable hearing aids introduced to the middle ear have been described and undergone limited trials (Snik *et al.*, 1998). They have used piezoelectric or electromagnetic devices to stimulate the ossicular chain. The only one to attain any widespread use has been the Vibrant Soundbridge, which uses an electromagnetic system (Mosnier *et al.*, 2008).

It has been proposed that these be used in patients with severe otitis externa or those dissatisfied with existing hearing aids because of sound quality, feedback or occlusion effect. It has also been used in some patients with ossicular chain defects (Colletti *et al.*, 2006).

However, recent studies have indicated deterioration of hearing in the operated ear and no improved speech recognition compared with standard hearing aids (Schmuziger *et al.*, 2006; Verhaegen *et al.*, 2008). The feedback problems and occlusion effects can also be addressed in a range of ways in modern hearing aids. The consensus, therefore at the present time would appear to be that such a device may be useful in patients with intractable otitis externa and moderate to severe hearing impairment. Those with otitis externa and less severe impairment can generally be helped with a BAHA, which does not threaten the residual hearing.

Cochlear implants

Cochlear implants are devices comprising a hearing-aid-like speech processor, which usually takes the form of a BTE hearing aid, linked to an electrode which is surgically inserted via the mastoid, middle ear and round window into the scala tympani of the cochlea, where it can stimulate the fibres of the cochlear nerve. A schematic diagram of the components is shown in Figure 11.3.

The aim is to bypass the non- or partially functional cochlea and to provide a meaningful electroauditory input to the auditory nervous system. While introduced clinically in the 1960s with single channel systems (House and Urban, 1973), since the development and introduction of multichannel systems in the 1980s (Tong *et al.*, 1982) such an approach has revolutionised the prosthetic approach for people with profound and total hearing impairment.

Initially, the implants were used only with totally deafened adults and, indeed, the single-channel systems provide only a supplement to speechreading and an awareness of environmental sounds. However, with the development of multichannel systems and more sophisticated signal processing techniques the criteria have been extended to individuals with severe hearing impairments. A common criterion has been that people with open-set speech recognition scores of 30% or worse with optimal hearing aids can be considered candidates, although certain centres have adopted a more liberal approach since the development of better signal processing systems. Indeed, the best performing patients achieve 100% speech recognition in the quiet and significant speech recognition in background noise.

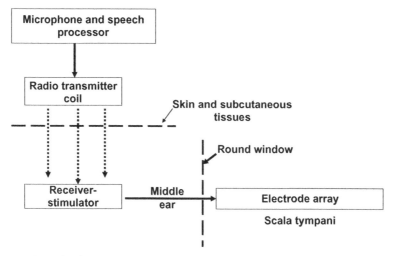

Figure 11.3 Schematic diagram of the cochlear implant system.

In addition, there have been studies examining a dual approach of hearing aid plus short cochlear implants for patients with relatively good low to mid-frequency hearing, dropping off precipitately in the mid-frequencies (von Ilberg *et al.*, 1999; Gantz and Turner, 2003). Vermeire *et al.* (2008) emphasise the importance of the frequency settings of both implant and hearing aid in such patients in order to provide the best speech recognition.

While cost-benefit studies of cochlear implantation as a whole are very positive (Summerfield *et al.*, 1994), there remains a question mark as to the criteria to be adopted to give most effective results and with regards to the cost benefit of bilateral cochlear implants in adults (Summerfield *et al.*, 2006). In addition, as most profound acquired hearing impairment occurs in older people, there are health constraints in terms of their undergoing a long and non-life-saving surgical procedure. Furthermore, some patients are reluctant to undergo such surgery, and others with long-standing hearing impairment are unlikely to obtain much benefit from such an intervention.

Brainstem and mid-brain implants

Brainstem implants were developed for patients who have no cochleas or whose cochlear nerves had been destroyed by the bilateral Schwannomas found in neurofibromatosis 2 (NF2). Implantation began with a single-channel system placed in the lateral recess of the fourth ventricle adjacent to the dorsal cochlear nucleus (Hitselberger *et al.*, 1984). Subsequently, multichannel systems were used (Laszig *et al.*, 1991) but have given very variable and limited results in terms of speech recognition performance (Nevison *et al.*, 2002). Colletti and Shannon (2005) suggest that this may be due in part to the trauma and anatomical changes consequent to the removal of the tumours, as they found better results in patients without tumours.

Such problems have led to the exploration of mid-brain implants inserted into the inferior colliculus (Lim *et al.*, 2007). These authors argue that this is more accessible surgically and less likely to be affected by surgery for the tumour removal. Elsewhere, Lim *et al.* (2008) suggest that implantation on to the central nucleus of the inferior colliculus appears to give the best results. However, at the present time, this is at a very early stage of development and, as with the brainstem implant, is applicable to only a tiny minority of patients with hearing difficulties.

Tactile aids

These devices, which are based on providing a representation of the acoustical signal by tactile stimulation, use either vibratory or electrical stimulation. They were used fairly extensively with profoundly hearing impaired children and adults up to the 1990s but, with the widespread introduction of multichannel cochlear implants, their role in the enablement process declined considerably. This decline came after a number of studies (e.g. Miyamoto *et al.*, 1995) indicated that cochlear implants resulted in markedly superior speech recognition and required less training in order to obtain such a performance.

The devices available ranged from a single-channel vibrotactile device, which provided little more than environmental awareness and some timing cues to supplement speechreading, to multichannel vibrotactile and electrotactile devices such as the Tickle Talker (Galvin *et al.*, 2000), which provided some open-set speech recognition after some 12–33 hours of training. Rönnberg *et al.* (1998) emphasise the importance of particular cognitive skills of the patient in the context of response to such training.

At the present time, in the enablement of hearing impaired adults, the role of such tactile devices is limited to those patients who are unable to have cochlear implants but need specific information about their environmental background and a supplement to their speechreading. Training has still to be extensive and the optimal techniques involved for any individual will depend on their cognition and specific needs.

General instrumentation

This category comprises devices that may be used by a range of individuals rather than being specific to one. An illustration of the most common needs and applications is shown in Figure 11.4. Figure 11.5 shows the percentage of patients fitted with different types of environmental aids in Norway in 1985, where they are available free of charge to patients (Warland, 1990). Figures for the percentage of different environmental aids used by people with hearing impairments in the United States in 1994 are shown in Figure 11.6, which excludes those using hearing aids or interpreters (Russell *et al.*, 1997).

These devices may be considered in two categories, following the classification of ICF (WHO, 2001), *products for use in daily living* (e.g. alarm clocks, doorbells) and *products for communication* (e.g. telephones, television). The approaches towards overcoming the activity limitations used within each category are broadly similar and will be considered in such a context. One of the main differences between the two categories is that in the context of daily living the emphasis is on increasing audibility or detectability of any signals, while in communication, it is more a question of improving the signal/noise ratio and comprehensibility of the signal. While ICF includes hearing aids and cochlear implants within the context of products for communication, they are excluded in the present consideration, being regarded as personal aids to hearing.

Products for use in daily living

These may be regarded as devices to potentiate alerting and warning signals, including door and telephone bells, smoke alarms, alarm clocks, baby monitors etc. The different approaches which may be used are shown in Table 11.2.

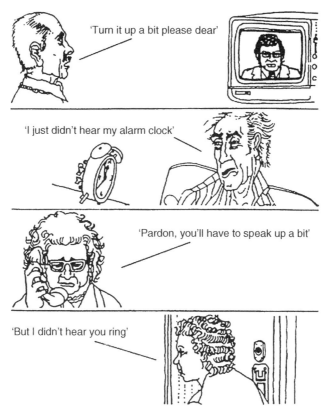

Figure 11.4 Common needs for general instrumentation.

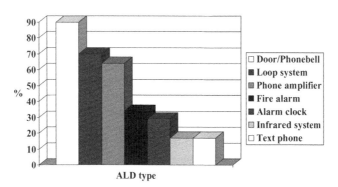

Figure 11.5 The commonest types of environmental aids distributed in Norway. (*Source:* based on data from Warland, 1990.)

The first approach is concerned with making the signals more audible. This may be approached by bringing them more within the range of hearing of the individual, whether in terms of the frequency of the stimulus or its loudness. Thus, as in the majority of people with hearing impairments, the high frequencies are most affected, hence simply using a low-frequency signal such as a buzzer for a doorbell or alarm clock can make it audible, whereas high-frequency rings will not be so.

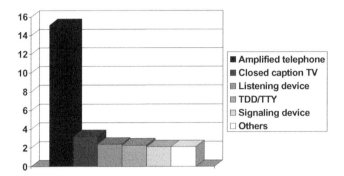

Figure 11.6 Environmental aids used by people with hearing impairment in the United States (1994). TDD = Telecommunication Device for the Deaf; TTY = Teletype. (*Source:* based on data from Russell *et al.*, 1997.)

Table 11.2 Approaches used in aids to daily living.

Approach	Examples
Auditory	Low frequency
	Loud
	Via extensions
	Via mobile devices
Visual	Built-in
	Strobe
	Linked to house lights
Tactile	Mobile vibrator
	Fan

Signals may be made louder for the patient either by amplifying them or by bringing them closer to the individual concerned. The latter can be done either by having extension bells or by linking them to the listener through a hard-wiring system within the house or by a radio link system to a receiver worn or carried by the person. Such systems are continually developing and the reader is referred to a range of commercial catalogues or web sites shown in the web site accompanying this book (http://www.wiley.com/go/stephens).

The other approaches entail the use of sensory substitution, using visual or vibrotactile systems, replacing or supplementing auditory signals. Most commonly now, strobe light systems linked to alarms or doorbells may be used as well as more traditional warning lights built into the devices or linked to the house lighting system.

Besides these, a range of vibratory systems are available, particularly for use under the pillow at night and linked to alarm clocks and baby monitors. Some of the more sophisticated approaches include wearable vibrotactile monitors, which provide different stimuli according to whether a doorbell or telephone bell or another alerting device has been activated. One study, however, has indicated that strobe lights have limited effectiveness in awakening people (Bruck and Thomas, 2009).

A range of other approaches to sensory stimulation including a fan alongside the bed blowing cold air onto the individual when the alarm rings have been used in the past but are rare nowadays.

Products for communication

This field has been revolutionised in recent years by technological developments. However, the general principle is to increase the information content of the signal, either by improving the signal/noise ratio or by providing visual information. The general approaches used are shown in Table 11.3. These apply to radios, telephones, TVs, computer communications and videos as well as communication and information provision in public palaces, such as banks, ticket offices, shops, cinemas and theatres.

Extension speakers with or without additional amplification are particularly useful for televisions or video players, when the TV can be linked to a hi-fi system or a speaker positioned close to the customary chair of the person concerned. In addition, they can be used with telephones, and it may be seen that such devices are the most commonly used of all environmental aids in the United States and the third most commonly provided in Norway. The principle of both approaches is to make the signal louder and improve the signal/noise ratio, particularly in noisy places.

Loop systems, FM radio systems and infrared systems are all concerned with improving the signal/noise ratio at the patient's ears with or without their hearing aids, bringing the sound source closer to the listener. Electromagnetic loop systems have been in use for many years and remain invaluable in public places, where a range of listeners with hearing aids switched to one of the loop pick-up systems can use them. In addition, a range of telephones are available with incorporated electromagnetic fields, or individual systems linked to radios or televisions with a neck loop or a silhouette loop placed alongside the user's hearing aid can be used. These all have to be hard-wired. Double-loop systems have been advocated for use in auditoriums and similar public places where the field induced by a traditional loop is sometimes patchy (Alterovitz, 2004).

Infrared devices are frequently used in the context of simultaneous translation and are valuable for taking sounds to people with hearing difficulties. The sound quality is good but a transmitter and receiver are required, together with a connection

Table 11.3 Approaches used in products for communication.

Approach	Examples
Auditory – improving the signal/noise ratio	Extension speakers Amplifiers Loop systems Infrared systems FM radio
Visual	Subtitling Teletext Video telephone Signing Skype Text phones Fax e-mail

between the receiver and the hearing aid, where relevant. Furthermore, bright light can interfere with the transmission, which will be restricted to specific locations where the listener can be in the same field as the transmitter.

The most effective approach at the present time is the use of FM systems linking the sound source with the listener(s). These were developed in a classroom context, but are now finding application in a range of personal environments, although one of the main limitations would seem to be the cost of such devices (Chisholm *et al.*, 2007). They also need a transmitter and receiver, but the latter can be attached to the hearing aid, which will need an audio-input link for this purpose. Alternatively, the receiver can be body-worn and connected to a neck loop system so that the listener can receive it via their loop pick-up setting.

The availability of subtitling has improved with the development of digital technology, and many DVDs include subtitling in a range of languages, including that of the film. It is also becoming more widely used in television transmissions (Teletext page 888)

Signing may be used in the background of some news broadcasts on the television as well as in information provision, such as safety instructions shown in aircraft, although the latter is far from universal. And third-generation mobile phones with video camera inputs as well as Skype on the Internet enable those whose main language is sign language to communicate with each other. There have been a number of attempts to introduce such videophone systems on landlines, although these have met with limited success and uptake.

Faxes, e-mails and text telephones have all contributed to revolutionising the way some people with hearing impairments communicate with each other. Textphones, in particular, are almost universal among younger people and have been a particular boon to younger Deaf people (Akamatsu *et al.*, 2006).

Whatever system is used, it is important that it be introduced to meet the specific needs of the individual concerned and that they have sufficient training in its optimal use. It should be acceptable in principle to the individual. While it may be argued that for older people, with more limited activities and social contacts, the selection of appropriate environmental aids may be more appropriate than conventional hearing aids, Jerger *et al.* (1996) found that an overwhelming majority of their older subjects opted for conventional hearing aids rather than environmental aids or a combination of the two. The candidacy for such devices in older people has been discussed comprehensively by Lesner (2003), who considers other reasons for their rejection.

Strategy

This section is concerned with key behavioural changes aimed at minimising the difficulties experienced by people with hearing problems. It is summarised in Table 11.4. Traditionally, such behavioural changes have been associated with the term *hearing tactics*, but here we emphasise that they need to be put in an appropriate perspective, taking into account the specific goals which are being addressed and the underlying personality of the individual concerned.

Goal setting

At this stage, it is important to define and address the goals which the patient sees as particularly important at this stage and which the professional sees as attainable. This should take into account any instrumentation which is being fitted or provided.

Table 11.4 Components of strategy.

Main elements	Components
Goal-setting	
Personality and philosophy of life	
Significant others	
Hearing tactics	Manipulating social interaction
	Manipulating the physical environment
	Observation
	Self-advocacy

Such goal-setting will entail some degree of negotiation between the patient and professional to ensure that these are priorities for the patient and are likely to be achievable. Some preliminary discussion will already have taken place within the context of the 'Integration and decision making' stage (see Chapter Ten) and will have prepared the mindset of both patient and professional for further discussion. Such discussions will start on the basis of the patient's responses to their open-ended questionnaires sent before their clinic appointment (Barcham and Stephens, 1980; Stephens *et al.*, 2001) and elaboration on this during their clinical interview. They will then have been refined during the instrumental stage to highlight what the patient's expressed residual problems are likely to be following appropriate instrumentation.

Once the goals have been defined, the stages in their achievement can be outlined either on a formal or informal basis (Kiresuk and Sherman, 1968; McKenna, 1987) and the means of achieving these goals discussed with the patient. This is a key aspect of the enablement process, and the reader is referred to those publications for details of the process, which must take into account the patient's underlying philosophy of life and personality and the attitudes of their significant others, as discussed below, before specific tactics are decided.

Personality and philosophy of life

These are aspects of the patient that will define the particular tactics which are going to be relevant for them in order to achieve specific goals. Thus, the patient may be outward going and extraverted or shy and introverted. For some, saving face may be important, whereas others may be less concerned about the attitudes of outsiders towards them and their communication approaches.

It is important to remember that such feelings and reactions may be governed by the circumstances in which the individual patients find themselves. Hence, a professional person may be confident and relaxed with all-comers at a professional meeting, but the same person may be shy and reticent in an unfamiliar domain. Even within the context of professional meetings, their approach may well be different when it is a local meeting, where most of those known are familiar to the patient, from a national or international meeting, where the person may be overawed by some of the 'celebrities' present. All will require different approaches.

Significant others

The attitudes and approach of those around the patient to his or her hearing difficulties, and even to the important goals, may have an important relevance to the tactics recommended. However, it is essential that the patient's needs and feelings be given priority over those of the significant others, who may seek to control the patient.

Hallberg and Barrenäs (1993) discuss the different approaches which wives of men with hearing impairments used: *co-acting, mediating, minimising* and *distancing*. Hétu *et al.* (1993) argue that the reaction of male partners of women with hearing impairments is less supportive. They also discuss the interactive role of the audiologist with the couple, where the audiologist should act as a facilitator, interacting with both members of the couple rather than with just one.

However, at the same time, audiologists must remember that their prime responsibility is to their patient. Hence, initial discussions with the patient alone should precede those involving both the patient and their partner. In the latter discussions, the partner should be encouraged to take a more positive supportive role, which should help minimise the impact of the patient's hearing impairment on them. This is discussed further in Chapter 7.

Hearing tactics

These were first presented under this title by Von der Lieth (1972), who defined them as 'Those methods used by someone suffering from a hearing impairment to solve the problems of his daily life – the practical, technical and psychological problems caused by the handicap.' However, many of these have been used spontaneously by both hearing and hearing impaired people for millennia.

Field and Haggard (1989) propose a classification of such tactics, which, however, excludes one of the most frequently used tactics, that of *avoidance*, or withdrawal (Stephens *et al.*, 1999). This is one of three tactics (together with *pretend* and *interrupt*) that Demorest and Erdman (1986) consider to be 'maladaptive'. They define such processes as those which 'detract from or inhibit the communication process'. However, we would argue, on analysing patient responses, that such avoidance behaviour may be very important for the individual from the standpoint of saving face (Jaworski and Stephens, 1998). It does, however, need to be used selectively.

The range of tactics that may be used is shown in Table 11.5, in which the first four are universally regarded as *positive* tactics. The last three are often regarded as *maladaptive*, but we would argue that they can have an important role in saving face if used selectively.

A consecutive series of patients was given a questionnaire in which they were asked whether they used a particular tactic (Stephens *et al.*, 1999). The percentages of those using one particular tactic 'always' or 'often' are shown in Figure 11.7. From this, it may be seen that the 'maladaptive' tactic of avoidance was one of the two most commonly used, together with the 'positive' tactic of asking for repetition. Pretending to have heard and interrupting the speaker were less frequently used, although positioning oneself to hear better was also used only 24% of the time.

The respondents were also asked whether they used such tactics in a range of circumstances. Some of these are shown for the avoidance tactic in Figure 11.8. It may be seen that, on the whole, this was used quite selectively, being most used with the family, who were more tolerant of the individual's behaviour, and least used in work situations, where it could create problems for the individual concerned, and where it is important for them to be involved in any particular situation. This emphasises the fact that any tactic must be used carefully and selectively, according to the specific needs and orientation of the patient.

Table 11.5 Types of hearing tactics frequently used.

Category of tactics	Examples
Manipulation of social interaction	Ask talker to talk slowly Ask talker to rephrase a misheard sentence
Manipulating the physical environment	Ensure light on face of speaker Try to talk in a quiet room
Observation	Watch face of speaker Take note of context
Self-advocacy	Explaining to others ways of facilitating communication
Avoidance	General avoidance Avoid difficult listening situations
Interrupt speaker	When listening is difficult Try to dominate conversations
Pretend to have heard	When listener doesn't understand Not wanting to interrupt flow of conversation

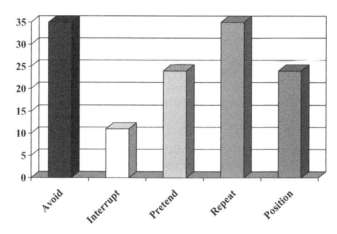

Figure 11.7 Degree of use of different tactics.

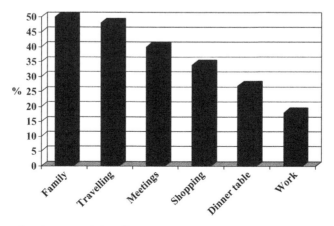

Figure 11.8 Use of avoidance tactic in different circumstances.

Table 11.6 Ancillary services to support the patient.

Ancillary service	Examples
Social services	Interpretation Environmental aid provision
Health services	Medical Psychological Physiotherapy
Education and training services	Educational support Environmental aid provision
Labour and employment services	Retraining Environmental aid provision
Voluntary organisations	Advocacy Local clubs with peer support Information provision

Ancillary help

This element of the process involves seeking additional help for the patient from outside professionals and bodies to address some of their problems that are beyond the knowledge and remit of the audiologist. This should be regarded as a way of complementing the audiologist's work, which continues, rather than handing over the management of the patient to a different type of professional. The elements of help which may be sought at this stage are shown in Table 11.6. For many patients, none of these may be either necessary or relevant, whereas for others they may play a key role in solving some of the problems arising from their hearing impairment.

Social services

The role of social services varies considerably from country to country. Within the United Kingdom, as well as providing general support with regard to housing and self-care, it has the responsibility for providing environmental aids. Such provisions, however, remain rather patchy, and vary from area to area. In some areas, there is a strong working relationship between audiology departments and the local social services, which avoids any duplication of effort and results in more relevant provisions for the patients.

In addition, many countries have specialised social workers for the Deaf, whose main role is to provide support and interpretation services for pre-lingually hearing impaired adults and children. Such support may include the establishment of clubs for Deaf people. Some such specialised social workers extend their remit to people with acquired hearing impairments, but normally their responsibility is primarily to the Deaf community.

More generally, they may have responsibility for the organisation of carers, which may be particularly necessary in older patients with balance problems in addition to their hearing difficulties. Such support may extend to those with a profound acquired hearing impairment and to arranging residential courses for such individuals.

Health service support

The needs for different aspects of this will depend on whether the audiology department includes medically and psychologically qualified personnel among its staff. The patient with hearing problems may, additionally, complain of tinnitus and balance difficulties, which will need investigation and treatment. They may be found to have untreated cognitive or more general health problems. In hearing aid fitting, they may have uncontrolled tremors, which may need a neurological opinion. The extent of referral or of internal management of these conditions will depend on the nature and interest of medical staff working in the department and, even with such staff, may require cross-referrals to other specialties.

In the course of the investigation and management of the patient, they may be found to have significant unmanaged psychological problems, which may or may not be related to their hearing difficulties. If the department does not include a qualified clinical psychologist, this will require cross-referral. In addition, for patients with more minor problems requiring relaxation and related training, referrals to physiotherapists can be helpful. Such physiotherapists will often provide a vestibular rehabilitation service as well.

Education and training services

Many countries have specifically trained educational counsellors who can support young people and adults going into further and higher education and, in recent years, there has been increasing emphasis on lifelong learning. To achieve such education effectively, the individual with hearing impairment needs ongoing support, and this can take the form of note-takers, liaison with the teachers/lecturers and the provision of FM systems. Distance learning via the Internet is a useful way to supplement or, in some cases, replace such an approach. In either case, appropriate counselling by a trained educationalist is essential if the individual is to appropriately pursue this path.

Labour and employment services

Since the 1980s, the emphasis in employment has moved markedly from agriculture and unskilled manufacturing to communication-based industries. This has had a significant impact on the employment of people of working age with hearing impairments (Danermark, 2005; this book Chapter 8).

To enable such individuals to manage optimally in such circumstances requires specific training and environmental aids including FM radio devices. In order to provide a coordinated approach in this respect, specific employment advisers for people with disabilities are necessary, who have a clear understanding of the difficulties faced by workers with hearing impairments and the needs of their environment. Such individuals may work for employment departments of local or central government and, in some countries, their work may be facilitated by government obligations on employers to include a certain proportion of individuals with disabilities in their workforce. For many employers, those with hearing disabilities may be more attractive than those with other disabilities, and they themselves may make a positive contribution in terms of provision of environmental aids and improving the work situation of the worker with a hearing impairment.

Voluntary organisations

Such bodies have several roles for people with hearing difficulties. They may provide information about hearing difficulties and what can be done to overcome these, they may organise local groups where the individual can meet others with similar problems and they may organise interpreters and other support for people with hearing difficulties. In addition, they have an important lobbying role in the context of both central and local government.

While all these roles may ultimately impact on the patient, a key area in the first instance is to provide contact with others with similar problems. This can have a major effect on individuals' acceptance of their own difficulties. Furthermore, many people with hearing difficulties will more willingly accept criticism and advice from others with such problems than from health professionals.

Audiology departments should provide their patients with a list of local organisations and their specific roles, indicating which may hold regular local meetings. Some web sites of appropriate organisations are shown on the web site related to this book (http://www.wiley.com/go/stephens).

Conclusion

This section of the enablement process covers choice of instrumentation, development of strategies and any referral to ancillary services. In essence, it should be covered in one or two sessions, although it may be necessary to return to components of this stage. The first element, instrumentation, covers both wearable, personalised instruments as well as environmental aids. The approach used in the latter will depend on whether they are addressing problems of communication or of other aspects of daily life. While personal instrumentation for the vast majority of individuals entails hearing aids, patients with specific needs may be considered for implantable aids, ranging from bone-anchored hearing aids through cochlear implants to mid-brain implants. In the selection of appropriate hearing aids, a range of factors, beyond electroacoustical characteristics, need to be taken into account.

Strategy entails defining the most appropriate tactics to be used to achieve the goals decided upon by the professional, the patient, with input as well from significant others. Referral to ancillary services with expertise beyond that of the clinic will be necessary in the case of many patients. This can provide additional medical and psychological help as well as support in the employment, educational and social service domains. Involvement of voluntary organisations should also be considered here. They can provide role models for the patient as well as advice and support in a number of different areas.

12 Enablement 3: Ongoing remediation and outcome assessment

Ongoing remediation

In essence, *ongoing remediation* is the process of integrating hearing impairment into one's life. It involves both instrumental and non-instrumental interventions, like training, hearing tactics, counselling, skill building and communication facilitation. The components of ongoing remediation are listed in Table 12.1. In the following section, we address the issue of applying ongoing remediation in the real world.

It is quite remarkable to observe that in most of the rehabilitation models, as described in the introduction of this book, the stage of ongoing remediation is considered as the follow-up to the instrumental stage. Once the stages of *evaluation*, *integration* and *instrumentation* have passed, the one considered *ongoing remediation* is next. It is debateable as to whether, in the process of enablement, this sequence is most effective, but research on this topic is largely lacking.

Another observation worth mentioning here is the terminology used by experts in the different stages of the enablement process. Whereas professionals in the instrumentation phase are usually concerned with *hearing'* and issues like the *perception of sounds, comfortable loudness level, listening comfort* and *speech in noise*, those who are involved in the ongoing remediation stage usually talk about *communication* and have a much broader and more holistic view of what communication comprises and what a patient may want to achieve. Communication requires the two-directional transfer of information, meaning or intent between two or more people and involves social interaction (Kiessling *et al.*, 2003).

The use of different terminology in different stages of the enablement process is also reflected in the choice of outcome measures in the different stages. Whereas measures of disability (i.e. *activity limitation*), including questions like 'Can you understand somebody talking to you in a quiet room?', may be most appropriate in the instrumentation phase, outcome measures in the ongoing remediation phase are usually concerned with *quality of life* and *participation restriction*.

It is clear that the *International Classification of Functioning, Disability and Health* (ICF; WHO, 2001) has had a great influence on the use of terminology in the different stages of the process of enablement. Within the context of ICF, *ongoing remediation* may be seen as part of 'participation' referring to 'involvement in life situations', including various domains. These are shown in Table 12.2.

The impact of hearing impairment in any of the areas shown in Table 12.2 has been described throughout the previous chapters of this book and, in particular, in Chapters 6 and 7. Counselling as to how to cope with hearing impairment in any of those areas may be needed. Various types of counselling exist, including individual or group

Table 12.1 Components of ongoing remediation.

Components	Areas covered
Information provision	Concerning the hearing impairment and aspects of the enablement process
Skill-building	In all aspects of the process including tactics, communication skills and optimal use of any instrumentation used
Instrument modification	Adjusting instrumentation in the light of auditory adaptation and the needs not met in short-term remediation
Counselling	The key area discussed below
Changes to the physical and cultural environment	Much may be implemented by the patient and professionals in the immediate environment, but other aspects require publicity and political action

Table 12.2 Domains of participation as defined by the ICF.

Code	Domain
d1	Learning and applying knowledge
d2	General tasks and demands
d3	Communication
d4	Mobility
d5	Self-care
d6	Domestic life
d7	Interpersonal interactions and relationships
d8	Major life areas
d9	Community, social and civic life

counselling, and a variety of intervention programmes, based either on group meetings or on home-based education, have become established and are detailed in the literature. The following section reports on each on these interventions as key approaches to ongoing remediation.

Individual counselling

The person in the clinic primarily responsible for the content and carrying out of ongoing remediation is usually the enablement (rehabilitation) worker. In different cases, an audiologist, hearing therapist, social worker or a psychologist fulfils that role. Of utmost importance in working with people with hearing impairment is the enablement worker's expression of empathy, validation and willingness to work cooperatively with the patient towards individual and creative solutions (Smith and Kampfe, 1997). Listening is an important skill. It is the enablement worker's task to determine what exactly the patient's problems and needs are. For that purpose, the worker's knowledge and experience of psychosocial aspects (see Chapter 6) are invaluable. In addition, the professional ought to know the patient's personal characteristics, and their personal and life circumstances. For example, it matters whether a patient still has an active working life or whether they have any family problems.

In other words, the whole picture is necessary for the enablement worker to develop strategies for individual patient situations. Thus, some patients may need one session only, whereas others may need a series of consultations.

The enablement worker may decide to include a visit to the patient's home to learn more about their family circumstances. Similarly, a visit to the workplace to educate the different stakeholders (e.g. employer, colleagues, occupational physician) may be highly relevant. In general, there is still an enormous lack of knowledge among those around the patient about what hearing impairment actually comprises and what its consequences are. The development of packages providing educational information, such as those described in Chapter 8, are of great importance.

The enablement worker may be consulted about a wealth of issues including acceptance of hearing loss, self-esteem, assertive expression, acceptance of hearing aids, energy conservation, environmental adaptations, motivation, obtaining support, control and compensation strategies. These issues may be dealt with in any of the domains listed in Table 12.2 as any of those areas may be affected. The concept of coping is essential in each domain.

Coping

Coping is a broad concept. It is defined as 'the process of managing external or internal demands that are appraised as taxing or exceeding the resources of the person' (Lazarus and Folkman, 1984). Coping strategies are ways to handle the problem and these are conscious processes. Unconscious automatic behaviour cannot be regarded as 'coping' according to Lazarus and Folkman (1984). Hallberg and Carlsson (1991) found that the major driving force behind using coping strategies was the individual's effort to maintain a positive (normal) self-image and to avoid being stigmatised (regarded as deviant in interactions with others).

A distinction can be made between practical (or behavioural) approaches and emotional strategies to manage the demands. When applying the issue of coping to hearing impairment, the use of hearing aids may be regarded as a practical approach. Other examples within this category are the acquisition of environmental aids, adjustment of the room acoustics, redelegation of tasks (e.g. at work), rearrangement of furniture and providing light in the room (see also Chapter 8).

Behavioural coping strategies include positioning oneself to hear the speaker, avoiding social events, facing the speaker, asking for repetition, asking for support and visiting a clinic or a professional. Demorest and Erdman (1986) additionally make a distinction between *verbal* and *non-verbal* strategies, the first category referring to strategies where speech is required (e.g. asking for repetition), whereas in the latter no speech is used (e.g. positioning yourself, facing the speaker). Avoidance and request for repetition seem to be the tactics most commonly used in social events (Stephens *et al.*, 1999).

Examples of emotional coping strategies are given throughout the previous sections of this book. Any of the emotional reactions towards hearing impairment (e.g. anger, distress, feelings of depression) may be regarded as a coping strategy as these may be very important in the process of adjusting to hearing impairment and accepting it. An individual with auditory difficulties may go through different stages in their journey to accept their hearing impairment, seek help for it, to obtain and use a hearing aid or consult a professional. Any stage may be accompanied by different emotional states.

The process of coping

It is for this reason that Andersson and Willebrand (2003) disagree with an a priori static classification of coping strategies into *adaptive* or *maladaptive* strategies, such as for example proposed by Demorest and Erdman (1986). Maladaptive strategies include avoidance behaviour, pretending to hear, guessing what was said, dominating conversations and ignoring others.

Andersson and Willebrand (2003) regard a classification into *adaptive* and *maladaptive* as too simplistic as one can only consider emotional states or certain behaviours as adaptive or maladaptive when these are seen in the context of time and seen along the process of adjusting to hearing impairment. For example, in the short term, avoidance behaviour may be crucial when one is trying to alleviate and regulate stressful circumstances and periods.

Comparable conclusions are drawn by Hallberg and Carlsson (1991). In their qualitative study, the participants appeared to use strategies *to avoid the social scene* and *to control the social scene* alternately, depending on how demanding the auditory situation was.

Andersson and Willebrand's view is in line with Jaworski and Stephens's (1998) report on *silence* as a face-saving strategy used by people with hearing impairment. Whereas avoidance of communication (silence) is typically seen as a negative and maladaptive strategy, their study shows that for many people with hearing impairment silence (or the avoidance of communication) can function as a means of managing the relationship with their communication partner, particularly in acoustically demanding situations (e.g. high levels of background noise). Asking for repetition in such circumstances may be more embarrassing than just keeping silent. Another example refers to inadequate positioning of another person (e.g. speaking from behind). Non-talk may be used to prevent what is likely to be an unsuccessful attempt at verbal interaction.

In other words, just assigning a positive (adaptive) or a negative (maladaptive) label to a certain coping strategy is not justified as context and time are not taken into account. Nonetheless, persistence of behaviour typically classified as maladaptive in the longer term may be inadequate and even counter-productive.

Studies of the dynamic process of adjusting to hearing impairment, taking the time component into account, are scarce. An example is a study by Engelund (2006), who conducted in-depth interviews with 14 people who had had normal hearing but were experiencing hearing problems at the time of the interview.

Engelund identifies four stages of 'consciousness of hearing problems' in the process of adjusting to hearing impairment, prior to help-seeking and interprets those as:

- attracting attention
- becoming suspicious
- sensing tribulation
- jeopardising the fundamental self.

The stages are illustrated in Figure 12.1.

The sequence of stages is characterised by the extent to which a person with hearing impairment is aware of their problems and their actions:

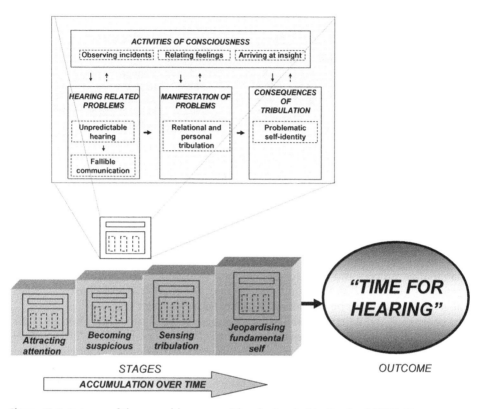

Figure 12.1 Outcome of the recognising process 'Time for hearing' by Engelund (2006). (*Source:* reproduced by permission from Engelund, 2006.)

1. In the first stage, the person with the hearing impairment is not aware of their limitations, and the hearing problems are mainly pointed out by others.
2. In the second stage, more and more episodes of misunderstanding occur and people start to use tactics to compensate for their hearing problems.
3. The third stage is characterised by more frequent use of withdrawal and avoidance behaviour, and people no longer attribute the problems to others, but rather to themselves. Annoyance may arise as well as anger, frustration and feelings of incompetence. People start to experience withdrawal as a better option than using tactics, as these no longer suffice. It finally leads to stage 4 (jeopardising the fundamental self).
4. It is at stage 4 where too many aspects in a person's life, both externally as well as internally, change. Feelings of insecurity about self-identity may arise and, at this stage, emotional reactions may result in negative outcomes. The growing discrepancy between who the person is at that stage and who they want to be makes the person seek help. Based on the work of Miller and Rollnick (2002), Engelund (2006) argues that it is when things are sufficiently discrepant from the desired or expected ideal that motivation for change begins. Only when people take ownership of a disability are they motivated to change the situation.

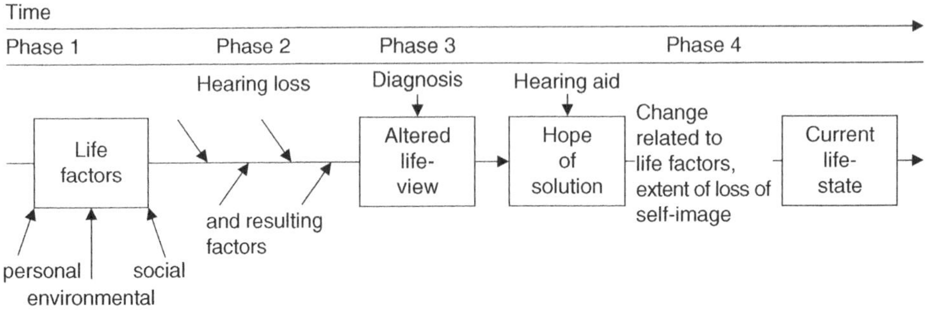

Time

| Phase 1 | Phase 2 | Phase 3 | Phase 4 |

Figure 12.2 Temporal overview of the progress of hearing impairment (Figure 13.2 in Jones *et al.*, 1987, p. 218. (*Source:* reproduced by permission of Taylor & Francis Books.)

Engelund's study is an interesting illustration as to how coping and coping mechanisms may change over time. Jones *et al.* (1987) recognise the issue of time in the rehabilitation process and introduce a temporal overview of the progress of hearing impairment (Figure 12.2). Engelund's stages may be seen as parts of Phase 2 of Jones *et al.*'s model. They can be considered as a further refinement.

In conclusion, while coping skills may not always be thoroughly effective, they nonetheless form part of a process that constitutes adjustment. In other words, adjustment to hearing impairment is a process incorporating the possibility of change and transition. The challenge for the future is to identify the type of interventions and services most effective at each stage in the adjustment process, prior to and post help-seeking and prior to and post diagnosis and intervention.

Returning to individual counselling given by an enablement worker, we find that traditional audiological counselling, with one or two individual sessions with a therapist as part of hearing aid fitting, may not be adequate for every individual to promote lasting lifestyle, coping and attitude changes. Some patients may need additional interventions to reach that goal. Examples of other forms of therapy are perceptual (or auditory) training, training in speechreading, clear speech, communication repair, home-based communication training and group counselling. Each of those intervention types is addressed in the following sections.

Auditory training/perceptual training

Most people with hearing impairment using amplification by hearing aids or cochlear implants discover that their auditory perceptions are both impoverished and different from those experienced before the hearing impairment or before using hearing aids or cochlear implants (Boothroyd, 2007). Auditory training helps people to adapt or to acclimatise to the 'new' sound perceptions or auditory sensations. It aims to improve their discrimination of vowels and other phonemes so that they can make the most use of their residual hearing and better understand sounds and speech.

Whereas adaptation may occur in the context of everyday communication, there are a range of programmes developed that help people to learn to deal with these new sensations (Sweetow and Palmer, 2005). Training usually requires daily sessions of about half an hour involving the repetitive presentation of stimuli (sounds, phonemes, words) over a period of days or weeks. Programmes have been developed for different clinical populations, such as cochlear implant users, adults, children with auditory processing disorders and older individuals with compromised cognitive skills (Kricos and McCarthey, 2007). It is widely accepted that auditory training can improve performance on the trained task (Rubinstein and Boothroyd, 1987; Amitay *et al.*, 2005; Sweetow and Palmer, 2005; Burk and Humes, 2008).

LACE

An example of a programme entailing auditory training is LACE (Listening and Communication Enhancement) (Sweetow and Sabes, 2006). LACE is an interactive home-based computer program. It aims to help people with hearing impairment to learn skills and strategies that help them to become better listeners, build their confidence and, consequently, increase the amount of speech they understand. It also addresses cognitive changes characteristic of the ageing process. While the program engages people with hearing impairment in the hearing aid fitting process, it is also applicable to those who do not use hearing aids.

For four weeks, a user spends half an hour, five days a week, working with the computer program to help enhance listening skills. The program provides a variety of interactive and adaptive tasks, which are divided into three main categories:

1. better comprehension of degraded speech
2. enhancement of cognitive skills
3. improvement of communication strategies.

The types of exercise include speech in babble, time-compressed (i.e. fast) speech, competing speakers, auditory working memory, use of contextual information (linguistics) and interactive communication strategies (i.e. helpful hints) (Table 12.3).

The user receives immediate feedback with regard to correct comprehension and can monitor their improvement from the beginning of therapy. The difficulty level of all exercises is adaptive, based on the accuracy of the patient's response to the previous trial. It means that if a task is accomplished correctly, the next one will be more difficult and, conversely, if a task is performed incorrectly, the next one will be easier.

In addition, the patient's audiologist can observe progress via a computer modem at a remote location.

Sweetow and Sabes (2006) conducted a study to evaluate the effectiveness of LACE. Sixty-five patients (aged 28–85 years) participated with pre- and post-test measures. They were randomly assigned to two groups, one receiving LACE immediately

Table 12.3 The proportion of exercises in LACE.

Type of task	Percentage of LACE
Better comprehension of degraded speech	
Speech in babble	30
Time-compressed (i.e. fast) speech	20
Competing speaker	20
Enhancement of cognitive skills	
Auditory working memory	15
Contextual information/linguistics (missing words)	15
Interactive communication strategies (helpful hints)	Shown throughout LACE

following baseline testing and one serving as a control for one month and then receiving LACE as a crossover group. Both objective and subjective outcome measures were used including a speech-in-noise (SPIN) test (i.e. hearing-in-noise test; HINT), QuickSin (quick speech-in-noise test), the Hearing Handicap Inventory for the Elderly (HHIE), the Communication Scale for Older Adults (CSOA), Stroop Color Word test and a listening span test measuring working memory. Significant improvement after training was observed on all outcomes, except for HINT. The results indicate that at least at the short term (immediately after training) the training is effective. In a subsequent study, Henderson *et al.* (2007) observed that participants with the poorest scores on the baseline tests, particularly those with the greatest degree of hearing impairment, had the poorest scores on measures of degraded and competing speech, and those with the highest hearing handicap scores were more likely to have greater improvement overall. It is unclear yet whether the improvements obtained with LACE remain stable over time.

Speechreading

Along with auditory (perceptual) training, training in speechreading (or lipreading) is regarded as an important part of the enablement process (Kricos, 2006; Boothroyd, 2007). Speechreading is a skill that aids communication. It is *seeing the sound of spoken language* and thus occurs in situations where the listener can both hear and see the speaker. The movements of the lips and tongue, together with facial expression and body language, are all cues for speechreading.

In general, people rely on visual cues to enhance their recognition of spoken language, in particular in adverse listening conditions or when an individual experiences difficulties in hearing. It is assumed that only 30% of the spoken language can be 'seen', as many letters and words are difficult to distinguish when they are pronounced. For example, the words *bad, mad* and *pad* look the same.

Nevertheless, speechreading has been acknowledged as an important skill and various studies have demonstrated that speech recognition significantly improves when visual cues are available. Such improvement occurs not only when the auditory speech signals are degraded (owing to noise, reverberation or hearing impairment) (Grant *et al.*, 1998) but also when the speech signals are intact (Reisberg *et al.*, 1987). In the study by Grant *et al.* (1998), all participants benefited from combining the auditory and visual cues in a sentence recognition task, even though large variations between participants were found. However, while some people seem to be natural speechreaders, others need to be taught how to speechread and need considerable training. The authors argue that the variability may reflect differences in the ability to use lexical, semantic and grammatical constraints and the ability to allocate top-down cognitive processes such as memory skills and processing speed, factors that are important in the comprehension of speech (see also Chapter 5). As mentioned in Chapter 4, visual acuity may also play a role in explaining interindividual differences in speechreading.

Middelweerd and Plomp (1987) applied the Speech-Reception-Threshold in noise (SRTn) test to young (19–28 years) and older (68–84 years) listeners. The authors compared two conditions: the sentences were presented in the auditory (A) and in the audiovisual (AV) condition. Compared to the auditory-alone (A) sentences, they observed an improvement of 4.6 dB in the score (i.e. the signal-to-noise ratio, defined as the threshold at which 50% of the sentences is repeated correctly) in the AV condition among the young listeners and an improvement of 4.0 dB among the older listeners. Since then, various studies confirmed the benefit of having visual cues available during speech recognition. However, people with hearing impairment do not exhibit better speechreading capacities than their normally hearing peers (Hygge *et al.*, 1992; Tye-Murray *et al.*, 2007).

A person's ability to speechread also depends on how well the speaker enunciates the speech sounds.

Clear speech

Clear speech is characterised by a slower rate, more frequent pauses, increased duration of phonemes, fuller differentiation between phonemes and good articulation. A number of studies have shown that speech produced in a clear manner is easier to understand than conversational speech (Gagné *et al.*, 1995; Schum, 1996). For example, Helfer (1997) presented words within nonsense sentences in the presence of background noise to normally hearing young listeners. Significant effects of speaking mode were found. Clear speech was easier to understand than was conversational speech, both in the auditory-alone condition and in the AV condition. Helfer's results demonstrate that speaking clearly and providing visual speech information offers complementary (rather than redundant) information. In addition, older participants showed more benefit from clear speech than younger participants (Helfer, 1998).

Speakers can be trained to produce clear speech (Schum, 1996; Kricos 2006). Talker training as an intervention for spouses, family members and friends of people with hearing impairment has therefore been advocated (Caissie *et al.*, 2005; Kricos, 2006). Minimising the speaker–listener distance is important to consider in this context (Erber *et al.*, 1998). Clear speech can be seen as an element of communication repair strategies.

Communication repair

Communication repair aims to give the communication partner an idea as to how they should actually modify their speech to ensure speech comprehension by the listener. In other words, communication repair concerns clarification of the precise reason the listener did not understand and 'repair' the utterances that have not been understood.

Conversations with people with hearing impairment are often characterised by communication breakdowns. These may occur when a person with hearing impairment just pretends to understand (bluffing) or simply says 'what' or 'huh', rather than attempting to repair the communication (Ross, 2002). Communication repair strategies focus on analysing *why* exactly the communication broke down. For example, if a person with hearing impairment missed only the last word in a sentence, but understood the rest, all that is necessary is to ask the speaker to repeat just that last word (or to spell it out) rather than to repeat the entire sentence. Another communication repair strategy is to now and then ask the *listener* with hearing impairment to repeat the last sentence. This is done to check the listener's comprehension and make sure that they are still following the conversation.

Alternative repair strategies are: 'Ask the speaker to talk a little slower', 'Ask the speaker to talk a little louder' and 'Ask the speaker to pronounce the sentence a little clearer' (Ross, 2002).

Training in communication repair strategies involves practice in rapidly applying the appropriate strategies in everyday communication. It also involves training and encouragement in becoming more assertive in applying communication repair strategies in day-to-day situations.

A group aural enablement programme is a typical setting in which speechreading, clear speech and communication repair strategies can be taught, trained and practised (Abrams *et al.*, 1992; Brewer, 2001; Kricos, 2006). Inclusion of significant others in such communication training programmes may be of particular importance (Preminger, 2003).

Communication strategies

Whereas speechreading, clear speech and communication repair may be considered as important strategies (or tactics) to enhance communication, there are a range of additional strategies than can be applied, both by the person with hearing impairment and their significant others. Many of these strategies have been mentioned throughout this and other chapters. Examples are the provision of light so that the speaker's face remains visible, positioning oneself so that the speaker's face is close and visible, try to get the attention of the person with hearing impairment before speaking, avoid talking from behind or from another room, reduce background noise (i.e. turn the radio off during conversations) and reduce reverberation with soft furnishings.

Home-based education

Whereas a group programme may be the most appropriate setting to train communication strategies (including speechreading), there are always a number of people who cannot be reached if this is the only service that is offered. The reasons for this are described later. Home-based education can serve as an alternative. Earlier, we reported on the home-based computer program LACE.

Kramer *et al.* (2005) developed a home-education programme focusing on communication strategies training. It is a self-administered intervention, comprising five videotapes (or DVDs) and an instruction booklet. Each videotape shows a short film representing an everyday situation familiar to most people. Adequate and inadequate coping behaviours of both the person with hearing impairment and the significant other are highlighted. The programme also incorporates speechreading exercises, information on how to use hearing aids and information about environmental aids. The films are sent by regular mail to the participants' homes, one at a time. People are encouraged to practise communication strategies with their significant others at home.

A randomised controlled trial was performed and a treatment group of people receiving hearing aid fitting and the home education was compared with a control group (hearing aid fitting only). An increased awareness of the benefits of speechreading and improved interaction with the significant other was observed only in the treatment group (Kramer *et al.*, 2005).

Group counselling

A wide variety of group programmes, specifically designed for aural enablement, exist. Examples are self-help groups, educational group intervention, peer discussion group intervention and support groups. An advantage of group programmes over individual intervention is that the group itself provides a situation for practising skills, interacting with others and learning from other group members (Hickson, 2007). It may also be used to appoint role models. As emphasised in Chapter 7, role modelling may be regarded as an important and useful strategy to enhance the enablement process focusing on the adjustment to hearing impairment. The audiological literature reports on a variety of group programmes that have been designed.

Self-help groups

Self-help groups are change-oriented organisations that are led by patients (Kurtz, 1997). Self-help groups are popular. In the United Kingdom, more than 2000 illness self-help groups exist. In the Netherlands and in other countries self-help groups are mostly overseen and facilitated by voluntary organisations.

The central issue with regard to self-help groups (and probably the issue of groups in general) is social comparison. Such comparison occurs between similar people or people with similar problems (Festinger, 1954). Self-help groups consist of just such people. Social comparison may seem to be a helpful and positive tool in the enablement process. However, it must be noted that social comparison can comprise a negative mechanism, depending on how one *interprets* the comparison (Buunk *et al.*, 1990). As illustrated in Chapter 7 of this book, role modelling (i.e. social comparison) may be interpreted positively or negatively. In fact, as described by Van der Zee *et al.* (1998) there seem to be four different categories:

1. Upward comparison interpreted positively ('When I compare myself with others who are experiencing fewer problems than me, I am pleased that things can get better')
2. Upward comparison interpreted negatively ('When I compare myself with others who are experiencing fewer problems than me, I find it threatening to notice that I am not doing so well')
3. Downward comparison interpreted positively ('When I compare myself with others who are experiencing more problems than me, I am relieved about my own situation')
4. Downward comparison interpreted negatively ('When I compare myself with others who are experiencing more problems than me, I experience fear that my health will decline')

Negative interpretations of comparisons, whether upwards or downwards, tend to be associated with avoidant coping behaviour (Van der Zee *et al.*, 1998), whereas positive interpretations seem to be related to adjusting coping behaviour. Dibb and Yardley (2006) confirmed these findings. They investigated the role of social comparison in the adjustment to Menière's disorder within a self-help group. Their study included 301 people with Menière's disorder. Controlling for the effects of disease severity and psychological factors that are known to influence both adjustment and the interpretation of social comparison information (i.e. self-esteem, control, optimism, age, sex), they observed that positive social comparison was indeed significantly related to better adjustment (as measured with functional and goal-oriented quality-of-life measures). They observed an adverse effect on quality of life at a 10-month follow-up among those who interpreted upward social comparison negatively and among those who very frequently and exhaustively compared themselves with others (associated with neuroticism and anxiety). Even though the results of a study solely including people with Menière's disorder cannot be generalised, the latter finding seems to suggest that personality is an essential factor determining whether one's participation in a self-help group will be successful. In particular, those who feel in control (high self-esteem) and are able to achieve positive social comparison may benefit, whereas those for whom making positive comparisons is difficult, self-help group participation may constitute a risk (Dibb and Yardley, 2006). For those people, support groups may be a better option.

Support groups

Support groups are led by one or more *facilitators* (sometimes used as synonymous with group leader or programme leader). It is the facilitator's role to get the patients to talk, to express their problems and feelings and talk about alternative ways of coping with hearing impairment. Working in a group requires special skills. It is not just organisation to bring the people together. The *process* of the group work itself is even more important. This process comprises the mechanisms by which the group acts as a unit rather than as a cluster of separate individuals. The facilitator needs to carefully manage the process so that the value of the group will not diminish or even be destroyed. As such, the group process can enhance the value of the group to be many times the sum of the worth of its individual participants. It is this *synergy* that makes a group work. Group work with people with hearing impairment is even more challenging as patient's hearing ability is an issue. It is therefore recommended to have two facilitators rather than one when people with hearing impairment are involved. Thus, one of the facilitators can lead the group discussion while the other sits at the side watching the process, making sure that every participant follows the group conversation, receives appropriate attention and is actively involved.

Preminger (2007) clearly indicates that no standard group programme exists, despite the fact that the majority of programmes in audiology have been designed in connection with hearing aid fitting (Hawkins, 2005). The aim is generally a problem-solving process. Different procedures are used in the provision of group services. These concern the material used, the frequency of the meetings, the length of the programme and the facilitator(s) (Preminger, 2007).

A review of the various programmes published in the literature reveals that whereas the time allocated to the different components may vary, the programmes usually cover:

▓ Educational lectures about the anatomy of the ear, types and degree of hearing impairment
▓ The communication process and listening devices, including hearing aids
▓ Training in speechreading and communication strategies
▓ Informational and psychosocial counselling
▓ Auditory training

> (Abrams *et al.* 1992; Kricos and Holmes, 1996; Beynon *et al.*, 1997;
> Brewer, 2001; Preminger, 2003).

Some courses also include relaxation techniques (Hétu and Getty, 1991; Norman *et al.*, 1995). Alternative programmes predominantly focus on one or two components, such as hearing tactics and coping (Andersson *et al.*, 1994).

Most group programmes have one- to two-hour weekly sessions over three or four consecutive weeks. Hétu and Getty (1991) offered an alternative option for those who could not attend the weekly sessions: an intensive session lasting one and a half days over the weekend. Their programme was primarily designed for workers with noise-induced hearing loss (NIHL).

Usually, there are about 10 participants in the group. A larger number would make the group too big to manage and conversations would become too noisy for people with hearing impairment. Some programmes allow significant others to participate (Hétu and Getty, 1991; Preminger, 2003). An advantage of including significant others in the programme is that patients can practise communication strategies with those with whom they communicate most often.

Community-based groups

All of the group programmes have one common characteristic: they were designed in relation to hearing aid fitting. There is, however, a huge number of people who suffer from hearing problems but have never visited an audiology clinic. Some of those people do not wish to wear hearing aids and, hence, decided to not seek help. Hickson and colleagues (2007a) designed a group intervention that may be seen as an alternative to hearing aid fitting as well as complementing hearing aid fitting. It is a group programme called Active Communication Education (ACE). An important feature of ACE is that it is conducted not in clinics but in community locations such as in senior citizens' centres or the public library. These locations are usually very accessible and user-friendly for older people. Many people who attend ACE have never been to an audiology clinic (Hickson, 2007a). The only prerequisite to participate in ACE is that a person has hearing or communication difficulties. It does not matter whether they use hearing aids or not.

ACE is an interactive group programme with six to eight people participating. The group meets for two hours a week for five weeks with a group facilitator. Significant others (e.g. close family and relatives) are also invited to come along.

ACE's approach is one of active problem-solving. The participant becomes active in the education process, collaborating with the facilitator (e.g. audiologist) and other group participants to find solutions to their problems. In the first session, the facilitator starts with a communication needs analysis. This is a crucial part, because the needs identified at this point become the topics that the group will work on over the following four sessions. Each participant is asked to answer the following question: 'What hearing/communication difficulties do you experience in everyday life as a result of your hearing impairment?'

Each group member has to state one difficulty. These are written on a board. Members continue to specify difficulties until all the problems they can think of are recorded. The facilitator then groups together all the difficulties that belong to the same category. In the next step, the participants are asked to rank them. The difficulties with the highest score become the topics covered in the sessions that follow. Hickson and colleagues argue that, in this way, no group member ends up dominating the group with their problems.

The ultimate aim of ACE is for group members to learn individual problem-solving skills that can be applied in a range of communication situations. It is a learning process, not just a few strategies.

Effectiveness of group programmes

With regard to the effectiveness of group interventions in the process of enablement, mixed findings have been reported. Hawkins (2005) conducted a systematic review of the effectiveness of adult group programmes and concludes that, at least in the short term (directly after the intervention), there are benefits. However, it is uncertain whether these effects remain stable in the long term (e.g. one year later), as there is a lack of studies with appropriate designs including long-term measurement. Two of the 13 studies that were reviewed by Hawkins (2005) used a longer period, one year (Chisholm et al., 2004) and two years (Andersson et al., 1995b). Both those studies observed a significant short-term benefit in the treatment group, but failed to find differences between the treatment and control group at the one-year (Chisholm et al., 2004) or two-year (Andersson et al., 1995b) follow-up assessments.

Hawkins (2005) raises the issue of what outcome measures should be used. Effects can only be found when the appropriate outcomes are used. The majority of researchers believe that a reduction in one's perception of *participation restriction* is the primary benefit that should be expected from group counselling. Nine of the 13 studies reviewed by Hawkins used questionnaires assessing participation restriction, the most common being the Hearing Handicap Inventory for the Elderly (HHIE), which focuses on emotional issues related to hearing impairment. The question remains, however, whether the HHIE or similar types of questionnaires assessing participation restriction, are the most appropriate. To illustrate this, Kricos and Holmes (1996) found an improvement in functioning as measured by the Communication Profile for the Hearing Impaired (CPHI, verbal and non-verbal strategies), but failed to detect a significant group difference (control vs treatment) using the HHIE. They argue that the CPHI is a more sensitive measure of the effects of communication training than the HHIE, even though Abrams et al. (1992) did find a significant treatment effect using the HHIE.

Andersson et al. (1994) found an improvement in several areas of activity (shopping, party, conversations) among those who were taught hearing tactics compared with controls who were not, but failed to find an effect in general emotional functioning measured by the Life Orientation Test (LOT). Similarly, Beynon et al. (1997) found a reduction in participation restriction for the 'communication' and 'vocational' subscales of the Quantified Denver Scale of Communication Function (QDS), but did not find an extra effect of their rehabilitation programme (speechreading, hearing tactics, use of hearing aids) on the 'self' (i.e. emotional response) and 'family' scales when comparing the scores with the results of the control group (hearing aid fitting only). Getty and Hétu (1991) found their participants (industrial workers) to be more confident in dealing with their hearing problems after participation in the group sessions. Follow-up results showed that the workers with hearing impairment judged their problems as being significantly less severe.

Preminger (2003) evaluated two types of groups. One comprised patients with hearing impairment. The second group comprised patients who attended the group along with their significant others. The results demonstrated that patients with hearing impairment in both groups showed a reduction in participation restriction (as measured with the HHIE) after the intervention. In addition, those attending the group with their significant others had a greater reduction than those who participated on their own.

The effectiveness of ACE was examined using a randomised controlled trial, in which 178 people (aged 53–94 years) participated (Hickson et al., 2007b). One group attended ACE and the other was in a 'placebo' group programme. It was a social programme with the same amount of group contact. To examine the benefit, a range of outcome measures was used, including the Client-Oriented Scale of Improvement (COSI). Among people allocated to ACE, Hickson *et al.* found a significant reduction in participation restriction as measured with the Hearing Handicap Questionnaire, and an improvement in their reported communication activities (QDS and the Self-Assessment of Communication). Further, an improvement in their general wellbeing (Ryff Psychological Well-being Scale) was observed. No improvements in generic quality of life (SF-36) were observed. Those who were allocated to the social programme also showed improvement, but there were fewer benefits.

With COSI it was found that 75% of participants in ACE reported some improvement on the primary goal they wished to achieve. In addition, the results were maintained after six months.

Further, to examine whether ACE results were better for some people than for others, the variables age, gender, degree of hearing impairment, hearing aid use, involvement of significant other in ACE and attitudes towards hearing impairment were investigated. The only personal variable that helped predict performance was *attitudes towards hearing impairment*. Those having more positive attitudes at the start of ACE showed better outcomes afterwards. Attitude seems to be a key ingredient. People who are more aware of their hearing impairment and more positive about enablement, have a greater success with treatment (Hickson, 2007a).

Arising from the above findings, a couple of remarks about the effectiveness of group enablement can be made:

- It may well be that hearing aid fitting per se positively influences emotional functioning, while extra enablement group programmes may be needed to get the individual with hearing impairment more involved in daily-life interactions and to enhance communication (as measured with the CPHI).
- The outcome measures used in most of the studies might have been limited with regard to their capacity to 'capture' the real effects of what group participation yields. It is known that the majority of patients who participated in a group programme are positive and report that it assisted with their understanding of their own situation.

A more patient-centred approach in outcome measurement, such as the COSI, may be more appropriate in this respect. Every patient has his or her unique problems that require unique solutions, and any evaluation of the outcomes should be performed with that in mind. As argued by Gagné (2003): 'Treatment effectiveness research should incorporate individualized outcome measures. That is, a unique set of outcome measures should be identified for each of the persons who participate in the treatment program. Further, each outcome measure should make it possible to document changes related to each participant's involvement in the specific activity identified in the objective of the intervention program.' The Hickson *et al.* (2007b) study may be an example of good practice in this respect.

Furthermore, the results reported by Preminger (2003) are promising, indicating the importance of having the significant other involved in the enablement process. Finally, as indicated by Hawkins (2005), the group facilitator may have an effect on the outcome. This issue has not been addressed in any of the studies described above.

The ongoing enablement process should include the most appropriate interventions for the individual, whether as a home-based programme, group or individual intervention or as a self-help group. In addition, the topics may be dependent on the life stage of the participants, whether they are working or retired.

Tailoring the enablement process to individual needs implies that any option of intervention should depend on the patient's choice. For example, it is known that many people are not keen on attending group meetings for various reasons, such as mobility problems, ill health, lack of time or distance. From the professional point of view, a complicating factor may be the need for resources to organise and run a group programme. Not only is accommodation required, but also personnel with specific expertise. These complicating factors may be the reason for the limited application of group interventions in regular audiological care. Home-based education programmes (if available) should be offered as an alternative.

Outcome assessment

Measures of outcomes have many functions, and different measures are appropriate for different needs. Such needs will be discussed briefly in this section, but the emphasis will be on the individual patient.

Cox *et al.* (2000) list the main functions of outcome measures and these are summarised in Table 12.4, which includes additional suggested uses and examples.

The uses of these and other measures as well as their characteristics are extensively reviewed by Noble (1998) and Bentler and Kramer (2000). The uses relating to inter-

Table 12.4 Uses of outcome measures with examples.

Use	Circumstances	Possible measures
Assessing outcome for a particular patient	Patient-oriented enablement	COSI; visual analogue scales; significant other measures; personalised satisfaction measures
Assessing effectiveness of a particular service	Comparison of different audiological centres	Satisfaction measures: SADL, GHABP; Changes in other measures: IOI-HA, IOI-SO, IOI-AI
Assessing a new technology or intervention	Comparisons of a new hearing aid processing system with more traditional systems	Speech-in-noise measures: SHAPIE, GHABP; Other tests to investigate the anticipated specific benefits of the new intervention: IOI-HA, IOI-SO, IOI-AI
Assessing effects on quality of life	Comparison of cost-effectiveness of audiological versus other medical or related interventions	SF-36, EuroQol, HUI
Research	Determination of which factors influence outcome	Any appropriate measures dependent on circumstances

(COSI = Client-Oriented Scale of Improvement (Dillon *et al.*, 1997); SADL = Satisfaction with Amplification in Daily Life (Cox and Alexander, 1999); IOI-HA = International Outcome Inventory for Hearing Aids (Cox *et al.*, 2000); IOI-SO, IOI-AI are the applications of the last to significant others and non-instrumental enablement (Noble, 2002); GHABP = Glasgow Hearing Aid Benefit Profile (Gatehouse, 1999); SHAPIE = Shortened Hearing Aid Performance Inventory for the Elderly (Dillon, 1994); SF-36 = Short-form Health Survey (Brazier *et al.*, 1998); HUI = Health Utilities Index (Torrance, 1986); EuroQol (http://www.euroqol.org)

ventions will not be discussed further here, and interested readers are referred to Cox (2000) for a general discussion of these.

With regards to the individual passing through the enablement process, there are a number of considerations which need to be taken into account:

1. What are their real problems and how severe are they? This forms a basis for measuring the effectiveness of the process by before and after measures.
2. What problems does the individual have after intervention?
3. How satisfied are they with the intervention?
4. Has the intervention benefited their significant others and the patient's relationships with them?
5. How well do they accept their residual problems?

Patient problems and their changes

Determination of the individual's hearing difficulties has been outlined in earlier sections and chapters. We would suggest that it is useful to send an open-ended questionnaire (e.g. the Life Effects questionnaire; Stephens *et al.*, 2001) to the patient prior to their appointment so that they can think about it and be better able to discuss their specific problems when they come to the clinic. On that occasion, the audiologist can pick up on the difficulties listed and seek clarification of particular points as well as asking whether the patient has any further problems.

Once sure that the main problems have been articulated, the audiologist can ask the patient either to rate their problems in order of importance, giving them a numerical score out of 10 or 100, or mark the importance of each on a visual analogue scale. The most important questions can then be entered onto the first part of the COSI form (Dillon *et al.*, 1997) for use when the main part of the enablement process is complete. Alternatively, the scores can be noted separately for further comparison.

When the patient indicates at the end of the process that they are managing well and are about to be discharged, these will be retrieved and the patient asked to indicate any changes in the individual complaints (worse, same, slightly better, better, much better) and how much of a problem they still have with their complaint. In this way, the professional can determine whether any of these difficulties needs further attention.

At this stage, it is important to ask the patient whether they have any additional complaints (as discussed by Louise Hickson in the Appendix). This is a key point, given that in any enablement process we are dealing with a dynamic and changing condition and series of experiences. The broad pattern of complaints at the repeat assessment tends to become more specific and more oriented towards weaknesses of certain aspects of the intervention received, such as hearing aids. This is shown in Figure 12.3 from the Cardiff arm of the study described by Hickson.

Similarly, if the individual has scored the severity of their problems prior to the enablement process, this scoring can be repeated after the process, the results compared in the same way (Bai and Stephens, 2005; Zhao *et al.*, 2008), and judgements made, following discussion with the patient, as to whether any further intervention is necessary. This process can then be repeated on subsequent occasions, together with probing for new problems and their rating in the same way as the others. Figure 12.4 shows representative responses from one of their patients with a cochlear implant

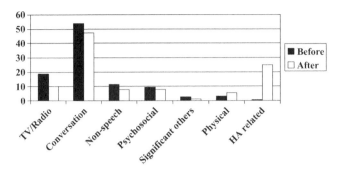

Figure 12.3 Patient complaints at the beginning and end of intervention.

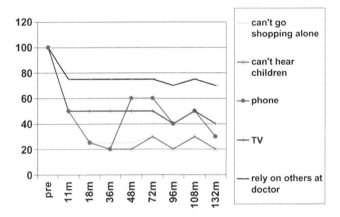

Figure 12.4 Ratings of different problems by a patient before cochlear implantation and up to 11 years post-implantation.

over a period of 11 years post-implantation. However, this figure does not include new complaints, specified post-implantation, and their ratings.

It may be seen that, for this individual, some complaints such as hearing her children and going shopping improve quite rapidly and dramatically, whereas others, such as the need for help when visiting her doctor, change very little and require attention in other ways, such as other organisation of deaf awareness training in the medical centre that she attends.

When this process is complete to the satisfaction of the patient and professional, the patient may either be discharged, with the opportunity of returning should they have any further problems, or be given a long-term appointment (e.g. 1–2 years) for a further check.

Patient-defined satisfaction

This can be tapped in a number of ways, and the approach used by Tyler and Kelsay (1990) and independently by Stephens and Meredith (1991b) has been to ask the patients to list the benefits and shortcomings of their intervention, post-enablement. Tyler and Kelsay (1990) use the terms *advantages* and *disadvantages*, but their results

Table 12.5 An example of benefit and shortcomings responses from a patient after cochlear implantation.

Benefits	Shortcomings
Obviously the restoring of sound. My grandson is 10 years old and I never heard him speak until this year.	No indication of battery life
Conversation restored with family and friends	Not getting as familiar with sound scales as I should be
Birdsong in the garden	When digging and perspiring, the appliance slips off the back of my ear
Road traffic where before I was dependent on others and using my eyes	Eating (i.e. chewing of food is loud)
Not using subtitles on the TV, which irritated the family	
Using telephone and not text	

were essentially the same with their patients with cochlear implants as those described by Stephens *et al.* (2008).

Stephens and Meredith (1991) analysed their results in terms of *acoustical, psychosocial, practical* and *medical* benefits and shortcomings and later Kennedy *et al.* (2008) used an analysis based on ICF (WHO, 2001). This approach has been applied to patients with cochlear implants, hearing aids and BAHAs but not, so far, to those receiving a programme of non-instrumental enablement.

An example of results from a patient listing both benefits and shortcomings in a patient with a cochlear implant is shown in Table 12.5.

It may be seen that for the audiologist, it is the shortcomings that are most important and indicate the areas which require more attention in further enablement booster sessions. Some problems will not, however, be resolved, and the patient will need to be helped to accept them (see below).

Significant others

Essentially similar approaches can be used with significant others of patients as with the patients themselves. Thus, we have used the Problem Questionnaire with significant others prior to intervention. Thus, Lormore and Stephens (1994) asked the significant others to list the problems which the patient has as a result of their hearing loss, so tapping into the significant others' perceptions and understanding of the patient's difficulties. Such results can then be compared with those reported by the patient and can give valuable information to be used in counselling sessions involving both patient and significant others.

In addition, significant others can be asked to list the problems which they experience themselves as a result of the patient's hearing loss (Stephens *et al.*, 1995). The areas highlighted are reports of frustration and of the fact that the patient is dependent on them. The latter is particularly important in the female partners of hearing impaired men (see Chapter 7). At the present time, no quantitative analyses/ratings appear to have been performed combined with such an approach in order to assess the impact of the enablement programme on the views of significant others, although, in practice, this could be easily done using a modified version of COSI.

Kelsay and Tyler (1996) gave their advantages/disadvantages questionnaire to the parents of children with cochlear implants to tap into their perceptions of their

Table 12.6 Significant other's responses for patient whose own responses are shown in Table 12.5.

Benefits	Shortcomings
Having proper conversations	For myself, family and
Everyday life is less stressful, there's a lot less arguments	friends there are no
Previously avoided long journeys because of conversation problems	problems or shortcomings
Don't have to make phone calls for him	because his quality of life
Don't have to use my daughter to get messages to him	has improved, which in
He'll now go out on his own to deal with any problems	turn means ours has
His confidence has improved:	improved. This can only
	get better and better.
▪ Joins in conversations when we are out socially	
▪ Able to go and see our grandson in school concerts	

children's benefits and shortcomings and to compare these with the previously rated anticipations of benefits and shortcomings. We have used a similar approach with significant others of adults with cochlear implants (Stephens *et al.*, 2008) and have attempted to separate the significant others' responses into those applying to the patient and those applying to the significant others themselves (Kennedy *et al.*, 2008). That study had asked the significant others to 'list the benefits you have noticed since your relative/friend has had their cochlear implant', and the same for shortcomings. This wording did not clearly separate the effects on the patient from those on the significant other, so the results included both and had to be separated on a *post hoc* basis. Such results for the wife of the patient whose results were shown in Table 12.5 are shown above in Table 12.6.

These responses very much reflect those for the total patient group studied by Kennedy *et al.* (2008), who report: 'Improved quality of life was reported for both partners. Reported shortcomings predominantly involved the cochlear implant and were device related.' However, some shortcomings may be highlighted by the significant other, such as 'Others still address me first' and may be used in further stages of the enablement programme.

Coping with residual problems

This is a domain of assessment which has been barely touched upon up to the present, although facilitating such coping may be regarded as one of the key areas of the ongoing enablement process. Some pointers may be obtained from studies of positive experiences associated with hearing impairment, in which a 'resignation' factor emerged in two analyses (Stephens and Kerr, 2003). In addition, such coping factors have emerged from studies on positive experiences associated with tinnitus and vertigo (Kentala *et al.*, 2008) and with Menière's disorder (Stephens *et al.*, 2007; 2009b).

In the study specifically on hearing problems, the two relevant questions which loaded on a 'resignation' factor were 'I am now a more patient person' and 'I have my own ways of coping'. The second of these was rated as often or sometimes true by 75% of the respondents (Stephens and Kerr, 2003).

Among patients with tinnitus, spontaneous comments have included 'Now I quite like my tinnitus. When I'm out with someone and they're talking about something I'm not interested in, I can just listen to my tinnitus instead.' In addition, from an open-ended questionnaire study, areas of response have included 'It could be worse' and 'I'm not alone when I have tinnitus' (Kentala *et al.*, 2008).

In Menière's disorder, this area of coping is even more marked. Thus, among responses to open-ended questioning, we find the comment 'I have learnt to take a more relaxed view of the disorder, not to panic' (Stephens *et al.*, 2007). When such individuals were studied using a structured questionnaire, two separate factors entailing coping loaded significantly in an analysis of positive experiences resulting in less impact of the condition. The first entailed responses to the two statements 'There are many worse diseases' and 'I have learnt to live with Menière's disorder'. The second covered the perspective as reflected in 'Menière's disorder is not present all the time' and 'Menière's disorder has led to a healthy life' (Stephens *et al.*, 2009b).

In the absence of any existing measure, it might be reasonable in the first instance to take the two statements used in the Stephens and Kerr (2003) paper and ask the patient to rate them. This should be done at the end of the main programme of enablement, and could be done using either the scaling 'often–sometimes–rarely–never true', used in that study or a visual analogue scale. However, much further research is needed in this field and the results obtained in patients with Menière's disorder may contribute to the development of more robust or personalised measures. The ideal under these circumstances should be a measure which can be tailored to the individual patient. It is possible that the inclusion of a third outcome measure in addition to the two currently used in COSI could provide such an answer. However, this would need to be restricted to those initial problems that had not been alleviated by the intervention.

Conclusion

Ongoing remediation mainly covers non-instrumental interventions and involves issues like auditory training, hearing tactics, speechreading, counselling, skill-building and communication facilitation. The concept of *coping* is essential. It is argued that the process of coping should be seen as a dynamic concept which evolves over time along the process of adjusting to hearing impairment. It means that a certain *maladaptive* strategy may turn into an *adaptive* strategy at a certain point in time, depending on the circumstances of the individual. Ongoing remediation may be organised in individual or in group settings. Home-based programmes do exist as well.

Group counselling may be divided into self-help groups, support groups and community-based groups. Several studies have described the effectiveness of the different types of non-instrumental interventions and are presented in this chapter. The inclusion of significant others in the process of ongoing remediation is recommended.

In any enablement process, we are dealing with a dynamic and changing condition and series of experiences. Therefore, throughout the process, the use of outcome measures should be considered. The assessment of the efficacy of the enablement process must be focused on the extent that it has helped the particular patient and minimised their problems.

Finally, tailoring the enablement process to individual needs implies that any option of intervention should depend on the patient's choice.

13 Overall conclusions

Throughout this book, we have shown that the impact of hearing impairment on an individual can be wide-ranging but, at the same time, such impact may vary considerably from person to person. The aim of the process of enablement is to minimise this impact both on the patient and on those around them. It is very much a patient-centred process, which aims to reduce any such impact where that can be achieved and to help the individual to adjust to and cope with the impact when it cannot.

In addition, it is important to remember that the effect of the condition is very much a dynamic process which can change as a result of alterations in the individual's environment and also within themselves in terms of attitudes and psychological states, as well as with changes in the severity of the underlying condition. Thus, changes in the environment (environmental contextual factors) will most commonly entail aspects of relationships with those around the person and of new relationships as well as new work and other challenges in such domains. Within the person (personal contextual factors), there may be changes in mood, such as in anxiety or depression related to factors other than their hearing impairment, which can have a major effect on the impact of their hearing impairment.

Initially, we considered the question of help-seeking by individuals with a hearing impairment. While many studies have indicated that less than a quarter of those with hearing impairments have had help, there are many factors behind such a lack of help and these are relevant to the current interest in hearing screening in older people. About a quarter of older individuals with such a hearing impairment are not aware of their impairment and it is ethically questionable as to whether or not they should be made aware of such a deficit in an impairment-based (hearing test) screening procedure. It is more justified in those who are aware of hearing difficulties and who have done nothing about it or have complained to their primary physician about their problems and not been referred for enablement. Such screening, therefore, should be based on a question tapping disability rather than impairment and we would advocate the use of the simple question 'Do you have any difficulty with your hearing – yes or no?' as a first stage in any such screening. This question has emerged well from comparative assessments in a large-scale study by Davis *et al.* (2007). Again, this should not be done unless an appropriate intervention of enablement can be offered to those detected by such a screen. Such intervention should be patient-centred.

The next two chapters dealing with types of hearing impairment and with other factors indicate a number of elements which may affect the severity and nature of the problems experienced by the individual with a hearing impairment and which need to be taken into account in the assessment of their needs. This does not, however, mean that they explain all the person's problems, but rather that they may account in part for the severity of such problems and need to be considered in the course of the enablement process. Thus, for example, patients with a severe hearing impairment and poor speech recognition will generally have more pronounced psychological problems than those with less severe impairments, although by no means all of such severely impaired patients will be so affected. In addition, the presence of disturbing tinnitus may have important ramifications for the enablement programme and those with deafblindness will need a wholly different approach. However, even such dually impaired patients will have a range of very different problems depending upon environmental and personal factors interacting with their impairments.

The next two chapters deal with the effects of hearing impairment on communication and on the social and emotional life of the individual. While we highlight Ramsdell's (1947) early work on the impacts of hearing impairment, it is clear that communication is the key area affected by hearing impairment. Much of what has been considered important in the enablement process over the years has focused on this domain. This can, however, be influenced by cognitive and other factors and the severity of its impact will be influenced by the environmental needs, both human and otherwise, of the patient. Indeed, communication entails interaction with other people and the role of significant others (family, friends, work colleagues and others) and must be addressed.

The psychological, social and emotional aspects of hearing impairments are key elements in the quality of life of the individual. While they interact with and are dependent upon the patient's communication abilities, they are also modulated by a range of other factors such as other disabilities experienced by the individual as well as their personality and underlying psychological state. All of these can have a major influence on the approach to be adopted in the enablement process.

In turn, both the patient's communication ability and their emotional state will impact on the topics of the next two chapters dealing with the family and with work situations. Most communication takes place within these circumstances, with work playing a major part in the life of the younger patients. The attitudes and understanding of those around the patient from their partner outwards has an important influence on the problems experienced by the patient and on their subsequent resolution. While psychological factors within the patient affected will influence relationships within both the family and the workplace, the patient's emotional state can in turn be influenced in either positive or negative ways by those around them.

The question of role models, particularly within the family, can be important here in terms of the patient's acceptance of their condition and in terms of early help-seeking. In the work environment, the nature of the person's work and responsibilities can be very important. In this and other contexts, it is essential for enablement professionals to remember that patients' problems are not static or simply affected by interventions, but that changes in the patient's environment and their perception of their difficulties can have a major impact on the problems experienced. In this respect, it is incumbent on the professionals always to gently enquire as to whether the individual has run into any new problems.

Leisure activities, the subject of the next chapter, are very variable in their nature as is the extent to which they may be affected by the patient's hearing impairment. Some, such as chess playing with a well-known partner, may be unaffected by hearing difficulties in one or both of the participants. Others, such as participation in local politics in noisy halls, may be found to be almost impossible. However, by the patient articulating their specific problems, the professional can generally work with them to ameliorate the problems, and to provide supportive counselling to help the patient's acceptance when continuing in such an activity is no longer going to be possible.

The final three chapters aim to draw all these elements together to develop an appropriate programme of enablement for the patient. It was developed to be non-prescriptive and applicable to patients with all types of hearing impairment within any sociomedical health care system. In the first of these chapters, we have high-lighted those aspects of the patient's background which need to be considered and which influence the approaches to intervention which might be appropriate to the individual patient. We highlight it as a problem-solving process aimed at reducing those difficulties which can be reduced and enhancing the patient's acceptance of those which cannot. The outcomes of this evaluation process must be drawn together and decisions made, in conjunction with the patient, as to the appropriate course of management. The 'one size fits all' approach is no longer acceptable.

The first stage of intervention entails processes which can be dealt with in one or two sessions. These include the choice and fitting of appropriate instrumentation, the development with the patient of an appropriate strategy, as well as the possible involvement of other agencies.

For those with major persistent problems which are not simply resolved, a more intensive and ongoing process of enablement will be necessary. This will particularly entail skill-building and counselling, as well as modifications to the instrumentation fitted at the previous stage. Possible programmes to provide this are discussed in which we have also considered the importance of involving those close to the patient in the enablement process. This will generally facilitate the process and, at the same time, reduce the impact of the patient's problems on them. Again, it is vital to remember that this is a dynamic process and that solving one problem can highlight others.

Assessment of the efficacy of the enablement process must be focused on the extent that it has helped the particular patient and minimised their problems. Such a process will entail alleviating the various problems as well as facilitating the acceptance of residual difficulties, in terms of both the patient and of their family. The changing nature of the problems has been largely neglected in the past and we provide pointers as to how this may be developed. In addition, while the alleviation of problems can be relatively easily assessed within both the patient and in those around them, there is a dearth of approaches to the assessment of their acceptance of any persistent problems. This area is important to the development of more patient-centred enablement.

Such enablement seen as teamwork between the professionals, the patient and their family in an ever-changing environment using any techniques which may be relevant is necessary to ensure the happiness and contentment of the individual with hearing impairment. That remains very much our goal.

Appendix Longitudinal change in enablement needs of older people with hearing impairment

Louise Hickson

This appendix contains a summary of a research project undertaken by an International Collegium of Rehabilitative Audiology (ICRA) working group comprising Louise Hickson, Sophia Kramer and Dafydd Stephens. The findings reported here were presented by the three collaborators at the 2005 International Collegium of Rehabilitative Audiology meeting in Gainsville, Florida.

Background

This project was undertaken in response to a research need identified at the 2001 Eriksholm Workshop 'Candidature and delivery of audiological services: Special needs of older people' (Kiessling *et al.*, 2003). The aim of the project was to investigate the longitudinal change in enablement needs of older people. The study aimed to address the question 'How do goals change over time?' Specifically, the group planned to evaluate changes in goals subsequent to initial enablement such as hearing aid fitting and/or participating in other forms of enablement (e.g. group communication programmes, individual communication training).

This issue is important because goal-setting has become a central aspect of hearing enablement, with the acceptance and use of such measures as the Client-Oriented Scale of Improvement (COSI; Dillon *et al.*, 1997) and the Glasgow Hearing Aid Benefit Profile (GHABP; Gatehouse, 1999). Goal-setting typically occurs at the initial assessment appointment and the outcomes of the process are measured subsequent to enablement. Goals are not revisited and this study was motivated by the concern that the failure to do this may mean that the overall service being provided to clients is not meeting their needs.

Procedure

Data collection was undertaken in Australia, the Netherlands and Wales. Initially, demographic details of participants were collected, including audiological information and type of enablement undertaken.

The Australian sample consisted of 24 people (12 males and 12 females; mean age = 71.9 years) with a mean pure tone average at frequencies 0.5, 1, 2 and 4 kHz in the better ear of 45 dBHL. All participants were undertaking a group enable-ment programme called Active Communication Education (ACE; Hickson, 2007).

Participants from the Netherlands comprised 20 adults (10 male and 10 females; mean age = 69 years) fitted with bilateral hearing aids. The mean pure tone average hearing loss for that group was 48 dBHL.

The Welsh sample consisted of 43 participants with a mean age of 69.7 years (24 males and 19 females) and a pure tone average of 38 dBHL. The vast majority (41/43) were fitted with hearing aids, and the remainder received hearing therapy.

Each patient was seen for at least two sessions and in some cases three sessions and the process employed is outlined below.

Session 1

1. Ask the patient to tell you about the problems that they have with hearing in everyday life – any particular circumstances, any particular people?

For example, 'I can't hear when my wife speaks to me from three rooms away.'

2. Ask the patient to consider each of the problems and discuss with them whether they would like these problems to be goals for enablement.

For example, 'Would you like to hear what your wife is saying?'

3. Then, look at goals and prioritise – so which of these is most important for you at the moment?

For example, 'Is hearing your wife better the most important thing for you at the moment?'

Session 2 (optional)

4. If the patient returns shortly after enablement (2–4 weeks post fitting) for a follow-up appointment, ask them to rate outcomes using the COSI ratings for degree of change.

Session 3

5. Contact the person 3–6 months after enablement – do not tell them at first what their original goals were. Ask them about the problems that they are having with hearing in everyday life NOW … go through the same process as in step 2, session 1. After that, say these were the original goals that you had – are any of them still a problem for you? If so, include them. Rate the outcome again in relation to the original goal using the COSI goals.

6. Repeat step 3 from session 1, prioritizing *all* goals.

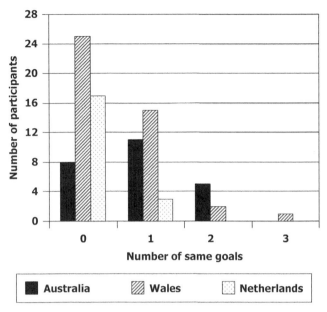

Figure A1 Number of participants who identified the same goals at session 3 compared to session 1.

Results

In the Australian sample, the mean number of goals identified at session 1 was 2.75, compared to 3.6 in the Welsh and 3.9 in the Dutch participants. The lower figure in the Australian sample is probably due to the nature of the intervention offered. Many of the participants who joined the group communication education programme (ACE) did so because they did not believe they had sufficient hearing difficulties to warrant hearing aid fitting. Thus, on average, they reported fewer difficulties initially than participants in Wales and the Netherlands who had chosen aid fitting did.

At the session 3 follow-up, the mean number of goals for Australian participants showed a slight increase to 2.9; however, the Welsh and Dutch participants had fewer goals at follow-up (1.6 for the Dutch and 2.2 for the Welsh).

Importantly, many participants identified new goals at follow-up. For example, in Figure A1 it can be seen that, of the 43 Welsh participants, 25 of them identified completely different goals at the follow-up (column labelled 0 on the x axis 'number of same goals') compared to the initial session. On average, the Welsh participants identified 1.8 completely new goals at follow-up. A feature of these new goals in all cohorts was that the new goals at follow-up tended to be more specific in nature than the original goals. An example of a general goal was 'Learning ways to overcome hearing difficulty', compared to the more specific goal of 'To hear my grandchildren during conversations without having to ask them to repeat something or speak louder'.

Another important aspect of these findings for enablement is that many participants continued to have the same goals as they had initially, even after the intervention had occurred. This indicates that they required further additional assistance of some kind. This occurred despite the fact that the outcomes of enablement, as measured by the COSI change scores, were very positive.

Conclusion

The main finding was that the nature of goals changed over time subsequent to initial enablement. Thus, it is essential that clinicians reassess the goals that clients want to work on and not assume that if original goals are met then that is all that the older person with hearing impairment requires. Additional enablement may be necessary to address the changing needs of older clients and ensure long-term satisfaction with enablement.

This preliminary study highlighted a number of other issues in this area that need to be addressed in future research and clinical work:

▨ Goal-setting tools exist in audiology but should guidelines (such as those suggested in this study) be developed to ensure the validity of the process?
▨ Are goals negotiated with clients or are they clinician-dominated?
▨ Is there any need to prioritise goals at all?
▨ Are clients given a chance to reconsider goals subsequent to enablement?

References

Please note that the entries for Stephens, D. and Stephens, S.D.G. are for the same author and so are listed together.

Abrams, H.B., Hnath-Chisolm, T., Guerreiro, S.M., Ritterman, S.I. (1992) The effects of intervention strategy on self-perception of hearing handicap. *Ear and Hearing* 13: –7.

Aguayo, M.O., Coady, N.F. (2001) The experience of deafened adults: implications for rehabilitative services. *Health and Social Work* 26: 269–76.

Ahmad, W., Darr, A., Jones, L., Nisar, G. (1998) *Deafness and Ethnicity: Services, policy and politics*. The Policy Press, Bristol.

Akamatsu, C.T., Mayer, C., Farrelly, S. (2006) An investigation of two-way text messaging use with deaf students at the secondary level. *Journal of Deaf Studies and Deaf Education* 11: 120–131.

Akeroyd, M.A. (2008) Are individual differences in speech reception related to individual differences in cognitive ability? *International Journal of Audiology* 47 (Suppl. 2): S53–S71.

Allen, N.H., Burns, A., Newton, V. *et al.* (2003) The effects of improving hearing in dementia. *Age and Ageing* 32: 189–93.

Alpiner, J.G. (1978) Adult rehabilitative audiology: an overview. In: *Handbook of Rehabilitative Audiology*, (ed. J.G. Alpiner), pp. 1–16. Williams and Wilkins, Baltimore.

Alpiner, J.G., Hansen, E.M., Kaufman, K.J. (2000) Transition: rehabilitative audiology into the new millennium. In: *Rehabilitative Audiology: Children and Adults*, 3rd edn, (eds J.G. Alpiner, P.A. McCarthy), pp. 3–26. Lippincott, Williams & Wilkins, Baltimore.

Alterovitz, G. (2004) Electrical engineering and nontechnical design variables of multiple inductive loop systems for auditoriums. *Journal of Deaf Studies and Deaf Education* 9: 202–209.

American Speech-Language-Hearing Association (ASHA) (2005) (Central) Auditory Processing Disorders, http://www.asha.org/members/deskref-journals/deskref/default, accessed 28 November 2007.

Amitay, S., Hawkey, D.J., Moore, D.R. (2005) Auditory frequency discrimination learning is affected by stimulus variability. *Perception & Psychophysics* 67 (4): 691–8.

Anderson, D.L., Noble, W. (2005) Couple's contributions about behaviours modulated by hearing impairment: links with relationship satisfaction. *International Journal of Audiology* 44: 197–205.

Andersson, G., Willebrand, M. (2003) What is coping? A critical review of the construct and its application in audiology. *International Journal of Audiology* 42: S97–S103.

Andersson, G., Melin, L., Scott, B., Lindberg, P. (1994) Behavioural counselling for subjects with acquired hearing loss. *Scandinavian Audiology* 23: 249–56.

Andersson, G., Melin, L., Scott, B., Lindberg, P. (1995a) A two-year follow-up examination of a behavioural treatment approach. *British Journal of Audiology* 29: 347–54.

Andersson, G., Melin, L., Scott, B., Lindberg, P. (1995b) An evaluation of a behavioural treatment approach to hearing impairment. *Behavioural Research and Therapy* 33: 283–92.

Andersson, G., Lindvall, N., Hursti, T., Carlbring, P. (2002) Hypersensitivity to sound (hyperacusis): a prevalence study conducted via internet and post. *International Journal of Audiology* 41: 545–54.

Andersson, G., Baguley, D.M., McKenna, L., McFerran, D. (2005) *Tinnitus*. Whurr, London.

Anon (1982) *Dorland's Pocket Medical Dictionary*, 23rd edn. Saunders, Philadelphia.

Argyle, M. (1988) *Bodily Communication*, 2nd edn. International Universities Press, Madison.

Armstrong, D.F., Wilcox, S. (2003) Origins of sign languages. In: *Oxford Handbook of Deaf Studies, Language and Education*, (eds Marschark, M., Spencer P.E.), pp. 305–318. Oxford University Press, Oxford.

Audran-McGovern, J., Hughes, C., Patterson, F. (2003) Effecting behavior change: awareness of family history. *American Journal of Preventive Medicine* 24: 183–9.

Austin, S., Coleman, E. (2004) Controversy in deafness: animal farm meets brave new world. In: *Deafness in Mind: Working psychologically with deaf people across the lifespan*, (eds S. Austin, S. Crocker), pp. 2–30. Whurr, London.

Austin, S., Crocker, S. (eds) (2004) *Deafness in Mind: Working psychologically with deaf people across the lifespan*. Whurr, London.

Baddeley, A. (1998) Working memory. *Comptes Rendus de l'Academie des Sciences*. Series III 321: 167–73.

Bai, Z., Stephens, D. (2005) Subjective outcome measures after cochlear implantation: overall measures. *Audiological Medicine* 3: 212–19.

Bamiou, D.E., Musiek, F.E., Luxon, L.M. (2003) The insula (island of Reil) and its role in auditory processing: literature review. *Brain Research: Brain Research Reviews* 42: 143–54.

Baran, J.A. (2007) Managing (central) auditory processing disorders in adolescents and adults. In: *Handbook of (Central) Auditory Processing Disorder*, Vol. 2, (eds G.D. Chermak, F.E. Musiek), pp. 243–72. Plural, San Diego.

Baran, J.A., Musiek, F. (2003) Central auditory disorders. In: *Textbook of Audiological Medicine: Clinical aspects of hearing and balance*, (eds L. Luxon, J.M. Furman, A. Martini, D. Stephens), pp. 495–511. Martin Dunitz, London.

Barcham, L.J., Stephens, S.D.G. (1980) The use of an open-ended problems questionnaire in auditory rehabilitation. *British Journal of Audiology* 14: 49–54.

Barfod, J. (1979) Speech perception processes and fitting of hearing aids. *Audiology* 18: 430–41.

Barlow, J.H., Turner, A.P., Hammond, C.L., Gailey, L. (2007) Living with late deafness: insight from between worlds. *International Journal of Audiology* 46: 442–8.

Batteau, D.W. (1967) The role of the pinna in human localisation. *Proceedings of the Royal Society B* 168: 158–80.

Bazargan, J., Baker, S., Bazargan, S.H. (2001) Sensory impairments and subjective well-being among aged African American persons. *Journal of Gerontology, Psychological Sciences* 56B: 268–78.

Békésy, G. von. (1947) A new audiometer. *Acta Oto-laryngologica* 35: 411–22.

Bench, J., Bamford, J. (eds) (1979) *Speech-hearing Tests and the Spoken Language of Hearing-impaired Children*. Academic Press, London.

Bennett, D., Byers, V. (1967) Increased intelligibility in the hypacusic by slow-play frequency transposition. *Journal of Auditory Research* 7: 107–18.

Bentler, R.A., Kramer, S.E. (2000) Guidelines for choosing a self-report outcome measure. *Ear and Hearing* 21: S37–S49.

Bergman, M. (1950) A manual for planning a clinic for the rehabilitation of the acoustically handicapped. *Acta Oto-laryngologica* Suppl. 89.

Berlin, C.I. (1999) *The Efferent Auditory System: Basic science and clinical applications*. Singular, San Diego.

Bess, F.H. (2000) The role of generic health-related quality of life measures in establishing audiological rehabilitation outcomes. *Ear and Hearing* 21: S74–S79.

Bess, F.H., Lichtenstein, M.J., Logan, S.A., Burger, M.C., Nelson, E. (1989) Hearing impairment as a determinant of function in the elderly. *Journal of the American Geriatrics Society* 37: 123–28.

Beynon, G.J., Thornton, F.L., Poole, C. (1997) A randomized, controlled trial of the efficacy of a communication course for first time hearing aid users. *British Journal of Audiology* 31: 345–51.

Bilger, C., Nuentzeq, J.M., Rabinowitz, W.M., Rzeczkowski, C. (1984) Standardization of a test of speech perception in noise. *Journal of Speech and Hearing Research* 27: 32–48.

Blauert, J. (1983) *Spatial Hearing: The psychophysics of human sound localization*. MIT Press, Cambridge, MA.

Bocca, E. (1958) Clinical aspects of cortical deafness. *Laryngoscope* 68: 301–9.

Booth, J.B. (1997) Sudden and fluctuant sensorineural hearing loss. In: *Scott-Brown's Otolaryngology*, Vol. 3, (ed. J.B. Booth), 6th edn, 17/1–82.

Boothroyd, A. (1968) Developments in speech audiometry. *Sound* 2: 3–10.

Boothroyd, A. (2007) Adult aural rehabilitation. What is it and does it work? *Trends in Amplification* 11: 63–71.

Borg, E. (2003) Assessment of communicating systems on the basis of an ecological conceptual framework. *International Journal of Audiology* 42: S23–S33.

Borg, E., Stephens, D. (2003) King Kopetzky syndrome in the light of an ecological conceptual framework. *International Journal of Audiology* 42: 312–18.

Borg, E., Bergkvist, C., Olsson, I., Wikström, C., Borg, B. (2008) Communication as an ecological system. *International Journal of Audiology* 47 (Suppl. 2): S131–S138.

Bosman, A.J., Snik, A.F.M., Van der Pouw, C.T.M., Mylanus, E.A.M., Cremers, C.W.R.J. (2001) Audiometric evaluation of bilaterally fitted bone-anchored hearing aids. *Audiology* 40: 158–67.

Branson, J., Miller, D., Marsaja, I.G. (1996) Everyone here speaks sign language, too: a deaf village in Bali, Indonesia. In: *Multicultural Aspects of Sociolinguistics in Deaf Communities*, (ed. C. Lucas), pp. 39–57. Gallaudet University Press, Washington DC.

Brantberg, K., Verrecchia, L. (2008) Testing vestibular-evoked myogenic potentials with 90-dB clicks is effective in the diagnosis of superior canal dehiscence. *Audiology and Neurotology* 14: 54–8.

Brazier, J., Usherwood, T., Harper, R., Thomas, K. (1998) Deriving a preference-based single index from the UK SF-36 Health Survey. *Journal of Clinical Epidemiology* 51: 1115–28.

Bregman, A.S. (2004) *Auditory Scene Analysis: The perceptual organization of sound*. MIT Press, Cambridge, MA.

Brewer, D.M. (2001) Considerations in measuring effectiveness of group audiologic rehabilitation classes. *Journal of the Academy of Rehabilitative Audiology* 43: 53–60.

Brooks, D. (1989) Counselling for the first-time user. In: *Adult Aural Rehabilitation*, (ed. D.N. Brooks), pp. 116–31. Chapman and Hall, London.

Brooks, D.N. (1976) The use of hearing aids by the hearing impaired. In: *Disorders of Auditory Function II*, (ed. S.D.G. Stephens), pp. 255–63. Academic Press, London.

Brooks D.N., Johnson D.I. (1981) Pre-issue assessment and counselling as a component of hearing-aid provision. *British Journal of Audiology* 15: 13–19.

Brooks, D.N., Hallam, R.S., Mellor, P.A. (2001) The effects on significant others of providing a hearing aid to the hearing-impaired partner. *British Journal of Audiology* 35: 165–71.

Bruck, D., Thomas, I.R. (2009) Smoke alarms for sleeping adults who are hard-of-hearing: comparison of auditory, visual and tactile signals. *Ear and Hearing* 30: 73–80.

Bumin, G., Uyanik, M., Aki, E., Kayihan, H. (2002) An investigation of risk factors for frail elderly people in a Turkish rest home. *Aging Clinical Experience Research* 14: 192–96.

Bunch, C.C. (1943) *Clinical Audiometry*. Mosby, St Louis.

Burk, M.H., Humes, L.E. (2008) Effects of long-term training on aided speech-recognition performance in noise in older adults. *Journal of Speech Language and Hearing Research* 51: 759–71.

Buunk, B.P., Collins, R.L., Taylor, S.E., Van Yperen, N.W., Dakof, G.A. (1990) The affective consequences of social comparison: either direction has its ups and downs. *Journal of Personality and Social Psychology* 59: 1238–49.

Byrne, D., Tonisson, W. (1976) Selecting the gain of hearing aids for persons with sensorineural hearing impairments. *Scandinavian Audiology* 5: 51–9.

Cacciatore, F., Napoli, C., Abete, P., Marciano, E., Triassi, M., Rengo, F. (1999) Quality of life determinants and hearing function in an elderly population: Osservatorio Geriatrico Campano Study Group. *Gerontology* 45: 323–8.

Caissie, R., Campbell, M.M., Frenette, W.L., Scott, L., Howell, I., Roy, A. (2005) Clear speech for adults with a hearing loss: does intervention with communication partners make a difference? *Journal of the American Academy of Audiology* 16: 157–71.

Carabellese, C., Appollonio, I., Rozzini, R. *et al.* (1993) Sensory impairment (visual & hearing) and quality of life in a community elderly population. *Journal of the American Geriatrics Society* 41: 401–7.

Carlsson, A.H., Bjorvatn, C., Engebretsen, L.F., Berglund, G., Natvig, G.K. (2004) Psychosocial factors associated with quality of life among individuals attending genetic counselling for hereditary cancer. *Journal of Genetic Counselling* 13: 425–45.

Carlsson, P., Danermark, B. (2006) Early childhood hearing impairment and family history: a long-term perspective. In: *The Effects of Genetic Hearing Impairment in the Family*, (eds D. Stephens, L. Jones), pp. 43–54. John Wiley & Sons, Chichester.

Carlsson, P.U. (1990) On direct bone conduction hearing devices. *Technical Report No 195*, Chalmers University of Technology, Göteborg, Sweden.

Chee, G.H., Goldring, J.E., Shipp, D.B., Ng, A.H.C., Chen, J.M., Nedzelski, J.M. (2004) Benefits of cochlear implantation in early-deafened adults: the Toronto experience. *Journal of Otolaryngology* 33: 26–31.

Chermak, G.D., Musiek, F.E. (eds) (2007) *Handbook of (Central) Auditory Processing Disorder*. Plural, San Diego.

Chia, E.M., Wang, J.J., Rochtchina, E., Cumming, R.R., Newall, P., Mitchell, P. (2007) Hearing impairment and health related quality of life: the Blue Mountains hearing study. *Ear and Hearing* 28: 187–95.

Chiossoine-Kerdel, J.A., Baguley, D.M., Stoddart, R.L., Moffat, D.A. (2000) An investigation of the audiologic handicap associated with unilateral sudden sensorineural hearing loss. *American Journal of Otology* 21: 645–51.

Chisholm, T.H., Abrams, H.B., McArdle, R. (2004) Short- and long-term outcomes of adult audiological rehabilitation. *Ear and Hearing* 25: 464–77.

Chisholm, T.H., Noe, C.M., McArdle, R., Abrams, H. (2007) Evidence for the use of hearing assistive technology by adults: the role of the FM system. *Trends in Amplification* 11: 73–89.

Chung, S.M., Stephens, S.D.G. (1986) Factors influencing binaural hearing aid use. *British Journal of Audiology* 20: 129–40.

Coles, R., Davis, A., Smith, P. (1990) Tinnitus: its epidemiology and management. In: *Presbyacusis and Other Age Related Aspects*, (ed. J.H. Jensen), pp. 377–402, Jensen, Copenhagen.

Colledge, A.L., Johns, R.E., Thomas, M.H. (1999) Functional ability assessment: guidelines for the workplace. *Journal of Occupational Environmental Medicine* 41: 172–80.

Colletti, V., Shannon, R.V. (2005) Open set speech perception with auditory brainstem implant? *Laryngoscope* 115: 1974–8.

Colletti, V., Soli, S.D., Carner, M., Colletti, L. (2006) Treatment of mixed hearing losses via implantation of a vibratory transducer on the round window. *International Journal of Audiology* 45: 600–608.

Coniavitis Gellerstedt, L., Danermark, B. (2003) Hearing impairment, working life conditions, and gender. *Scandinavian Journal of Disability Research* 6: 225–44.

Conrad, R. (1979) *The Deaf Schoolchild*. London: Harper & Row.

Cornett, O. (1967) Cued speech. *American Annals of the Deaf* 112: 3–13.

Costa, P.T., McCrae, R.R. (1992) *NEO-PI-R Professional Manual*. Psychological Assessment Resources, Odessa, FL.

Coulson, S. (2006) The impact that a family history of late onset hearing impairment has on those with the condition themselves. In: *The Effects of Having a Family History of Hearing Impairment*, (eds D. Stephens, L. Jones), pp. 95–116. John Wiley & Sons, Chichester.

Courtois, J., Berland, O. (1972) Ipsi-lateral no-mould fitting of hearing aids. *Scandinavian Audiology* 1: 177–95.

Cox, R. (ed.) (2000) Proceedings of the (1999) Audiological workshop at Eriksholm, Denmark. *Ear and Hearing* 21: S1–S115.

Cox, R.M., Alexander, G.C. (1995) The abbreviated profile of hearing aid benefit. *Ear and Hearing* 16: 176–86.

Cox, R.M., Alexander, G.C. (1999) Measuring satisfaction with amplification in daily life: The SADL scale. *Ear and Hearing* 20: 306–20.

Cox, R.M., Alexander, G.C., Gilmore, C. (1987) Development of the connected speech test (CST) *Ear and Hearing* 8: S119– S126.

Cox, R.M., Alexander, G.C., Gray, G. (1999) Personality and the subjective assessment of hearing aids. *Journal of the American Academy of Audiology* 10: 1–13.

Cox, R., Hyde, M., Gatehouse, S. *et al.* (2000) Optimal outcome measures, research priorities and international cooperation. *Ear and Hearing* 21: S106– S115.

Cox, R.M., Alexander, G.C., Gray, G. (2005) Who wants a hearing aid? Personality profiles of hearing aid seekers. *Ear and Hearing* 26: 12–26.

Craig, E. (1973) The Paget Gorman sign system. *Journal of the Society of Teachers of the Deaf* 14: 24–7.

Cuijpers, M., Lautenbach, H. (2006) *Disabled Employees*. Report of the Dutch Ministry of Social Affairs and Employment.

Dalton, D.S., Cruickshanks, K.J., Klein, B.E., Klein, R., Wiley, T.L., Nondahl, D.M. (2003) The impact of hearing loss on quality of life in older adults. *Gerontologist* 43: 661–8.

Daneman, M., Carpenter, P.A. (1980) Individual differences in working memory and reading. *Journal of Verbal Learning and Verbal Behavior* 19, 450–66.

Daneman, M., Merikle, P.M. (1996) Working memory and language comprehension: a meta-analysis. *Psychonomic Bulletin and Review* 3: 422–33.

Danermark, B. (2005) review of the psychosocial effects of hearing impairment in the working-age population. In: *The Impact of Genetic Hearing Impairment*, (eds D. Stephens, L. Jones), pp. 106–136. Whurr, London.

Danermark, B., Coniavitis Gellerstedt, L. (2004) Psychosocial work environment, hearing impairment and health. *International Journal of Audiology* 43: 383–9.

Danermark, B.D., Möller, K. (2008) Deafblindness, ontological security and social recognition. *International Journal of Audiology* 47: S119–S123.

Davis, A. (1995) *Hearing in Adults*. Whurr, London.

Davis, A. (1997) Epidemiology. In: *Scott-Brown's Otolaryngology*, Volume 2, (ed. D. Stephens), 6th edn. pp. 2/3/1–38. Butterworth-Heinemann, Oxford.

Davis, A., Fortnum, H.M., Coles, R.R.A., Haggard, M.P., Lutman, M.E. (1985) *Damage to Hearing Arising from Leisure Noise: A Review of the Literature*. HMSO, London.

Davis, A., Stephens, D., Rayment, A., Thomas, K. (1992) Hearing impairments in middle age: the acceptability, benefit and cost of detection (ABCD). *British Journal of Audiology* 26: 1–14.

Davis, A., Smith, P., Ferguson, M., Stephens, D., Gianopoulos, I. (2007) Acceptability, benefit and costs of early screening for hearing disability: a study of potential screening tests and models. *Health Technology Assessment* 11: 1–294.

Declau, F., Van de Heyning, P. (2007a) Otosclerosis: a genetic update. In: *Genes, Hearing and Deafness,* (eds A. Martini, D. Stephens, A.P. Read), pp. 111–19. Informa, London.

Declau, F., Van de Heyning, P. (2007b) Diagnosis and management strategies in congenital middle and external ear anomalies. In: *Genes, Hearing and Deafness* (eds A. Martini, D. Stephens, A.P. Read), pp. 239–51. Informa, London.

DeFilippo, C.L., Scott, B.L. (1978) A method for training and evaluating the reception of ongoing speech. *Journal of the Acoustical Society of America* 63: 1186–92.

De Graaf, R., Bijl, R. (2002) Determinants of mental distress in adults with a severe auditory impairment: differences between prelingual and postlingual deafness. *Psychosomatic Medicine* 64: 61–70.

De Jager, H.J., Goedegebure, A. (2003) Het expertise centrum gehoor en arbeid voor slechthorende werknemers (Dutch). *Tijdschrift voor Bedrijfs- en Verzekeringsgeneeskunde* 11: 14–15.

De Jong Gierveld, J. (1987) Developing and testing a model of loneliness. *Journal of Personality and Social Psychology* 53: 119–28.

Demorest, M.E., Erdman, S.A. (1986) Scale composition and item analysis of the communication profile for the hearing impaired. *Journal of Speech and Hearing Research* 29: 515–35.

Detaille, S.I., Haafkens, M.A., Van Dijk, F.J.H. (2003) What employees with rheumatoid arthritis, diabetes mellitus and hearing loss need to cope at work. *Scandinavian Journal of Work and Environmental Health* 29: 134–42.

Dibb, B., Yardley, L. (2006) How does social comparison within a self-help group influence adjustment to chronic illness? A longitudinal study. *Social Science & Medicine* 63: 1602–13.

Diener, E., Emmons, R.A., Larsen, R.J., Griffin, S. (1985) The satisfaction with life scale. *Journal of Personal Assessment* 41, 71–5.

Dillon, H. (1994) Shortened hearing aid performance inventory for the elderly (SHAPIE): a statistical approach. *Australian Journal of Audiology* 16: 37–48.

Dillon, H. (2001) *Hearing Aids.* Sydney, Boomerang.

Dillon, H., James, A., Ginnis, J.A. (1997) The Client-Oriented Scale of Improvement (COSI) and its relationship to several other measures of benefit and satisfaction provided by hearing aids. *Journal of the American Academy of Audiology* 8: 27–43.

Drossman, D.A. (1998) Presidential address: gastrointestinal illness and the biopsychosocial model. *Psychosomatic Medicine* 60: 258–67.

Duijvestijn, J.A., Anteunis, L.J., Hoek, C.J., Van den Brink, R.H., Chenault, M.N., Manni, J.J. (2003) Help-seeking behaviour of hearing-impaired persons aged > or = 55 years: effect of complaints, significant others and hearing aid image. *Acta Oto-laryngologica* 123: 846–50.

Dye, M., Kyle, J. (2001) *Deaf People in the Community: Hearing and disability.* Deaf Studies Trust, Bristol.

Edgett, L.M.D. (2002) *Help-seeking for advanced rehabilitation by adults with hearing loss: an ecological model.* PhD Thesis, University of British Columbia.

Edwards, B. (2007) The future of hearing aid technology. *Trends in Amplification* 11: 31–46.

Engelund, G. (2006) *'Time for hearing': recognising process for the individual.* PhD Thesis, University of Copenhagen.

Erber, N.P., Holland, J., Osborn, R.R. (1998) Communicating with elders: effects of speaker–listener distance. *British Journal of Audiology* 32: 135–8.

Erdman, S.A., Demorest, M.E. (1998a) Adjustment to hearing impairment I: description of a heterogeneous clinical population. *Journal of Speech, Language and Hearing Research* 41: 107–22.

Erdman, S.A., Demorest, M.E. (1998b) Adjustment to hearing impairment II: audiological and demographic correlates. *Journal of Speech, Language and Hearing Research* 41: 123–36.

Eriksson-Mangold, M., Carlsson, S.G. (1991) Psychological and somatic distress in relation to perceived hearing disability, hearing handicap and hearing measurements. *Journal of Psychosomatic Research* 35: 729–40.

Eriksson-Mangold, M.M., Erlandsson, S.I. (1984) The psychological importance of nonverbal sounds: an experiment with induced hearing deficiency. *Scandinavian Audiology* 13: 243–49.

Ewertsen, H.W. (1974) Pilot study auditory and audiovisual speech perception related to auditory disorders. *Scandinavian Audiology* (Suppl. 4): 76–82.

Ewertsen, H.W. (1976) The history of Danish medical audiology 1951–(1976) In: *Danish Audiology 1951–(1976)*, (eds O. Bentzen, H.W. Ewertsen, G. Salomon,), Nyt Nordisk forlag Arnold Busck, Copenhagen.

Ewing, I.R. (1944) *Lipreading and Hearing Aids*, 2nd edn. Manchester University Press, Manchester.

Fellinger, J., Holzinger, D., Dobner, U. *et al.* (2005) Mental distress and quality of life in a deaf population. *Social Psychiatry and Psychiatric Epidemiology* 40: 737–42.

Fellinger, J., Holzinger, D., Gerich, J., Goldberg, D. (2007) Mental distress and quality of life in the hard of hearing. *Acta Psychiatrica Scandinavica* 115: 243–5.

Ferman, L., Verschuure, J., Van Zanten, B. (1993) Impaired speech perception in noise in patients with a normal audiogram. *Audiology* 32 (1): 49–54.

Festinger, L. (1954) A theory of social comparison processes. *Human Relations* 7: 117–40.

Field, D.L., Haggard, M.P. (1989) Knowledge of hearing tactics: (I) assessment by questionnaire and inventory. *British Journal of Audiology* 23: 349–54.

Fischel-Ghodsian, N., Bykhovskaya, Y., Yaylor, K. *et al.* (1997) Temporal bone analysis of patients with presbyacusis reveals high frequency of mitochondrial mutations. *Hearing Research* 110: 147–54.

Fisher, K., Kettl, P. (2005) Aging with mental retardation: increasing population of older adults with MR require health interventions and prevention strategies. *Geriatrics* 60: 26–9.

Foo, C., Rudner, M., Rönnberg, J., Lunner, T. (2007) Recognition of speech in noise with new hearing instrument compression release settings requires explicit cognitive storage and processing capacity. *Journal of the American Academy of Audiology* 18: 618–31.

Fooks, L., Morgan, R., Sharma, P., Adekoke, A., Turnbull, C.J. (2000) The impact of hearing on communication. *Postgraduate Medicine* 76: 92–5.

Forchammer, G. (1903) *Orm Nodvendigheden af Sikre Meddelelsesmidler i Døvestummeundervisningen.* Frimodt, Copenhagen.

Fortnum, H., Barton, G., Stephens, D., Stacey, P., Summerfield, A.Q. (2006) The impact for children of having a family history of hearing impairment in a UK-wide population study. In: *The Effects of Having a Family History of Hearing Impairment*, (eds D. Stephens, L. Jones), pp. 29–42. John Wiley & Sons, Chichester.

Foster, J.R., Summerfield, A.Q., Marshall, D.H., Palmer, L., Ball, V., Rosen, S. (1993) Lip-reading the BKB sentence lists: corrections for list and practice effects. *British Journal of Audiology* 27: 233–46.

Fourcin, A.J. (1980) Speech pattern audiometry. In: *Auditory Investigation: The scientific and technological basis*, (ed. H.A. Beagley), pp. 170–208. Oxford University Press, Oxford.

Fourcin, A.J., Stephens, S.D.G., Hazan, V., Irwin, J., Ball, V., Delmont, J. (1985) Audiological rehabilitation of patients with brainstem disorders. *British Journal of Audiology* 19: 29–42.

Fransen, P.M.L., Bültmann, U., Kant, I.J., Amelsvoort, L.G.P.M. (2003) The association between chronic diseases and fatigue in the working population. *Journal of Psychosomatic Research* 54: 339–44.

French St George, M., Barr-Hamilton, R. (1975) Relief of the occluded ear sensation to improve earmould comfort. *Journal of the American Auditory Society* 4: 30–5.

Friedman, R., Van Laer, L., Huentelman, M.J. *et al.* (2009) *GRM7* variants convey susceptibility to age-related hearing impairment, (in preparation).

Gagné, J.P. (2003) Treatment effectiveness research in audiological rehabilitation: fundamental issues related to dependent variables. *International Journal of Audiology* 42 (Suppl. 1): S104–S111.

Gagné, J.P., Masterson, V., Munhall, K.G., Bilida, N., Querengesser, C. (1995) Across talker variability in auditory, visual and audiovisual speech intelligibility for conversational and clear speech. *Journal of the Academy of Rehabilitative Audiology* 27: 135–58.

Galvin, K.L., Blaney, P.J., Cowan, R.S., Oerlemans, M., Clark, G.M. (2000) Generalization of tactile perceptual skills to new context following tactile-alone word recognition training with the Tickle Talker. *Journal of the Acoustical Society of America* 108: 2969–79.

Gantz, B.J., Turner, C.W. (2003) Combining acoustic and electric hearing. *Laryngoscope* 113: 1726–30.

Garstecki, D.C., Erler, S.F. (1999) Older adult performance on the Communication Profile for the hearing impaired: gender difference. *Journal of Speech Language Hearing Research* 42: 785–96.

Gatehouse, S. (1990) Determinants of self-reported disability in older subjects. *Ear and Hearing* 11: S57–S65.

Gatehouse, S. (1991) The role of non-auditory factors in measured and self-reported disability. *Acta Otolaryngologica* 476: S249–S256.

Gatehouse, S. (1992) The time course and magnitude of perceptual acclimatization of frequency responses: evidence from monaural fitting of hearing aids. *Journal of the Acoustical Society of America* 92: 1258–68.

Gatehouse, S. (1994) Components and determinants of hearing aid benefit. *Ear and Hearing* 15: 30–49.

Gatehouse, S. (1999) The Glasgow Hearing Aid Benefit Profile: derivation and validation of a client-centred outcome measure for hearing aid services. *Journal of the American Academy of Audiology* 10: 80–103.

Gatehouse, S., Gordon, J. (1990) Response times to speech stimuli as measures of benefit from amplification. *British Journal of Audiology* 24: 63–8.

Gatehouse, S., Noble, W. (2004) The Speech, Spatial and Qualities of Hearing Scale (SSQ). *International Journal of Audiology* 43: 85–9.

Gatehouse, S., Naylor, G., Elberling, C. (2006a) Linear and nonlinear hearing aid fittings: 1. Patterns of benefit. *International Journal of Audiology* 45: 130–52.

Gatehouse, S., Naylor, G., Elberling, C. (2006b) Linear and nonlinear hearing aid fittings: 2. Patterns of candidature. *International Journal of Audiology* 45: 153–71.

Gates, G.A., Couropmitree, N.N., Myers, R.H. (1999) Genetic associations in age-related hearing thresholds. *Archives of Otolaryngology – Head and Neck Surgery* 125: 654–9.

Gates, G.A., Anderson, M.L., Feeney, M.P., McCurry, S.M., Larson, E.B. (2008) Central auditory dysfunction in older persons with memory impairment or Alzheimer dementia. *Archives of Otolaryngology* 134: 771–7.

Gelfand, S. (2004) *Hearing: An introduction to psychological and physiological acoustics*, 4th edn. Informa, London.

George, E.L.J., Zekveld, A.A., Kramer, S.E., Goverts, S.T., Festen, J.M., Houtgast, T. (2007) Auditory and nonauditory factors affecting speech reception in noise by older listeners. *Journal of the Acoustical Society of America* 121: 2362–75.

Getty, L., Hétu, R. (1991) Development of a rehabilitation program for people affected with occupational hearing loss: 2. Results from group intervention with 48 workers and their spouses. *Audiology* 30 (6): 317–29.

Gianopoulos, I., Stephens, D. (2002) Opting for two hearing aids: a predictor of long-term use among adult patients fitted after screening. *International Journal of Audiology* 41: 518–26.

Gianopoulos, I., Stephens, D. (2005) General considerations about screening and their relevance to adult hearing screening. *Audiological Medicine* 3: 165–74.

Gilhome Herbst, K. (1983) Psychosocial consequences of disorders of hearing in the elderly. In: *Hearing and Balance in the Elderly*, (ed. R. Hinchcliffe), pp. 174–200. Edinburgh, Churchill Livingstone.

Gilhome Herbst, K.R., Humphrey, C.M. (1980) Hearing impairment and mental state in the elderly living at home. *British Medical Journal* 281: 903–5.

Gilhome Herbst, K., Meredith, R., Stephens, S.D.G. (1991) Implications of hearing impairment for elderly people in London and Wales. *Acta Oto-laryngologica* 476: S209–S214.

Goebel, G., Floezinger, U. (2008) Pilot study to evaluate psychiatric co-morbidity in tinnitus patients with and without hyperacusis. *Audiological Medicine* 6: 78–84.

Golabek, W., Nowakowska, M., Siwiek, H., Stephens, S.D.G. (1989) Problems of the hearing impaired in Poland. *British Journal of Audiology* 23: 73–5.

Goldstein, D.P., Stephens, S.D.G. (1980) *Audiological Rehabilitation: Management model, I.* Technical Memorandum 1. Royal National Throat Nose and Ear Hospital, Audiological Rehabilitation Centre, London.

Goldstein, D.P., Stephens, S.D.G. (1981) Audiological Rehabilitation: management model, I. *Audiology* 20: 432–52.

Graneheim, U.H., Lundman, B. (2004) Qualitative content analysis in nursing research: concepts, procedures and measures to achieve trustworthiness. *Nurse Education Today* 24 (2): 105–12.

Grant, K.W., Walden, B.E., Seitz, P.F. (1998) Auditory-visual speech recognition by hearing-impaired subjects: consonant recognitions, sentence recognition, and auditory-visual integration. *Journal of the Acoustical Society of America* 103: 2677–90.

Griggs, M. (1998) *Deafness and mental health: perceptions of health within the deaf community.* PhD thesis, University of Bristol.

Griggs, M. (2004) Deaf wellness explored. In: *Deafness in Mind: Working psychologically with deaf people across the lifespan,* (eds S. Austen, S. Crocker), pp. 115–26. Whurr, London.

Grimby, A., Ringdahl, A. (2000) Does having a job improve the quality of life among post-lingually deafened Swedish adults with severe-profound hearing impairment? *British Journal of Audiology* 34: 187–95.

Groce, N. (1985) *Everyone Here Spoke Sign Language.* Harvard University Press, Cambridge, MA.

Gussekloo, J., de Bont, L.E.A., von Faber M *et al.* (2003) Auditory rehabilitation of older people from the general population: the Leiden 85+ study. *British Journal of General Practice* 53: 536–40.

Gussekloo, J., de Craen, A.J., Oduber, C., van Boxtel, M.P., Westendorp, R.G. (2005) Sensory impairment and cognitive functioning in oldest-old subjects: the Leiden 85+ study. *American Journal of Geriatric Psychiatry* 13: 781–6.

Guttmacher, A.E., Collins, F.S., Carmona, R.H. (2004) The family history: more important than ever. *New England Journal of Medicine* 351: 2333–6.

Håkansson, B., Tjellström, A., Rosenhall, U., Carlsson, P. (1985) The bone-anchored hearing aid: principal design and psychoacoustical evaluation. *Acta Oto-laryngologica* 100: 229–39.

Hall, D.A., Hart, A.C., Johnsrude, I.S. (2003) Relationships between human auditory cortical structure and function. *Audiology and Neurootology* 8: 1–18.

Hallam, R.S., Stephens, S.D.G. (1985) Vestibular disorder and emotional distress. *Journal of Psychosomatic Research* 29: 407–13.

Hallam, R., Ashton, P., Sherbourne, K., Gailey, L. (2006) Acquired profound hearing loss: mental health and other characteristics of a large sample. *International Journal of Audiology* 45: 715–23.

Hallberg, L.R.-M. (1996) Occupational hearing loss: coping and family life. *Scandinavian Audiology* 25 (Suppl. 43): S25–S33.

Hallberg, L.R.-M. (1999) Hearing impairment, coping and consequences on family life. *Journal of the Academy of Rehabilitative Audiology* 32: 45–9.

Hallberg, L.R.-M., Barrenäs, M.L. (1993) Living with a male with noise-induced hearing loss: experiences from the perspective of spouses. *British Journal of Audiology* 27: 253–61.

Hallberg, L.R.-M., Barrenäs, M.L. (1995) Coping with noise-induced hearing loss: experiences from the perspective of middle-aged male victims. *British Journal of Audiology* 29: 219–30.

Hallberg, L.R.-M., Carlsson, S.G. (1991) A qualitative study of strategies for managing a hearing impairment. *British Journal of Audiology* 25: 201–11.

Hallberg, L.R.-M., Jansson, G. (1996) Women with noise-induced hearing loss: an invisible group? *British Journal of Audiology* 30: 340–5.

Hällgren, M., Larsby, B., Lyxell, B., Arlinger, S. (2005) Speech understanding in quiet and noise, with and without hearing aids. *International Journal of Audiology* 44: 574–83.

Hardick, E.J., Oyer, H.J., Irion, P.E. (1970) Lipreading performance as related to measurements of vision. *Journal of Speech and Hearing Research* 13: 92–100.

Harford, E., Barry, J. (1965) A rehabilitation approach to the problems of unilateral hearing impairment: the Contralateral Routing of Signals (CROS). *Journal of Speech and Hearing Disorders* 30: 121–38.

Hatfield, N. (1982) Sign language assessment. In: *Deafness and Communication*, (eds D.G. Sims, G.G. Walter, R.L. Whitehead), pp. 187–198. Williams and Wilkins, Baltimore.

Hawkins, D.B. (2005) Effectiveness of counselling-based adult group aural rehabilitation programs: a systematic review of the evidence. *Journal of the American Academy of Audiology* 16: 485–93.

Hawthorne, G. (2008) Perceived social isolation in a community: its prevalence and correlates of people's lives. *Social Psychiatry and Psychiatric Epidemiology* 43: 140–150.

Heine, C., Browning, C.J. (2002) Communication and psychosocial consequences of sensory loss in older adults: overview and rehabilitation directions. *Disability and Rehabilitation* 24: 763–73.

Helfer, K. (1997) Auditory and auditory-visual perception of clear and conversational speech. *Journal of Speech, Language and Hearing Research* 40: 32–443.

Helfer, K. (1998) Auditory and auditory-visual recognition of clear and conversational speech by older listeners. *Journal of the American Academy of Audiology* 9: 234–43.

Henderson Sabes, J., Sweetow, R.W. (2007) Variables predicting outcomes on listening and communication enhancement (LACE) training. *International Journal of Audiology* 46: 374–83.

Herth, K. (1998) Integrating hearing loss into one's life. *Qualitative Health Research* 8: 207–223.

Hétu, R. (1994) Mismatches between auditory demands and capacities in the industrial work environment. *Audiology* 33: 1–14.

Hétu, R. (1996) The stigma attached to hearing impairment. *Scandinavian Audiology* 25 (Suppl. 43): S12–S24.

Hétu, R., Getty, L. (1991) Development of a rehabilitation program for people affected with occupational hearing loss: 1. A new paradigm. *Audiology* 30 (6): 305–16.

Hétu, R., Lalonde, M., Getty, L. (1987) Psychosocial disadvantages associated with occupational hearing loss as experienced in the family. *Audiology* 26: 141–52.

Hétu, R., Riverin, L., Lalande, N., Getty, L., St-Cyr, C. (1988) Qualitative analysis of the handicap associated with occupational hearing loss. *British Journal of Audiology* 22: 251–64.

Hétu, R., Jones, L., Getty, L. (1993) The impact of acquired hearing impairment on the intimate relationship: implications for rehabilitation. *Audiology* 32: 363–81.

Hétu, R., Getty, L., Philibert, L., Desilets, F., Noble, W., Stephens, D. (1994) Mise au point d'un outil clinique pour la mesure d'incapacités auditives et de handicaps. *Journal of Speech-Language Pathology and Audiology* 18: 83–95.

Hickson, L. (2007) Pull out an 'ACE' to help your patients become better communicators. *Hearing Journal* 60 (1): 10–17.

Hickson, L., Worrall, L., Scarinci, N. (2007a) *Active Communication Education (ACE): A program for older people with hearing impairment*. Speechmark, London.

Hickson, L., Worral, L., Scarinci, N. (2007b) A randomized controlled trial evaluating the Active Communication Education program for older people with hearing impairment. *Ear and Hearing* 28: 212–30.

High, W.S., Fairbanks, G., Glorig, A. (1964) Scale for self-assessment of hearing handicap. *Journal of Speech and Hearing Disorders* 29: 215–30.

Higson, J.M., Haggard, M.P., Field, D.L. (1994) Validation of parameters for assessing Obscure Auditory Dysfunction: robustness of determinants of OAD status across samples and test methods. *British Journal of Audiology* 28 (1): 27–39.

Hinchcliffe, R. (1992) King-Kopetzky syndrome: an auditory stress disorder? *Journal of Audiological Medicine* 1: 89–98.

Hines, J. (2000) Communication problems of hearing impaired patients. *Nursing Standards* 14: 33–7.

Hipskind, N.M. (2007) *Visual stimuli in communication. In: Introduction to Audiological Rehabilitation,* (eds R.L. Schow, M.A. Nerbonne), 7th edn. pp. 151–96. Pearson, Boston.

Hirsh, I.J., Davis, H., Silverman, S.R., Reynolds, E.G., Eldert, E., Benson, R.W. (1952) Development of materials for speech audiometry. *Journal of Speech and Hearing Disorders* 17: 321–37.

Hitselberger, W.E., House, W.F., Edgerton, B.J., Whitaker, S. (1984) Cochlear nucleus implants. *Otolaryngology – Head and Neck Surgery* 92: 52–4.

Hodgson, W.R., Skinner, P.H. (1977) Hearing aid assessment and use in audiologic habilitation. Williams and Wilkins, Baltimore.

Hoeks, B. (1995) The pupillary response as a measure of processing load. Thesis. Katholieke Universiteit Nijmegen, The Netherlands.

Holder, W. (1669) *Elements of Speech.* Martyn, London.

Holt, J.A. (1994) Stanford Achievement Test, 8th edn. Reading comprehension subgroup results. *American Annals of the Deaf* 138: 172–5.

Hough, J., McGee, M., Himelick, T., Vernon, J. (1986) The surgical technique for the implantation of the temporal bone stimulator (AUDIANT ABC). *American Journal of Otology* 7: 315–21.

House, W.F., Urban, J. (1973) Long-term results of electrode implantation and electric stimulation of the cochlea in man. *Annals of Otology, Rhinology and Laryngology* 82: 504–17.

Houtgast, T., Festen, J.M. (2008) On the auditory and cognitive functions that may explain an individual's elevation of the speech reception threshold in noise. *International Journal of Audiology* 47: 287–95.

Houtgast, T., Steeneken, H.J.M. (1973) The modulation transfer function in room acoustics as a predictor of speech intelligibility. *Acoustica* 28: 66–73.

Hudson, D. (1958) *Sir Joshua Reynolds.* Bles, London.

Humes, L.E., Christopherson, L. (1991) Speech identification difficulties of hearing-impaired elderly persons: the contribution of auditory processing deficits. *Journal of Speech, Language and Hearing Research* 34: 686–93.

Humes, L.E., Burk, M.H., Coughlin, M.P., Busey, T.A., Strauser, L.E. (2007) Auditory speech recognition and visual text recognition on younger and older adults: similarities and differences between modalities and the effects of presentation rate. *Journal of Speech, Language, and Hearing Research* 50: 283–303.

Humphrey, C., Gilhome Herbst, K., Faruqi, S. (1981) Some characteristics of the hearing impaired elderly who do not present themselves for rehabilitation. *British Journal of Audiology* 15: 25–30.

Hutchinson, S.L., Loy, D.P., Kleiber, D.A., Dattilo, J. (2003) Leisure as a coping resource: variations in coping with traumatic injury and illness. *Leisure Sciences* 25: 143–61.

Huygen, P.L.M., Pauw, R.J., Cremers, C.W.R.J. (2007) Audiometric profiles associated with genetic non-syndromal hearing impairment: a review and phenotype analysis. In: *Genes, Hearing and Deafness,* (eds A. Martini, D. Stephens, A.P. Read), pp. 185–204. Informa, London.

Hyde, M.L., Riko, K. (1994) A decision-analytic approach to audiological rehabilitation. *Journal of the Academy of Rehabilitative Audiology* 26: S337–S374.

Hygge, S., Ronnberg, J., Larsby, B., Arlinger, S. (1992) Normal hearing and hearing impaired subjects' ability to follow conversation in competing speech, reversed speech, and noise backgrounds. *Journal of Speech and Hearing Research* 35: 208–5.

von Ilberg, C., Kiefer, J., Tillien, J. *et al.* (1999) Electric-Acoustic-Stimulation (EAS) of the Auditory System: new technology against severe hearing loss. *Journal for Oto-Rhino-Laryngology and its Related Specialties* 61: 334–40.

Itard, J.M.G. (1821) *Traité des maladies de l'oreille et de l'audition,* Vol. 2. Mequignon-Marvis, Paris.

Jacob, R.G., Furman, J.M., Cass, S.P. (2003) Psychiatric consequences of vestibular dysfunction. In: *Textbook of Audiological Medicine: Clinical aspects of hearing and balance*, (eds L. Luxon, J.M. Furman, A. Martini, D. Stephens), pp. 869–87. Martin Dunitz, London.

Jacobs, J.W., Beinhard, M.E., Delgado, A. (1977) Screening for organic mental syndromes in the medically ill. *Annals of Internal Medicine* 86: 40–46.

Jahrsdoerfer, R.A., Yeakley, J.W., Aguilar, E.A., Cole, R.R., Gray, L.C. (1992) Grading system for the selection of patients with congenital aural atresia. *American Journal of Otology* 13: 6–12.

Jakes, S. (1997) Otological symptoms and emotional disturbance. In: *Scott-Brown's Otolaryngology*, Vol. 2, (ed. D. Stephens), 6th edn. pp. 2/4/1–23. Butterworth-Heinemann, Oxford.

Janisse, M.P. (1977) *Pupillometry: The Psychology of the Papillary Response*. John Wiley & Sons, Washington.

Jaworski, A. (1993) *The Power of Silence: Social and pragmatic perspective*. Sage, Newbury Park, CA.

Jaworski, A., Stephens, D. (1998) Self-reports on silence as a face-saving strategy by people with hearing impairment. *International Journal of Applied Linguistics* 8: 61–80.

Jerger, J. (1964) Auditory tests for disorders of the central auditory mechanism. In: *Neurological Aspects of Auditory and Vestibular Disorders*, (eds W.S. Fields, B.R. Alford), pp. 77–86. Charles Thomas, Springfield, IL.

Jerger, J., Musiek, F. (2000) Report of the consensus conference on the diagnosis of auditory processing disorders in school-aged children. *Journal of the American Academy of Audiology* 11: 467–74.

Jerger, J., Chmiel, R., Florin, E., Pirozzolo, F., Wilson, N. (1996) Comparison of conventional amplification and an assistive listening device in elderly persons. *Ear and Hearing* 17: 490–504.

Johnson, N.E. (2004a) Nonmetro residence, hearing loss, and its accommodation among elderly people. *Journal of Rural Health* 20: 136–41.

Johnson, N.E. (2004b) Nonmetro residence and impaired vision among elderly Americans. *Journal of Rural Health* 20: 142–50.

Jones, L. (1997) Living with hearing loss. In: *Adjustment to Acquired Hearing Loss: Analysis, change and learning*, (ed. J.G. Kyle), pp. 126–39. Antony Rowe, Chippenham.

Jones, L., Kyle, J., Wood, P.L. (1987) *Words Apart*. Tavistock, London.

Jones, L., Mir, G., Khan, R. (2006) Ethnicity, spirituality and genetics services. In: *The Effects of Genetic Hearing Impairment in the Family*, (eds D. Stephens, L. Jones), pp. 297–319. John Wiley & Sons, Chichester.

Jordan, O., Greisen, O., Bentzen, O. (1967) Treatment with binaural hearing aids. *Archives of Otolaryngology* 85: 319–26.

Kacker, S.K., Hinchcliffe, R. (1970) Unusual Tullio phenomena. *Journal of Laryngology and Otology* 94: 155–66.

Kahneman, D., Beatty, J. (1966) Pupil diameter and load on memory. *Science* 154: 1583–5.

Kalikow, D.N., Stevens, K.N., Elliott, L.L. (1977) Development of a test of speech intelligibility in noise using sentence material with controlled word predictability. *Journal of the Acoustical Society of America* 61: 1337–51.

Karlsson, K.K., Harris, J.R., Svartengren, M. (1997) Description and primary results from an audiometric study of male twins. *Ear and Hearing* 18: 114–20.

Karlsson-Espmark, A.-K., Rosenhall, U., Erlandsson, S., Steen, B. (2002) the two faces of presbyacusis: hearing impairment and psychosocial consequences. *International Journal of Audiology* 41: 125–35.

Karlsson-Espmark, A.-K., Hansson-Scherman, M. (2003) Hearing confirms existence and identity: experiences from persons with presbyacusis. *International Journal of Audiology* 42: 106–15.

Kates, J.K. (2008) *Digital Hearing Aids*. Plural, San Diego.

Katz, D.I., Mills, V.M., Cassidy, J.W. (1997) The neurologic rehabilitation model in clinical practice. In: *Neurologic Rehabilitation: A guide to diagnosis, prognosis, and treatment planning*, (eds V.M. Mills, J.W. Cassidy, D.I. Katz), pp. 1–27. Blackwell, Malden, MA.

Keller, F. (1971) *Hörgeräteanspassung in Klinische Sicht*. Universitätsklinik HNO Freiburg.

Kelsay, D.M., Tyler, R.S. (1996) Advantages and disadvantages expected and realized by pediatric cochlear implant recipients as reported by their parents. *American Journal of Otolaryngology* 17: 866–73.

Kennedy, V., Stephens, D., Fitzmaurice, P. (2008) The impact of cochlear implants from the perspective of significant others of adult cochlear implant users. *Otology and Neurotology* 29: 607–14.

Kentala, E., Wilson, C., Pyykkö, I., Varpa, K., Stephens, D. (2008) Positive experiences associated with tinnitus and balance problems. *Audiological Medicine* 6: 55–61.

Kerr, P.C., Cowie, R.I.D. (1997) Acquired deafness: a multi-dimensional experience. *British Journal of Audiology* 31: 177–88.

Kerr, P.C., Stephens, D. (1997) The use of an open-ended questionnaire to identify positive aspects of acquired hearing loss. *Audiology* 36: 19–28.

Kerr, P.C., Stephens, D. (2000) Understanding the nature and function of positive experiences in living with auditory disablement. *Scandinavian Journal of Disability Research* 2: 21–38.

Kiessling, J., Pichora-Fuller, M.K., Gatehouse, S. (2003) Candidature for and delivery of audiological services: special needs of older people. *International Journal of Audiology* 42 (Suppl. 2): S92–S101.

Killion, M. (1981) Earmold options for wideband hearing aids. *Journal of Speech and Hearing Disorders* 46: 10–20.

Kim, Y., Duhamel, K.N., Valdimarsdottir, H.B., Bovbjerg, D.H. (2005) Psychological distress among healthy women with family histories of breast cancer: effects of recent life events. *Psycho-Oncology* 14: 555–63.

King, K., Stephens, D. (1992) Auditory and psychological factors in 'Auditory Disability with Normal Hearing'. *Scandinavian Audiology* 21: 109–14.

Kiresuk, T., Sherman, R. (1968) Goal attainment scaling: a general method for evaluating comprehensive mental health programmes. *Community Mental Health Journal* 4: 443–53.

Knutson, J.F., Lansing, C.R. (1990) The relationship between communication problems and psychological difficulties in persons with profound acquired hearing loss. *Journal of Speech and Hearing Disorders* 55: 656–64.

Koenig, W. (1950) Subjective effects in binaural hearing. *Journal of the Acoustical Society of America* 22: 61–2.

Kramer, S. (2005) The psychosocial impact of hearing loss among elderly people: a review. In: *The Impact of Genetic Hearing Impairment*, (eds D. Stephens, L. Jones), pp. 137–164. Whurr, London.

Kramer, S.E. (ed) (2006) *Hearing at work: how do we deal with that? CD-ROM information package for professionals, patients and significant others*. Report. VU University Press, Amsterdam.

Kramer, S.E. (2008) Hearing impairment, work and vocational enablement. *International Journal of Audiology* 47 (Suppl. 2): S124–S130.

Kramer, S.E., Kapteyn, T.S., Festen, J.M., Tobi, H. (1996) The relationships between self-reported hearing disability and measurements of auditory disability. *Audiology* 35: 277–87.

Kramer, S.E., Kapteyn, T.S., Festen, J.M., Kuik, D.J. (1997) Assessing aspects of auditory handicap by means of pupil dilatation. *Audiology* 36: 155–64.

Kramer, S.E., Kapteyn, T.S., Festen, J.M. (1998) The self-reported handicapping effect of hearing disabilities. *Audiology* 37: 302–12.

Kramer, S.E., Kapteyn, T.S., Kuik, D.J., Deeg, D.J.H. (2002) The association of hearing impairment and chronic diseases with psychosocial health status in older age. *Journal of Aging and Health* 14: 122–37.

Kramer, S.E., Allessie, G.H.M., Dondorp, A.W., Zekveld, A.A., Kapteyn, T.S. (2005) A home education program for older adults with hearing impairment and their significant others: a randomized trial evaluating short- and long-term effects. *International Journal of Audiology* 44: 255–64.

Kramer, S.E., Zekveld, A.A., Stephens, D. (2006a) Effects of a family history on late onset hearing impairment: results of an open-ended questionnaire. In *The Effects of Having a Family History of Hearing Impairment*, (eds D. Stephens, L. Jones), pp. 71–80. John Wiley & Sons, Chichester.

Kramer, S.E., Stephens, D., Espeso, A. (2006b) The awareness of having a family history of hearing problems and the impact on those with hearing difficulties themselves: a structured questionnaire. *Audiological Medicine* 4: 179–90.

Kramer, S.E., Kapteyn, T.S., Houtgast, T. (2006c) Comparing normally hearing and hearing impaired employees using the Amsterdam Checklist for Hearing and Work. *International Journal of Audiology* 45: 503–12.

Kramer, S.E., Zekveld, A.A., Houtgast, T. (2009) Measuring cognitive factors in speech comprehension: the value of using the Text Reception Threshold test as a visual analogue of the SRT test. *Scandinavian Journal of Psychology* (in press).

Kricos, P.B. (2000) The influence of nonaudiological variables on audiological rehabilitation outcomes. *Ear & Hearing* 21: S7–S14.

Kricos, P.B. (2006) Audiologic management of older adults with hearing loss and compromised cognitive/ psychoacoustic auditory processing capabilities. *Trends in Amplification* 10 (1): 1–28.

Kricos, P.B., Holmes, A.E. (1996) Efficacy of audiologic rehabilitation for older adults. *Journal of the American Academy of Audiology* 7 (4): 219–29.

Kricos, P.B., McCarthey, P. (2007) From ear to there: a historical perspective on auditory training. *Seminars in Hearing* 28: 89–98.

Kujala, U.M., Kaprio, J., Sarna, S., Koskenvuo, M. (1998) Relationship of leisure-time activity and mortality. *Journal of the American Medical Association* 279: 440–444.

Kurtz, L.F. (1997) *Self-help and Support Groups: A handbook for practitioners*. Sage, Thousand Oaks, CA.

Lane, H., Bahan, B. (1998) Ethics of cochlear implantation in young children: a review and reply from a Deaf-World perspective. *Otolaryngology – Head and Neck Surgery* 119: 297–313.

Larsby, B., Hällgren, M., Lyxell, B., Arlinger, S. (2005) Cognitive performance and perceived effort in speech processing tasks: effects of different noise backgrounds in normal hearing and hearing-impaired subjects. *International Journal of Audiology* 44: 131–43.

Laszig, R., Kuzma, J.A., Seifert, V., Lenhardt, E. (1991) The Hannover auditory brainstem implant: a multiple electrode prosthesis. *European Archives of Oto-Rhino-Laryngology* 248: 420–421.

Lazarus, R.S., Folkman, S. (1984) Coping and adaptation. In: *Handbook of Behavioral Medicine* (ed. W.D. Gentry), pp. 282–325. Guilford Press, New York.

Lee, D.J., Gómez-Marin, O., Lee, H.M. (1996) Sociodemographic correlates of hearing loss and hearing aid use in Hispanic adults. *Epidemiology* 7: 443–6.

Lee, P., Smith, J.P., Kington, R. (1999) Relationship of self-rated vision and hearing to functional status and well-being among seniors 70 years and older. *American Journal of Ophthalmology* 127: 447–52.

Lehmann, R.R. (1954) Bilateral sudden deafness. *New York State Journal of Medicine* 54: 1481–5.

Lesinski, A., Kempf, H.G., Lenarz, T. (1998) Tullio Phänomen nach Kochlearimplantation. *Hals-Nasen-Ohrenärzte* 46: 692–4.

Lesner, S.A. (2003) Candidacy and management of assistive listening devices: special needs of the elderly. *International Journal of Audiology* 42 (Suppl. 2): S68–S76.

Lewis, J.E., Stephens, S.D.G., McKenna, L. (1994) Tinnitus and suicide. *Clinical Otolaryngology* 19: 50–54.

Libby, E.R. (1982) A new acoustic horn for small ear canals. *Hearing Instruments* 33 (9): 48.

Lim, D.P., Stephens, S.D.G. (1991) Clinical investigation of hearing loss in the elderly. *Clinical Otolaryngology* 16: 288–93.

Lim, H.H., Lenarz, T., Anderson, D.J., Lenarz, M. (2008) The auditory midbrain implant: effects of electrode location. *Hearing Research* 242: 74–85.

Lim, H.H., Lenarz, T., Joseph, G. *et al.* (2007) Electrical stimulation of the midbrain for hearing restoration: insight into the functional organization of the human central auditory system. *Journal of Neuroscience* 27: 13541–51.

Lindenberger, U., Baltes, P.B. (1994) Sensory functioning and intelligence in old age: a strong connection. *Psychology and Aging* 9: 339–55.

Lindenberger, U., Scherer, H., Baltes, P.B. (2001) The strong connection between sensory and cognitive performance in old age: not due to sensory acuity reductions operating during cognitive assessment. *Psychology and Aging* 16: 196–205.

Lindley, G. (1999) Adaptation to loudness: implications for hearing aid fittings. *Hearing Journal* 52 (11): 50, 52, 56–7.

Lipowski, Z.J. (1988) Somatization: the concept and its clinical application. *American Journal of Psychiatry* 145: 1358–68.

Lloyd, K.M., Auld, C.J. (2002) The role of leisure in determining quality of life: issues of content and measurement. *Social Indicators Research* 57: 43–71.

Lormore, K.A., Stephens, S.D.G. (1994) Use of the open-ended questionnaire with patients and their significant others. *British Journal of Audiology* 28: 81–9.

Lundborg, T., Linzander, S., Rosenhamer, H., Lindström, B., Svärd, I., Fransson, A. (1973) Experience with hearing aids in adults. *Scandinavian Audiology* (Suppl. 3): 9–46.

Lunner, T. (2003) Cognitive function in relation to hearing aid use. *International Journal of Audiology* 42: S49–S58.

Lunner, T., Sundewall-Thorén, E. (2007) Interactions between cognition, compression and listening conditions: effects on speech-in-noise performance on a two-channel hearing aid. *Journal of the American Academy of Audiology* 18: 604–17.

Lupsakko, T.A., Kautiainen, H.J., Sulkava, R. (2005) The non-use of hearing aids in people aged 75 years and over in the city of Kuopio in Finland. *European Archives of Otorhinolaryngology* 262: 165–9.

Lutman, M.E., Brown, E.J., Coles, R.R.A. (1987) Self-reported disability and handicap in the population in relation to pure-tone threshold, age, sex and type of hearing loss. *British Journal of Audiology* 21: 45–58.

McFarland, D.J., Cacace, A.T. (1995) Modality specificity as a criterion for diagnosing central auditory processing disorders. *American Journal of Audiology* 4: 36–48.

McGurk, H., MacDonald, J. (1976) Hearing lips and seeing voices. *Nature* 264: 746–8.

McKenna, L. (1987) Goal planning in audiological rehabilitation. *British Journal of Audiology* 21: 5–11.

McMahon, C.M., Kifley, A., Rochtchina, E., Newell, P., Mitchell, P. (2008) The contribution of family history to hearing loss in an older population. *Ear and Hearing* 29: 578–84.

McMahon, S.B., Koltzenburg, M. (eds) (2005) *Wall and Melzack's Textbook of Pain*, 5th edn. Elsevier, London.

Mackenbach, J.P., Kunst, A.E., Cavelaars, A.E., Groenhof, F., Geurts, J.J. (1997) Socioeconomic inequalities in morbidity and mortality in Western Europe. The EU Working Group on Socioeconomic Inequalities in Health. *Lancet* 349: 1655–9.

Markides, A. (1977a) Rehabilitation of people with acquired deafness in adulthood. *British Journal of Audiology* Supplement 1.

Markides, A. (1977b) *Binaural Hearing Aids*. Academic Press, London.

Martini, A., Prosser, S., Mazzoli, M. *et al.* (1996) Contribution of age related factors to the progression of non-syndromic hereditary hearing impairment. *Journal of Audiological Medicine* 5: 141–56.

Martini, A., Milani, M., Rosignoli, M., Mazzoli, M., Prosser, S. (1997) Audiometric patterns of genetic non-syndromal sensorineural hearing loss. *Audiology* 36: 228–36.

Martini, A., Stephens, D., Read, A.P. (eds) (2007) *Genes, Hearing and Deafness*. Informa, London.

Maurer, J.F., Rupp, R.R. (1979) *Hearing and Aging: Tactics for intervention*. Grune & Stratton, New York.

May, J.J. (2000) Occupational hearing loss. *American Journal of Industrial Medicine* 37: 112–20.

Mayou, R., Farmer, A. (2002) ABC of psychological medicine: functional somatic symptoms and syndromes. *British Medical Journal* 325: 265–8.

Meehan, T., France, E.A., Stephens, S.D.G. (2002) The use of an open-ended questionnaire with parents of hearing-impaired teenagers: an exploratory study. *Journal of Audiological Medicine* 11: 46–59.

Mencher, G.T., Davis, A. (2006) Bilateral or unilateral amplification: is there a difference? *International Journal of Audiology* 45: S3–S11.

Meredith, R., Thomas, K.J., Callaghan, D.E., Stephens, S.D.G. (1989) A comparison of three types of ear-moulds in elderly users of post-aural hearing aids. *British Journal of Audiology* 23: 239–44.

Merluzzi, F., Hinchcliffe, R. (1973) Threshold of subjective auditory handicap. *Audiology* 12: 65–9.

Meyer-Bisch, C. (1990) Audioscan: a high-definition audiometry technique based on Meyer-Bisch, C. Audiometrie automatique de depistage preventif: le balayage frequentiel asservi (audioscan). *Cahiers de Notes Documentaires* 139: 335–45.

Meyer-Bisch, C. (1996) Audioscan: a high definition audiometry technique based on constant-level frequency sweeps: a new method with new hearing indicators. *Audiology* 35: 63–72.

Meyer-Bisch, C. (2007) *Guide de prevention du risqué auditif*. Association Française des Orchèstres, Paris.

Middelweerd, M.J., Plomp, R. (1987) The effect of speechreading on the speech-reception threshold of sentences in noise. *Journal of the Acoustical Society of America* 82: 2145–7.

Middleton, A., Jewison, J., Mueller, R.F. (1998) Attitudes of deaf adults toward genetic testing for hereditary deafness. *American Journal of Human Genetics* 63: 1175–80.

Middleton, A., Moumoulidis, I., Crossland, G. *et al.* (2006) Attitudes of adults with otosclerosis towards issues surrounding genetics and the impact of hearing loss. In: *The Effects of Having a Family History of Hearing Impairment*, (eds D. Stephens, L. Jones), pp. 237–43. John Wiley & Sons, Chichester.

Middleton, A., Lewis, P.A., Stephens, D. How can deaf people needing a special approach to genetic counselling be identified? (in press).

Miller, W.R., Rollnick, S. (2002) *Motivational Interviewing: Preparing people for change*. Guilford Press, New York.

Miyamoto, R.T., Robbins, A.M., Osberger, M.J., Todd, S.L., Riley, A.I., Kirk, K.I. (1995) Comparison of multichannel tactile aids and multichannel cochlear implants in children with profound hearing impairments. *American Journal of Otology* 16: 8–13.

Mokkink, L.B., Knol, D., Zekveld, A.A., Goverts, S.T., Kramer, S.E. (2009) Factor structure and reliability of the Dutch version of seven scales of the Communication Profile for the Hearing Impaired (CPHI). *Journal of Speech Language and Hearing Research* (in press).

Møller, A.R. (2006) *Hearing: Anatomy, physiology and disorders of the auditory system*, 2nd edn. Academic Press, New York.

Möller, K. (2005) The impact of combined vision and hearing impairment and of deafblindness. In: *The Impact of Genetic Hearing Impairment* (eds D. Stephens, L. Jones,), pp. 165–94. Whurr, London.

Möller, K., Danermark, B. (2007) Social recognition, participation, and the dynamic between the environment and personal factors of students with deafblindness. *American Annals of the Deaf* 152: 42–55.

Moore, B.C.J. (2007) *Cochlear Hearing Loss: Physiological, psychological and technical aspects*, 2nd edn. John Wiley & Sons, Chichester.

Moore, B.C.J., Huss, M., Vickers, D.A., Glasberg, B.R., Alcántara, J.I. (2000) A test for the diagnosis of dead regions in the cochlea. *British Journal of Audiology* 34: 205–24.

Moore, B.C.J., Glasberg, B.R., Stone, M.A. (2004) New version of the TEN test with calibrations in dB HL. *Ear and Hearing* 25: 478–87.

Morata, T.C., Themann, C.L., Randolph, R.F., Verbsky, B.L., Byrne, D.C., Reeves, E.R. (2005) Working in noise with a hearing loss: perceptions from workers, supervisors, and hearing conservation program managers. *Ear and Hearing* 26: 529–45.

Morgan-Jones, R.A. (2001) *Hearing Differently: The impact of hearing on family life.* Whurr, London.

Mosnier, I., Sterkers, O., Bouccara, D. *et al.* (2008) Benefit of the Vibrant Soundbridge device in patients implanted for 5 to 8 years. *Ear and Hearing* 29: 281–4.

Mulrow, C.D., Aquilar, C., Endicott, J.E. *et al.* (1990) Association between hearing impairment and the quality of life of elderly individuals. *Journal of the American Geriatrics Society* 38: 45–50.

Musiek, F.E., Baran, J.A. (2007) *The Auditory System: Anatomy, physiology and clinical correlates.* Allyn & Bacon, Boston, MA.

Musiek, F.E., Baran, J.A., Shinn, J.B., Guenette, L., Zaidan, E., Weihing, J. (2007) Central deafness: an audiological case study. *International Journal of Audiology* 46: 433–41.

Nachtegaal, J., Kuik, D.J., Anema, J.R., Goverts, S.T., Festen, J.M., Kramer, S.E. (2009a) The relationship between hearing status and need for recovery after work, psychosocial work characteristics, and sick leave: results from an Internet based National Survey on Hearing. *International Journal of Audiology* (in press).

Nachtegaal, J., Smit, J.H., Smits, J. *et al.* (2009b) The association between hearing status and psychosocial health before the age of 70 years: results from an Internet based National Survey on Hearing. *Ear and Hearing* 30 (3): 302–12.

Naramura, H., Nakansishi, N., Tatara, K., Ishiyama, M., Shiraishi, H., Yamamoto, A. (1999) Physical and mental correlates of hearing impairment in the elderly in Japan. *Audiology* 38: 24–9.

Neary, W.J., Ramsden, R.T., Evans, D.G.R., Baser, M.E. (2005) Psychosocial aspects of NF2. In: *The Impact of Genetic Hearing Impairment*, (eds D. Stephens, L. Jones), pp. 201–218. Whurr, London.

Nedzelnitsky, V. (1980) Sound pressures in the basal turn of the cat cochlea. *Journal of the Acoustical Society of America* 68: 1676–89.

Nelson, D.I., Nelson, R.Y., Concha-Barrientos, M., Fingerhut, M. (2005) The global burden of occupational noise-induced hearing loss. *American Journal of Industrial Medicine* 48: 446–58.

Nevison, B., Laszig, R., Sollman, W.P. *et al.* (2002) Results from a European clinical investigation of the Nucleus multichannel auditory brainstem implant. *Ear and Hearing* 23: 170–83.

Newman, C., Hug, G., Jacobson, G.P., Sandridge, S. (1997) Perceived hearing handicap of patients with unilateral or mild hearing loss. *Annals of Otology, Rhinology and Laryngology* 106: 210–214.

Nilsson, M., Soli, S.G., Sullivan, J.A. (1994) Development of the Hearing in Noise Test for the measurement of speech reception thresholds in quiet and in noise. *Journal of the Acoustical Society of America* 92: 1085–99.

Noback, C.R. (1985) Neuroanatomical correlates of central auditory function. In: *Assessment of Central Auditory Dysfunction: Foundations and clinical correlates*, (eds M.L. Pinheiro, F.E Musiek,), pp. 7–21. Williams and Wilkins, Baltimore.

Noble, W. (1983) Hearing, hearing impairment and the audible world: a theoretical essay. *Audiology* 22: 325–38.

Noble, W. (1998) *Self-assessment of Hearing and Related Functions.* Whurr, London.

Noble, W. (2002) Extending the IOI to significant others and to non-hearing-aid-based interventions. *International Journal of Audiology* 41: 27–9.

Noble, W., Atherley, G. (1970a) The Hearing Measurement Scale: a questionnaire for the assessment of auditory disability. *Journal of Auditory Research* 10: 229–50.

Noble, W., Atherley, G.R. (1970b) The hearing measurement scale as a paper–pencil form: preliminary results. *Journal of the American Audiological Society* 5: 95–106.

Noble, W., Gatehouse, S. (2004) Interaural asymmetry of hearing loss, Speech, Spatial and Qualities of hearing scale (SSQ), disabilities and handicap. *International Journal of Audiology* 43: 100–114.

Noble, W., Gatehouse, S. (2006) Effects of bilateral versus unilateral hearing aid fitting on abilities measured by the Speech, Spatial and Qualities of hearing scale (SSQ) *International Journal of Audiology* 45: 172–81.

Noble, W., Hétu, R. (1994) An ecological approach to disability and handicap in relation to impaired hearing. *Audiology* 33: 117–26.

Noble, W.G., Byrne, D., Lepage, B. (1994) Effects on sound localization of configuration and type of hearing impairment. *Journal of the Acoustical Society of America* 95: 992–1005.

Norman, M., George, C.R., Downie, A., Milligan, J. (1995) Evaluation of a communication course for new hearing aid users. *Scandinavian Journal of Audiology* 14: 63–9.

Olsen, W.O., Noffsinger, D., Kurdziel, S. (1975) Speech discrimination in quiet and in white noise by patients with peripheral and central lesions. *Acta Oto-laryngologica* 80: 375–82.

O Mahoney, C.F., Stephens, S.D.G., Cadge, B.A. (1996) Who prompts patients to consult about hearing loss? *British Journal of Audiology* 30: 153–8.

Palmer, K.T., Griffin, M.J., Sydall, H.E., Davis, A., Pannett, B., Coggon, D. (2002) Occupational exposure to noise and the attributable burden of hearing difficulties in Great Britain. *Occupational and Environmental Medicine* 59: 634–9.

Parving, A., Christensen, B. (1993) Training and employment in hearing-impaired subjects at 20–35 years of age. *Scandinavian Audiology* 2: 133–9.

Parving, A., Biering-Sorensen, M., Bech, B., Christensen, B., Sorensen, M.S. (1997). Hearing in the elderly >80 years of age: prevalence of problems and sensitivity. *Scandinavian Audiology* 26: 99–106.

Pauls, M.D., Hardy, W.G. (1948) Fundamentals in the treatment of communicative disorders caused by hearing disability. Part 2. *Journal of Speech and Hearing Disorders* 13: 97–105.

Petitot, C., Perrot, X., Collet, L., Bonnefoy, M. (2007) Maladie d'Alzheimer, troubles d'audition et apareillage auditive: une revue des données actuelles. *Psychologie & Neuropsychiatrie du Vieillissement* 5: 121–5.

Pichora-Fuller, M.K. (2003a) Processing speed and timing in aging adults: psychoacoustics, speech perception, and comprehension. *International Journal of Audiology* 42: S59–S67.

Pichora-Fuller, M.K. (2003b) Cognitive aging and auditory information processing. *International Journal of Audiology* 42 (Suppl. 2): S26–S32.

Pichora-Fuller, M.K., Singh, G. (2006) Effects of age on auditory and cognitive processing: implications for hearing aid fitting and audiologic rehabilitation. *Trends in Amplification* 10: 29–59.

Pichora-Fuller, M.K., Souza, P.E. (2003) Effects of aging on auditory processing of speech. *International Journal of Audiology* 42: S11–S16.

Pichora-Fuller, M.K., Schneider, B.A., Daneman, M. (1995) How young and old adults listen to and remember speech in noise. *Journal of the Acoustical Society of America* (1995) 97: 593–608.

Pichora-Fuller, M.K., Johnson, C.E., Roodenburg, K.E.J. (1998) The discrepancy between hearing impairment and handicap in the elderly: balancing transaction and interaction. *Journal of Applied Communication Research* 26: 99–119.

Piercy, S.K., Goldstein, D.P. (1994) Hearing aid rejection: the type III individual. *ASHA* 51–2.

Plant, G.L., Macrae, J.H., Pearce, J.L. (1980) Performance on a lipreading test by native and non-native speakers of English. *Australian Journal of Audiology* 2: 25–9.

Plomp, R., Mimpen, A.M. (1979a) Improving the reliability of testing the speech reception threshold for sentences. *Audiology* 18: 43–52.

Plomp, R., Mimpen, A.M. (1979b) Speech reception threshold for sentences as a function of age and noise level. *Journal of the Acoustical Society of America* 66: 1333–42.

Pope, S.K., Sowers, M. (2000) Functional status and hearing impairments in women at midlife. *Journal of Gerontology Series B: Psychological Sciences & Social Sciences* 55 (3): S190–S194.

Preminger, J.E. (2003) Should significant others be encouraged to join adult group audiologic rehabilitation classes? *Journal of the American Academy of Audiology* 14: 545–55.

Preminger, J.E. (2007) Issues associated with the measurement of psychosocial benefits of group audiologic rehabilitation programs. *Trends in Amplification* 11 (2): 113–23.

Prosser, S., Martini, A. (2007) Understanding the phenotype: basic concepts in audiology. In: *Genes, Hearing and Deafness: From molecular biology to clinical practice*, (eds A. Martini, D. Stephens, A.P. Read), pp. 19–38. Informa, London.

Pryce, H., Wainwright, D. (2008) Help-seeking for medically unexplained hearing difficulties: a qualitative study. *International Journal of Therapy and Rehabilitation* 15: 1–7.

Pyykkö, I., Ishizaki, H., Aalto, H., Starck, J. (1992) Relevance of the Tullio phenomenon in assessing perilymphatic leak in vertiginous patients. *American Journal of Otology* 13: 339–42.

Rakerd, B., Seits, P.F., Whearty, M. (1996) Assessing the cognitive demand of speech listening for people with hearing losses. *Ear and Hearing* 17: 97–106.

Ramsdell, D.A. (1947) The psychology of the hard-of-hearing and the deafened adult. In: *Hearing and Deafness: A guide for laymen*, (ed. H. Davis), pp. 392–418. Murray Hill, New York.

Reeve, K.J. (2003) *Children with mild and unilateral hearing impairment: current management and outcome measures*. PhD thesis, University of Nottingham.

Reisberg, D., McLean, J., Goldfield, A. (1987) Easy to hear but hard to understand: a speechreading advantage with intact stimuli. In: *Hearing by Eye: The psychology of lip-reading*, (eds R. Campbell, B. Dodd), pp. 97–113. Erlbaum, London.

Rendell, R.J., Stephens, S.D.G. (1988) Auditory disability with normal hearing. *British Journal of Audiology* 22: 223–4.

Ringdahl, A., Grimby, A. (2000) Severe-profound hearing impairment and health-related quality of life among post-lingual deafened Swedish adults. *Scandinavian Audiology* 29: 266–75.

Ringdahl, A., Brenstaaf, S., Simonsson, M. *et al.* (2001) A three-year follow-up of a four-week multidisciplinary audiological rehabilitation programme. *Journal of Audiological Medicine* 10: 142–57.

Roberts, P. (1992) *An ergonomic investigation into the design of a behind-the-ear (BTE) hearing aid to overcome handling difficulties experienced by elderly users*. Undergraduate dissertation, University of Glamorgan, Department of Mechanical Engineering.

Robinson, J.D., Baer, T., Moore, B.C.J. (2007) Using transposition to improve consonant discrimination and detection for listeners with severe high-frequency hearing loss. *International Journal of Audiology* 49: 293–308.

Rogers, M.T., Zhao, F., Harper, P.S., Stephens, D. (2002) Absence of hearing impairment in adult onset facioscapulohumeral muscular dystrophy. *Neuromuscular Disorders* 12: 358–65.

Rönnberg, J. (2003) Cognition in the hearing impaired and the deaf as a bridge between signal and dialogue: a framework and a model. *International Journal of Audiology* 42: S68–S76.

Rönnberg, J., Borg, E. (2001) A review and evaluation of research on the deaf-blind from perceptual, communicative and rehabilitative perspectives. *Scandinavian Audiology* 30: 67–77.

Rönnberg, J., Andersson, U., Lyxell, B., Spens, K. (1998) Vibrotactile speech tracking support: cognitive prerequisites. *Journal of Deaf Studies and Deaf Education* 3: 143–56.

Rönnberg, J., Samuelsson, E., Borg, E. (2002) Exploring the perceived world of the deafblind: on the development of an instrument. *International Journal of Audiology* 41: 136–43.

Rönnberg, J., Rudner, M., Foo, C., Lunner, T. (2008) Cognition counts: a working memory system for ease of language understanding. *International Journal of Audiology* 47 (Suppl. 2): S99–S105.

Ross, M. (2002) Tracking and communication repair strategies. Rehabilitation Engineering Research Center on Hearing Enhancement (RERC), Gallaudet University. Available from: http://www.hearingresearch.org.

Ruben, J.R. (2000) Redefining the survival of the fittest: communication disorders in the 21st century. *Laryngoscope* 110: 241–5.

Rubinstein, A., Boothroyd, A. (1987) The effect of two approaches to auditory training on speech recognition by hearing-impaired adults. *Journal of Speech and Hearing Research* 30: 153–60.

Rudner, M., Foo, C., Sundewall-Thorén, E., Lunner, T., Rönnberg, J. (2008) Phonological mismatch and explicit cognitive processing in a sample of 102 hearing-aid users. *International Journal of Audiology* 47 (Suppl. 2): S91–S98.

Russell, J.N., Hendershot, G.E., LeClere, F., Howie, L.J. (1997) *Trends and differential use of assistive technology devices: United States, (1994). Advance data from vital and health statistics* No. 292. National Center for Health Statistics, Hyattsville, MD.

Rustin, L., Kuhr, A. (1989) *Social Skills and the Speech Impaired*. Taylor & Francis, London.

Rutman, D., Boisseau, B. (1995) Acquired hearing loss: social and psychological issues in adjustment processes. *International Journal of Rehabilitation Research* 18: 313–23.

Saeed, S.R., Ramsden, R.T., Axon, P.R. (1998) Cochlear implantation in the deaf-blind. *American Journal of Otology* 19: 774–7.

Saglier, C., Perez-Diaz, F., Collet, L., Jouvent, R. (2004) Psychologie, psychopathologie des malentendants et aide auditive. *Les Cahiers de l'Audition* 17: 34–40.

Sakata, T., Esaki, Y., Yamano, T., Sueta, N., Nakagawa, T. (2008) A comparison between the feeling of ear fullness and tinnitus in acute sensorineural hearing loss. *International Journal of Audiology* 47: 134–40.

Sanchez, L., Stephens, S.D.G. (1997) A tinnitus problem questionnaire in a clinic population. *Ear and Hearing* 18: 210–217.

Sataloff, R.T. (1991) Hearing loss in musicians. *American Journal of Otology* 12: 122–7.

Sato-Minako, Ogawa-Kaoru, Saito-Hideyuki *et al.* (2005) (Evaluation of sudden deafness by HHIA and questionnaire.) (Medline abstract.) *Nippon Jibiinkoka Gakkai kaiho* 108: 1158–64.

Saunders, G., Haggard, M.P. (1989) The clinical assessment of 'obscure auditory function' (OAD): 1. Auditory and psychological factors. *Ear and Hearing* 10: 200–208.

Saunders, G.H., Haggard, M.P. (1992) The clinical assessment of 'Obscure Auditory Dysfunction' (OAD): 2. Case control analysis of determining factors. *Ear and Hearing* 13: 241–54.

Saunders, G.H., Haggard, M.P. (1993) The influence of personality-related factors upon consultation for two different 'marginal' organic pathologies with and without reports of auditory symptomatology. *Ear and Hearing* 14: 242–8.

Savikko, N., Routasalo, P., Tilvis, R.S., Strandberg, T.E., Pitkälä, K.H. (2005) Predictors and subjective causes of loneliness in an aged population. *Archives of Gerontology and Geriatrics* 41: 223–33.

SBU (2003) *Hearing Aids for Adults*. The Swedish Council on Technology Assessment in Health Care, Stockholm.

Scarinci, N., Worrall, L., Hickson, L. (2008) The effect of hearing impairment in older people on the spouse. *International Journal of Audiology* 47: 141–51.

Scherer, M.J., Frisina, D.R. (1998) Characteristics associated with marginal hearing loss and subjective well-being among a sample of older adults. *Journal of Rehabilitation, Research and Development* 35: 420–426.

Scherich, D.L., Mowry, R. (1997) Job accommodations in the workplace for persons who are deaf or hard of hearing: current practices and recommendations. *Journal of Rehabilitation* 62: 27–37.

Schmuziger, N., Schimmann, F., Wengen, D., Patscheke, J., Probst, R. (2006) Long-term assessment after implantation of the Vibrant Soundbridge device. *Otology and Neurotology* 27: 183–8.

Schneider, B.A., Daneman, M., Pichora-Fuller, M.K. (2002) Listening in aging adults: from discourse comprehension to psychoacoustics. *Canadian Journal of Experimental Psychology* 56: 139–52.

Schow, R.L. (2008). *Introduction to Audiologic Rehabilitation*, 5th edn. Allyn & Bacon, Boston.

Schow, R.L., Nerbonne, M.A. (1995) *Introduction to Audiologic Rehabilitation*, 3rd edn. Allyn & Bacon, Needham Heights, MA.

Schow, R.L., Nerbonne, M.A. (2007) *Introduction to Audiologic Rehabilitation*, 5th edn. Pearson, Boston.

Schum, D.J. (1996) Intelligibility of clear and conversational speech of young and elderly talkers. *Journal of the American Academy of Audiology* 7: 212–8.

Schwartz, M.D., Taylor, L., Willard, K.S. (1999) Distress, Personality and mammography utilization among women with a family history of breast cancer. *Health Psychology* 18: 327–32.

Shaw, E.A.G. (1974) Transformation of sound pressure level from the free field to the eardrum in the horizontal plane. *Journal of the Acoustical Society of America* 56: 1848–1861.

Sindhusake, D., Stephens, D., Newall, P., Mitchell, P. (2006) The impact of a family history of hearing loss in the Blue Mountain Study. In: *The Effects of Having a Family History of Hearing Impairment*, (eds D. Stephens, L. Jones), pp. 15–27. John Wiley & Sons, Chichester.

Singh, G., Pichora-Fuller, K., Hayes, D., Carnahan, H. (2008) The relationship between age, manual dexterity and successful hearing aid use. Poster presented at the 29th International Congress of Audiology, Hong Kong.

Singleton, J.L., Supalla, S.J. (2003) Assessing children's proficiency in natural signed languages. In: *Oxford Handbook of Deaf Studies, Language and Education*, (eds M. Marschark, P.E. Spencer), pp. 289–302. Oxford University Press, Oxford.

Sirimanna, T., Stephens, D., Board, T. (1996) Tinnitus and Audioscan notches. *Journal of Audiological Medicine* 5: 38–48.

Sixt, E., Rosenhall, U. (1997) Presbyacusis related to socio-economic factors and state of health. *Scandinavian Audiology* 26: 133–40.

Skamris, N. (1974) Assessment of lipreading ability of deafened persons. In: *Visual and Audiovisual Perception of Speech*, (eds H. Nielsen, E. Knapp), pp. 128–35. Almquist and Wiksell, Stockholm.

Sluiter, J.K., De Croon, E.M., Meijman, T.F., Frings-Dresen, M.H.W. (2003) Need for recovery from work related fatigue and its role in the development and prediction of subjective health complaints. *Occupational Environmental Medicine* 60 (Suppl. 1): S162–S170.

Smaldino, J., Traynor, R. (1982) Comprehensive evaluation of the older adult for audiological reconditioning. *Ear and Hearing* 3: 148–59.

Smith, S.M., Kampfe, C.M. (1997) Interpersonal relationship implications of hearing loss in persons who are older. *Journal of Rehabilitation* 63: 15–22.

Smits, C., Kapteyn, T.S., Houtgast, T. (2004) Development and validation of an automatic speech-in-noise screening test by telephone. *International Journal of Audiology* 43: 15–28.

Smits, C., Kramer, S.E., Houtgast, T. (2006a) Speech reception thresholds in noise and self-reported hearing disability in a general adult population. *Ear and Hearing* 27: 538–49.

Smits, C., Merkus, P., Houtgast, T. (2006b) How we do it: the Dutch functional hearing-screening tests by telephone and internet. *Clinical Otolaryngology* 31: 436–40.

Snik, A.F.M., Mylanus, E.A.M., Cremers, C.W.R.J. (1998) Implantable hearing devices for sensorineural hearing loss: a review of the audiometric data. *Clinical Otolaryngology* 23: 414–19.

Snik, A., Leijendeckers, J., Hol, M., Mylanus, E., Cremers, C. (2008) The bone-anchored hearing aid for children: recent developments. *International Journal of Audiology* 47: 554–9.

Snoeckx, R.L., Van Camp, G. (2007) Nonsyndromic hearing loss: cracking the cochlear code. In: *Genes, Hearing and Deafness*, (eds A. Martini, D. Stephens, A.P. Read), pp. 63–78. Informa, London.

Sorgdrager, B., Kramer, S.E., Dreschler, W.A. (2006) Terreinverkenning. In: *Trends in de bedrijfs- en verzekeringsgeneeskund*, (Trends in Occupational Health Care) (ed. A.N.H. Van Weel), pp. 10–11. Bohn Stafleu en Van Loghum, Houten, The Netherlands.

Speranza, F., Daneman, M., Schneider, B.A. (2000) How aging affects the reading of words in noisy backgrounds. *Psychology and Aging* 15: 253–8.

Stark, P., Hickson, L. (2004) Outcomes of hearing aid fitting for older people with hearing impairment and their significant others. *International Journal of Audiology* 43: 390–398.

St Claire, L., He, Y. (2009) How do I know if I need a hearing aid? *Applied Psychology* 58: 24–41.

Stephens, J. (2006) Longer-term aspects of the language development of children with cochlear implants. *Audiological Medicine* 4: 151–63.

Stephens, S.D.G. (1979) The role of electrophysiological tests in auditory rehabilitation. *Revue de Laryngologie* 100: 729–37.

Stephens, S.D.G. (1980) Evaluating the problems of the hearing impaired. *Audiology* 19: 205–20.

Stephens, S.D.G. (1982) Audiological rehabilitation: extending the model. *Auditory Rehabilitation Centre Technical Memorandum* No. 4. Royal National Throat, Nose and Ear Hospital, London.

Stephens, S.D.G. (1983a) Aetiology of hearing loss in adults. In: *Prevention of Deafness and Genetic Counselling*, (eds European Association of Audiophonological Centres), pp. 9–19. EAAC, Brussels.

Stephens, D. (1983b) Rehabilitation and service needs. In: *Hearing Science and Hearing Disorders*, (eds M.E. Lutman, M.P. Haggard), pp. 283–324. Academic Press, London.

Stephens, S.D.G. (1984) Hearing aid selection: an integrated approach. *British Journal of Audiology* 18: 199–210.

Stephens, S.D.G. (1987a) Audiological rehabilitation. In: *Scott-Brown's Otolaryngology*, Vol. 2 (ed. D. Stephens), 5th edn. pp. 446–80. Butterworth, London.

Stephens, S.D.G. (1987b) People's complaints of hearing difficulties. In: *Adjustment to Acquired Hearing Loss*, (ed. J.G. Kyle), pp. 37–47. Centre for Deaf Studies, Bristol.

Stephens, S.D.G. (1988) Management model for the rehabilitation of the profoundly deaf. *Quaderni di Audiologia* 4: 574–81.

Stephens, D. (1996) Hearing rehabilitation in a psychosocial framework. *Scandinavian Audiology* 24 (Suppl. 43): 57–66.

Stephens, D. (1997) Audiological rehabilitation. In: *Scott-Brown's Otolaryngology*, Vol. 2, (ed. D. Stephens), 6th edn, pp. 2/13/19–21. Butterworth-Heinemann, Oxford.

Stephens, D. (2001) Audiological terms. In: *Definitions, Protocols and Guidelines in Genetic Hearing Impairment*, (eds A. Martini, M. Mazzoli, D. Stephens, A. Read), pp. 9–14. Whurr, London.

Stephens, D. (2003) Audiological rehabilitation. In: *Textbook of Audiological Medicine: Clinical aspects of hearing and balance*, (eds L. Luxon, J.M. Furman, A. Martini, D. Stephens), pp. 513–31. Martin Dunitz, London.

Stephens, D. (2005) The impact of hearing impairment in children. In: *The Impact of Genetic Hearing Impairment*, (eds D. Stephens, L. Jones), pp. 73–105. Whurr, London.

Stephens, D. (2007) Psychosocial aspects of genetic hearing impairment. In: *Genes, Hearing and Deafness*, (eds A. Martini, D. Stephens, A.P. Read), pp. 145–61. Informa, London.

Stephens, S.D.G., Anderson, C.M.B. (1971) Experimental studies on the uncomfortable loudness level. *Journal of Speech and Hearing Research* 14: 262–70.

Stephens, S.D.G., Ballam, H.M. (1974) The sono-ocular test. *Journal of Laryngology and Otology* 88: 1049–59.

Stephens, D., Danermark, B. (2005) The international classification of functioning, disability and health as a conceptual framework for the impact of genetic hearing impairment. In: *The Impact of Genetic Hearing Impairment*, (eds D. Stephens, L. Jones,), pp. 54–67. Whurr, London.

Stephens, S.D.G., Goldstein, D.P. (1983) Auditory rehabilitation for the elderly. In: *Hearing and Balance in the Elderly*, (ed. R. Hinchcliffe), pp. 201–26. Churchill Livingstone, Edinburgh.

Stephens, D., Hétu, R. (1991) Impairment, disability and handicap in audiology: towards a consensus. *Audiology* 30: 185–200.

Stephens, D., Jones, L. (eds) (2005) *The Impact of Genetic Hearing Impairment*. Whurr, London.

Stephens, D., Jones, L. (eds) (2006) *The Effects of Genetic Hearing Impairment in the Family*. John Wiley & Sons, Chichester.

Stephens, D., Kerr, P. (1996) Handicap and its management in the elderly. In: *Proceedings of the European Conference on Audiology*, (eds R. Schoonhoven, T.S. Kapteyn, J.A.P.M. de Laat), pp. 348–52. Vereniging voor Audiologie, Leiden, The Netherlands.

Stephens, D., Kerr, P. (2003) The role of positive experiences in living with acquired hearing loss. *International Journal of Audiology* 42: S118–S127.

Stephens, D., Kramer, S.E. (2005) The impact of having a family history of hearing problems on those with hearing difficulties themselves: an exploratory study. *International Journal of Audiology* 44: 206–12.

Stephens, D., Lemkens, N. (2006) People's reaction to having a family history of Otosclerosis. In: *The Effects of Having a Family History of Hearing Impairment*, (eds D. Stephens, L. Jones), pp. 245–254. John Wiley & Sons, Chichester.

Stephens, D., McKenna, L. (2008) (eds) Tinnitus management. *Audiological Medicine* 6: 1–91.

Stephens, S.D.G., Meredith, R. (1991a) Physical handling of hearing aids by the elderly. *Acta Oto-laryngologica* 476: S281–S285.

Stephens, S.D.G., Meredith, R. (1991b) Qualitative reports of hearing aid benefit. *Clinical Rehabilitation* 5: 225–9.

Stephens, D., Meredith, R. (1991c) The Afan Valley audiological rehabilitation studies. In: *Presbyacusis and Other Age Related Aspects*, (ed. J. Hartwig-Jensen), pp. 323–37. Jensen, Copenhagen.

Stephens, S.D.G., Rendell, R.J. (1988) Auditory disability with normal hearing. *Quaderni di Audiologia* 4: 233–8.

Stephens, D., Zhao, F. (1996) Hearing impairment: special needs of the elderly. *Folia Phoniatrica et Logopaedica* 48: 137–42.

Stephens, D., Zhao, F. (2000) The role of a family history in King Kopetzky syndrome (Obscure auditory dysfunction). *Acta Oto-laryngologica* 120: 197–200.

Stephens, D., Zhao, F. (2002) Effectiveness of self-rating measures of auditory activity limitation and participation restriction in patients with hearing impairment. *Iranian Audiology* 1: 33–40.

Stephens, S.D.G., Blegvad, B., Krogh, H.J. (1977) The value of some suprathreshold auditory measures. *Scandinavian Audiology* 6: 213–21.

Stephens, S.D.G., Callaghan, D.E., Hogan, S., Meredith, R., Rayment, A., Davis A (1990a) Hearing disability in people aged 50–65: effectiveness and acceptability of rehabilitative intervention. *British Medical Journal* 300: 508–11.

Stephens, S.D.G., Lewis, P.A., Charny, M.D., Farrow, S.C., Francis, M. (1990b) Characteristics of self-reported hearing problems in a community survey. *Audiology* 29: 93–100.

Stephens, S.D.G., Meredith, R., Callaghan, D.E., Hogan, S., Rayment, A. (1991a) Early intervention and rehabilitation: factors influencing outcome. *Acta Oto-laryngologica* 476: S221–S225.

Stephens, S.D.G., Callaghan, D.E., Hogan, S., Meredith, R., Rayment, A., Davis, A. (1991b) Acceptability of binaural hearing aids: a cross-over study. *Journal of the Royal Society of Medicine* 84: 267–9.

Stephens, S.D.G., Lewis, P.A., Charny, M. (1991c) Assessing hearing problems within a community survey. *British Journal of Audiology* 25: 337–43.

Stephens, D., Lewis, P., Charny, M. (1991d) Are attitude and lifestyle important factors in the hearing disabled elderly? In: *Presbyacusis and Other Age Related Aspects*, (ed. J. Hartwig-Jensen), pp. 239–52. Jensen, Copenhagen.

Stephens, D., France, L., Lormore, K. (1995) Effects of hearing impairment on the patient's family and friends. *Acta Oto-laryngologica* 115: 165–7.

Stephens, D., Board, T., Hobson, J., Cooper, H. (1996) Reported benefits and problems experienced with bone-anchored hearing aids. *British Journal of Audiology* 30: 215–20.

Stephens, S.D.G., Jaworski, A., Lewis, P., Aslan, S. (1999) An analysis of communication tactics used by hearing-impaired adults. *British Journal of Audiology* 33: 17–27.

Stephens, D., Jones, G., Gianopoulos, I. (2000) The use of outcome measures to formulate intervention strategies. *Ear and Hearing* 21: S15– S23.

Stephens, D., Gianopoulos, I., Kerr, P. (2001) Determination and classification of the problems experienced by hearing-impaired elderly people. *Audiology* 40: 294–300.

Stephens, D., Lewis, P., Davis, A. (2003a) The influence of a perceived family history of hearing difficulties in an epidemiological study of hearing problems. *Audiological Medicine* 1: 228–31.

Stephens, D., Zhao, F., Kennedy, V. (2003b) Is there an association between noise exposure and King Kopetzky syndrome? *Noise and Health* 5: 55–62.

Stephens, D., Lewis, P., Davis, A. (2006) The impact of having a family history of hearing loss in elderly people. In: *The Effects of Having a Family History of Hearing Impairment*, (eds D. Stephens, L. Jones). pp. 3–13. John Wiley & Sons, Chichester.

Stephens, D., Kentala, E., Varpa, K., Pyykkö, I. (2007) Positive experiences associated with Menière's disorder. *Otology and Neurotology* 28: 982–7.

Stephens, D., Ringdahl, A., Fitzmaurice, P. (2008) Reported benefits and shortcomings of cochlear implantation by patients and their significant others. *Cochlear Implants International* 9: 186–98.

Stephens, D., Pyykkő, I., Varpa, K., Poe, D., Kentala, E. (2009a) Self-reported effects of Menière's disorder on the individual's life: a qualitative analysis, (in preparation).

Stephens, D., Pyykkö, I., Varpa, K., Kentala, E. (2009b) Relevant positive experiences reported by people with Menière's disorder: a quantitative study, (in preparation).

Stewart-Kerr, P. (1992) *The experience of acquired deafness: a psychological perspective*. PhD thesis, Belfast, Queen's University.

Strawbridge, W.J., Wallhagen, M.I., Schema, S.J., Kaplan, G.A. (2000) Negative consequences of hearing impairment in old age. *Gerontologist* 40: 320–6.

Sumby, W.H., Pollack, I. (1954) Visual contribution to speech intelligibility in noise. *Journal of the Acoustical Society of America* 25: 212–15.

Summerfield, A.Q., Marshall, D.H., Davis, A.C. (1994) Cochlear implantation: demand, costs and utility. *Annals of Otology, Rhinology and Laryngology* 104: 245–58.

Summerfield, A.Q., Barton, G.R., Toner, J. *et al.* (2006) Self-reported benefits from successive bilateral cochlear implantation in post-lingually deafened adults: randomised controlled trial. *International Journal of Audiology* 45: S99–S107.

Swan, I.R.C., Gatehouse, S. (1990) Factors influencing consultation for management of hearing disability. *British Journal of Audiology* 24: 155–60.

Sweetow, R., Palmer, C.V. (2005) Efficacy of individual auditory training in adults: a systematic review of the evidence. *Journal of the American Academy of Audiology* 16: 494–504.

Sweetow, R.W., Sabes, J.H. (2006) The need for and development of an adaptive listening and communication enhancement (LACE) program. *Journal of the American Academy of Audiology* 17: 538–58.

Tambs, K. (2004) Moderate effects of hearing loss on mental health and subjective well-being. *Psychosomatic Medicine* 66: 776–82.

Terluin B., van Marwijk, H.W., Adèr, H.J. *et al.* (2006) The Four-Dimensional Symptom Questionnaire (4DSQ): a validation study of a multidimensional self-report questionnaire to assess distress, depression, anxiety and somatization. *BMC Psychiatry* 22: 6–34.

Thomas, A., Gilhome Herbst, K. (1980) Social and psychological implications of acquired deafness for adults of employment age. *British Journal of Audiology* 14: 76–85.

Thomas, P.D., Hunt, W.C., Garry, P.J., Hood, R.B., Goodwin, J.M., Goodwin, J.S. (1983) Hearing acuity in a healthy elderly population: effects on emotional, cognitive and social status. *Journal of Gerontology* 38: 321–5.

Tillman, T.W., Carhart, R. (1966) *An expanded test for speech discrimination using CNC monosyllabic words: Northwestern University Auditory Test No 6*. Technical Report No. *SAM-TR-66-55*. USAF School of Aerospace Medicine, Brooks Air Force Base, Texas.

Tolson, D., Stephens, D. (1997) Age-related hearing loss in the dependent elderly population: a model for nursing care. *International Journal of Nursing Practice* 3: 224–30.

Tong, Y.C., Clark, G.M., Martin, L.F., Busby, P.A., Dowell, R.C. (1982) Psychophysical and speech perception studies on two multiple channel cochlear implant patients. *Journal of the Acoustical Society of America* 71: 153–60.

Toppila, E., Starck, J. (2004) The attenuation of hearing protectors against high-level shooting impulses. *Archives of Acoustics* 29: 275–83.

Toriello, H.V., Reardon, W., Gorlin, R.J. (eds) (2004) *Hereditary Hearing Loss and Its Syndromes*, 2nd edn. Oxford University Press, Oxford.

Torrance, G.W. (1986) Measurement of health state utilities for economic appraisal: a review. *Journal of Health Economics* 5: 1–30.

Trenberth, L., Drewe, P. (2002) The importance of leisure as a means of coping with work-related stress: an exploratory study. *Counselling Psychology Quarterly* 15: 59–72.

Trenberth, L., Drewe, P. (2005) An exploration of the role of leisure in coping with work related stress using sequential tree analysis. *British Journal of Guidance and Counselling* 33: 101–16.

Trychin, S. (2002) *Guidelines for providing mental health services to people who are hard of hearing*. Report No. *ED466082*. University of California, San Diego.

Tullio, P. (1929) *Das Ohr und die Enstehung der Sprache und Schrift*. Urban and Schwartzenberg, Munich.

Turner, O., Windfuhr, K., Kapur, N. (2007) Suicide in deaf populations: a literature review. *Annals of General Psychiatry* 6: 26.

Tye-Murray, N. (1998) *Foundations of Aural Rehabilitation*. Singular, San Diego.

Tye-Murray, N., Sommers, M.S., Spehar, B. (2007) Audiovisual integration and lipreading abilities of older adults with normal and impaired hearing. *Ear and Hearing* 28: 656–68.

Tyler, R.S. (1994) Advantages and disadvantages expected and reported by cochlear implant patients. *American Journal of Otology* 15: 523–31.

Tyler, R.S. (ed.) (2000) *Tinnitus Handbook*. Singular, San Diego.

Tyler, R.S., Baker, L.J. (1983) Difficulties experienced by tinnitus sufferers. *Journal of Speech and Hearing Disorders* 48: 150–54.

Tyler, R.S., Kelsay, D. (1990) Advantages and disadvantages reported by some of the better cochlear implant patients. *American Journal of Otology* 11: 282–9.

Tyler, R.S., Baker, L.J., Armstrong-Bednall, G. (1983) Difficulties experienced by hearing aid candidates and hearing aid users. *British Journal of Audiology* 17: 191–201.

Ubido, J., Huntington, J., Warburton, D. (2002) Inequalities in access to healthcare faced by women who are deaf. *Health and Social Care in the Community* 10: 247–53.

UK National Screening Committee (2003) Criteria for appraising the viability, effectiveness and appropriateness of a screening programme, http://www.nsc.nhs.uk/uk_nsc/uk_nsc_ind.htm, accessed 26 October 2007.

Unal, M., Yamer, L., Dogruer, Z.N., Yildrim, H., Vayisoglu, Y., Camdeviren, H. (2005) N-acetyltransferase 2 gene polymorphism and presbyacusis. *Laryngoscope* 115: 2238–41.

Utley, J. (1946) A test of lipreading ability. *Journal of Speech and Hearing Disorders* 11: 109–16.

Van Boxtel, M.P.J., Van Beijsterveldt, C.E.M., Houx, P.J. *et al.* (2000) Mild hearing impairment can reduce verbal memory performance in a healthy population. *Journal of Clinical and Experimental Neuropsychology* 22: 147–54.

Van Cruijsen, N., Dullaart, R.P., Wit, H.P., Albers, F.W. (2005) Analysis of cortisol and other stress-related hormones in patients with Ménière's disease. *Otology and Neurotology* 26: 1214–19.

Van den Brink, R.H.S. (1995) *Attitude and illness behaviour in hearing impaired elderly*. PhD thesis, University of Groningen.

Van den Brink, R.H.S., Wit, H.P., Kempen, G.I.J.M., Van Heuvelen, M.J.G. (1996) Attitude and help-seeking for hearing impairment. *British Journal of Audiology* 30: 313–24.

Van der Zee, K., Oldersma, F., Buunk, B., Bos, D. (1998) Social comparison preferences among cancer patients as related to neuroticism and social comparison orientation. *Journal of Personality and Social Psychology* 75: 801–10.

Van Eyken, E., Van Laer, L., Fransen, E. *et al.* (2006) KCNQ4 a gene for age related hearing impairment? *Human Mutations* 27: 1007–16.

Van Laer, L., Van Camp, G. (2007) Age-related hearing impairment: ensemble playing of environmental and genetic factors. In: *Genes, Hearing and Deafness*, (eds A. Martini, D. Stephens, A.P. Read), pp. 79–90. Informa, London.

Van Laer, L., Van Camp, G. (2008) Genetic aspects of age-related hearing impairment. Paper presented at *The XIV International Symposium in Audiological Medicine*, 18–21 September, Ferrara, Italy.

Van Laer, L., Van Eyken, E., Fransen, E. *et al.* (2008) The grainyhead like 2 gene (*GRHL2*), alias *TFCP2L3*, is associated with age-related hearing impairment. *Human Molecular Genetics* 17: 159–69.

Velmans, M. (1973) Speech imitation in simulated deafness, using visual cues and 'recoded' auditory information. *Speech and Language* 16: 224–36.

Verghese, J., Lipton, R.B., Katz, M.J. *et al.* (2003) Leisure activities and the risk of dementia in the elderly. *New England Journal of Medicine* 348: 2508–16.

Verhaegen, V.J., Mylanus, E.A., Cremers, C.W., Snik, A.F. (2008) Audiological application criteria for implantable hearing aid devices: a clinical experience at the Nijmegen ORL clinic. *Laryngoscope* 118: 1645–9.

Vermeire, K., Anderson, I., Flynn, M., Van de Heyning, P. (2008) The influence of different speech processor and hearing aid settings on speech perception outcomes in electric acoustic stimulation patients. *Ear and Hearing* 29: 76–86.

Vernon, M., Duncan, E. (1990) Advances in rehabilitation of deaf-blind persons. *Advances in Clinical Rehabilitation* 3: 167–84.

Vernon, M., Koh, S.D. (1970) Early manual communication and deaf children's achievement. *American Annals of the Deaf* 115: 527–36.

Verschuure, H., Homans, N., Van der Zwan, J. (2007) Satisfaction of use with a commercial array microphone hearing system. Paper presented at the *International Collegium of Rehabilitative Audiology* meeting, 20 June, Leuven, Belgium.

Vesterager, V., Salomon, G. (1991) Psychosocial aspects of hearing impairment in the elderly. *Acta Otolaryngologica* 476: S215–S220.

Vohr, B.R., Moore, P.E., Tucker, R.J. (2002) Impact of family health insurance and other environmental factors on universal hearing screen program effectiveness. *Journal of Perinatology* 22: 380–5.

Von der Lieth, L. (1972) Hearing tactics, I. *Scandinavian Audiology* 1: 155–60.

Wade, D. (2003) Enablement: The new rehabilitation! Paper presented to the *Royal Society of Medicine: Wales meeting, 'The power of belief'*, Cardiff, 12th May 2003.

Wade, D.T. (2005) Describing rehabilitation interventions. *Clinical Rehabilitation* 19: 811–18.

Wade, D.T. (2006a) Belief in rehabilitation: the hidden power for change. In: *The Power of Belief: Psychosocial influences on illness, disability and medicine*, (eds P.W. Halligan, M. Aylward), pp. 87–96. Oxford University Press, Oxford.

Wade, D.T. (2006b) Why *physical* medicine, *physical* disability and *physical* rehabilitation? We should abandon Cartesian dualism. *Clinical Rehabilitation* 20: 185–90.

Wade, D.T., Halligan, P. (2003) New wine in old bottles: the WHO ICF as an explanatory model of human behaviour. *Clinical Rehabilitation* 17: 349–54.

Wade, D.T., de Jong, B.A. (2000) Recent advances in rehabilitation. *British Medical Journal* 320: 1385–8.

Walden, B.E. (1980) Aural rehabilitation for adults. In: *Audiology for the Physician*, (ed. R.W. Keith), pp. 295–312. Williams and Wilkins, Baltimore.

Wallhagen, M.I., Strawbridge, W.J., Kaplan, G.A. (1996) 6-year impact of hearing impairment on psychosocial and physiologic functioning. *Nurse Practitioner* 21 (9): 11–14.

Warland, A. (1990) The use and benefits of assistive devices and systems for the hard-of-hearing. *Scandinavian Audiology* 19: 59–63.

Watson, C.S., Qiu, W.W., Chamberlain, M.M., Li, X. (1996) Auditory and visual perception: confirmation of a modality-independent source of individual differences in speech recognition. *Journal of the Acoustical Society of America* 100: 1153–62.

Watson, L.A. (1944) Certain fundamental principles in prescribing and fitting hearing aids. *Laryngoscope* 54: 531–58.

Werngren-Elgström, M., Dehlin, O., Iwarsson, S. (2003) Aspects of quality of life in persons with pre-lingual deafness using sign language: subjective well-being, ill-health symptoms, depression and insomnia. *Archives of Gerontology and Geriatrics* 37: 13–24.

Whetnall, E. (1951) Rehabilitation of the deaf. *Medical Practitioner* 222: 20.

WHO (1980) *International Classification of Impairments, Disabilities and Handicaps*. World Health Organization, Geneva.

WHO (1992) *International Statistical Classification of Diseases and Related Health Problems – 10th Revision*. World Health Organization, Geneva.

WHO (2001) *International Classification of Functioning, Disability and Health – ICF*. World Health Organization, Geneva.

Wingfield, A. (1996) Cognitive factors in auditory performance: context, speed of processing, and constraints of memory. *Journal of the American Academy of Audiology* 7: 175–82.

Wood, P.H.N. (1980) The language of disablement: a glossary relating to disease and its consequences. *International Rehabilitation Medicine* 2: 86–92.

Zekveld, A.A., George, E.L.J., Kramer, S.E., Goverts, S.T., Houtgast, T. (2007a) The development of the Text Reception Threshold test: A visual analogue of the Speech Reception Threshold test. *Journal of Speech, Language, and Hearing Research* 50: 576–84.

Zekveld, A.A., Deijen, J.B., Goverts, S.T., Kramer, S.E. (2007b) The relationship between nonverbal cognitive functions and hearing loss. *Journal of Speech, Language, and Hearing Research* 50: 74–82.

Zhao, F., Stephens, D. (1996a) Hearing complaints of patients with King-Kopetzky Syndrome (obscure auditory dysfunction). *British Journal of Audiology* 30: 397–402.

Zhao, F., Stephens, D. (1996b) Determinants of speech-hearing disability in King-Kopetzky syndrome. *Scandinavian Audiology* 25: 91–6.

Zhao, F., Stephens, D. (1999a) Audioscan testing in patients with King-Kopetzky syndrome. *Acta Otolaryngologica* 119: 306–10.

Zhao, F., Stephens, D. (1999b) Audioscan notches in patients with King-Kopetzky syndrome and a family history of hearing impairment. *Journal of Audiological Medicine* 8: 101–12.

Zhao, F., Stephens, D. (2000) Subcategories of patients with King-Kopetzky syndrome. *British Journal of Audiology* 34: 241–56.

Zhao, F., Stephens, S.D.G., Sim, S.W., Meredith, R. (1997) The use of qualitative questionnaires in patients having and being considered for cochlear implants. *Clinical Otolaryngology* 22: 254–9.

Zhao, F., Bai, Z., Stephens, D. (2008) The relationship between changes in self-rated quality of life after cochlear implantation and changes in individual complaints. *Clinical Otolaryngology* 33: 427–34.

Zwolan, T.A., Kileny, P.R., Telian, S.A. (1996) Self-report of cochlear implant use and satisfaction by prelingually deafened adults. *Ear and Hearing* 17: 198–210.

Index

Printed and bound by CPI Group (UK) Ltd, Croydon, CR0 4YY

27/10/2024

14580153-0001